Locating Zika

The emergence of Zika virus in 2015 challenged conventional ideas of mosquito-borne diseases, tested the resilience of health systems and embedded itself within local sociocultural worlds, with major implications for environmental, sexual, reproductive and paediatric health. This book explores this complex viral epidemic and situates it within its broader social, epidemiological and historical context in Latin America and the Caribbean. The chapters include a diverse set of case studies from scholars and health practitioners working across the region, from Brazil, Venezuela, Ecuador, Mexico, Colombia, the United States and Haiti. The book explores how mosquito-borne disease epidemics (not only Zika but also Chikungunya, Dengue and malaria) intersect with social change and health governance. By doing so, the authors reflect on the ways in which situated knowledge and social science approaches can contribute to more effective health policy and practice for mosquito-borne disease threats in a changing world.

Kevin Bardosh (PhD) is Research Assistant Professor of Anthropology, Environmental and Global Health and Emerging Pathogens at the University of Florida, USA.

Routledge Studies in Health and Medical Anthropology

Depression in Kerala
Ayurveda and Mental Health Care in 21st-Century India
Claudia Lang

Diagnosis Narratives and the Healing Ritual in Western Medicine
James P. Meza

The Anthropology of Epidemics
Christos Lynteris, Frédéric Keck and Ann H. Kelly

Haemophilia in Aotearoa New Zealand
Julie Park, Kathryn M. Scott, Deon York and Michael Carnahan

Locating Zika
Social Change and Governance in an Age of Mosquito Pandemics
Kevin Bardosh

www.routledge.com/Routledge-Studies-in-Health-and-Medical-Anthropology/book-series/RSHMA

Locating Zika

Social Change and Governance in an Age of Mosquito Pandemics

Edited by Kevin Bardosh

Routledge
Taylor & Francis Group
LONDON AND NEW YORK

First published 2020
by Routledge
2 Park Square, Milton Park, Abingdon, Oxon OX14 4RN

and by Routledge
52 Vanderbilt Avenue, New York, NY 10017

Routledge is an imprint of the Taylor & Francis Group, an informa business

British Library Cataloguing-in-Publication Data
A catalogue record for this book is available from the British Library

Library of Congress Cataloging-in-Publication Data
Names: Bardosh, Kevin, editor.
Title: Locating zika: social change and governance in an age of mosquito pandemics / [edited by] Kevin Bardosh.
Description: Milton Park, Abingdon, Oxon; New York, NY: Routledge, 2020. |
Series: Social change and governance in an age of mosquito pandemics |
Includes bibliographical references and index.
Identifiers: LCCN 2019029014 (print) | LCCN 2019029015 (ebook) |
ISBN 9781138315112 (hardback) | ISBN 9780429456558 (ebook)
Subjects: LCSH: Zika virus infection–Epidemiology–Latin America.
Classification: LCC RA644.Z56 L63 2020 (print) |
LCC RA644.Z56 (ebook) | DDC 614.5/885098–dc23
LC record available at https://lccn.loc.gov/2019029014
LC ebook record available at https://lccn.loc.gov/2019029015

ISBN: 978-1-138-31511-2 (hbk)
ISBN: 978-0-429-45655-8 (ebk)

Typeset in Times New Roman
by Deanta Global Publishing Services, Chennai, India

Contents

Figures

Tables

Contributors

Maria do Socorro Veloso de Albuquerque (PhD) is a researcher in the Department of Social Medicine, Health Sciences Center, Federal University of Pernambuco Brazil.

Sandra Valongueiro Alves (MD, PhD) is a Researcher in Public Health at the Federal University of Pernambuco, Brazil, where she works on maternal health.

Thália Velho Barreto de Araújo (MD, PhD) is an Associate Professor and coordinator of the Graduate Program in Public Health of the Federal University of Pernambuco, Brazil.

Kevin Bardosh (PhD) is Research Assistant Professor of Anthropology, Environmental and Global Health and Emerging Pathogens at the University of Florida.

Priscilla Bennett (PhD) is a Health Education Program Consultant at the Florida Department of Health in Monroe County. She received her PhD in Sociocultural Anthropology from Binghamton University, SUNY.

Mercy J. Borbor-Cordova (PhD) is an Associate Professor at Escuela Superior Politecnica del Litoral (ESPOL), Faculty of Marine Sciences, Biology & Oceanic Sciences, in Ecuador. She was Vice Minister of the Environment of Ecuador from 2010-2013.

Roberto Briceño-León (PhD) is Professor of Sociology at Central University of Venezuela, Director of the Social Science Laboratory (LACSO) and coordinator of the Venezuelan Violence Observatory. He has published 24 books in Spanish, English and Portuguese, and more than 200 scientific articles.

Mauricio Fuentes-Vallejo (MSc) is a Geographer and PhD candidate at University Paris 8 Vincennes Saint-Denis (Laboratory of Social Dynamics and Spatial Reconstruction) and the University Nacional de Colombia.

Yui Fujii is an undergraduate student at the University of Florida majoring in Public Health, Anthropology and Japanese.

Tatiana García-Betancourt (MSc) is a Social Science Researcher in the Division of Public Health at Fundación Santa de Bogotá in Colombia.

Héctor Gómez-Dantés (MD, MSC) is a Senior Researcher and Professor in the area of vector-borne disease epidemiology, based at the Instituto Nacional de Salud Pública, Mexico.

Catalina González-Uribe is an Associate Professor of Public Health at the School of Medicine of Universidad de los Andes, Bogota, Colombia. She is also the co-founder of Ensamble, a consultancy group that promotes social change through research on equity, inclusion and human, social and environmental wellbeing.

Milady Guevara (DVM) is a Veterinarian, Malariologist and Associate Professor of the Faculty of Health Sciences, University of Carabobo, Aragua Campus, Venezuela.

Rebecca Rose Henderson is an MD/PhD candidate at the University of Florida in cultural anthropology.

Naveed Heydari is a graduate with an MPH from the University of Colorado. He spent two years living in coastal Ecuador studying mosquito-borne illnesses and the social factors that contribute to their spread.

Tereza Maciel Lyra (MD, PhD) is a Research Professor at the Aggeu Magalhães Institute, FIOCRUZ and Professor in the Faculty of Medical Sciences of the University of Pernambuco, Brazil.

Pablo Manrique-Saide (Ph.D) is a Professor of Public Health Entomologist at the Universidad Autonoma de Yucatan, Mexico.

Gustavo Corrêa Matta (PhD) is a Senior Researcher in Public Health at the National School of Public Health at Oswaldo Cruz Foundation (ENSP/FIOCRUZ), Brazil. He is associate editor of PHYSIS (Journal of Collective Health) and the coordinator of Zika Social Science Network at FIOCRUZ.

Ana Paula Lopes de Melo is Professor of Public Health at Academic Center of Vitória, Federal University of Pernambuco and a PhD Candidate in Public Health at Aggeu Magalhães Institute, Fiocruz, Brazil.

Lenir da Silva Nascimento is a graduate with a medical degree from the Federal University of Rio de Janeiro, a Masters in Maternal and Child Health from the Fernandes Figueira Institute and a PhD in Public Policies and Human Education from the State University of Rio de Janeiro, Brazil.

Carolina de Oliveira Nogueira is currently a researcher and member of the Zika Social Science Network. She holds a PhD in Anthropology from National Museum, Federal University of Rio de Janeiro, Brazil.

Norma Pavía-Ruz (MD, MSC) is based at the Centro de Investigaciones Regionales, Unidad Biomédica, Universidad Autónoma deYucatán, Mexico.

Camila Pimentel (PhD) is a Sociologist and Public Health Researcher at Aggeu Magalhães Institute, Fiocruz. She is co-coordinator of the Zika Social Science Network, based at Fiocruz, Brazil.

Juliana Quintero is an Epidemiologist at the Division of Public Health at Fundación Santa de Bogotá in Colombia and a PhD candidate at the London School of Hygiene & Tropical Medicine.

María José Rafful-Ceballos is a cross-cultural health researcher based at the Universidad Nacional Autónoma de Mexico, Mexico.

Jimmy Emmanuel Ramos-Valencia (MSC) is a Social Anthropologist currently based at the Autonomous University of Baja California, Tijuana, México.

Anna M. Stewart-Ibarra (PhD, MPA) is a faculty member in the Department of Medicine and the Department of Public Health and Preventative Medicine at the State University of New York Upstate Medical University (SUNY UMU). She is also the Director of the Research Program on Latin America and the Caribbean at SUNY UMU, which focuses on the social and environmental determinants of infectious diseases.

Iris Terán (MD) is a Professor in the Faculty of Health Sciences, University of Carabobo, Aragua Campus, Venezuela.

Ligia Vera-Gamboa (MD, MSC) is a professor of sex education at the Universidad Autonoma de Yucatan, Mexico.

Josué Villegas-Chim is a Social Anthropologist based at the Universidad Autónoma de Yucatán, Mexico.

Acknowledgements

This book emerged from a symposium on the Zika response in the Americas held in May 2017 at the University of Florida. I would like to thank Prof. Glenn Morris, the director of the Emerging Pathogens Institute, for his support in organizing the event, and to all the participants for the lively presentations and discussion. Additional funding for this book project was provided by a Wellcome Trust Society and Ethics Fellowship. The Wellcome Trust generously covered the fees associated with making the manuscript open access, for which I am very grateful. I would like to thank my many co-authors, who have worked hard in bringing this book idea to fruition and have endured my editorial inputs and suggestions – it has really been a pleasure working with all of you. Lastly, I would like to thank my wife, Danica Thiessen, for her encouragement, support and intellectual camaraderie.

1 Understanding the global Zika response

Biographical sketches of an emergent pandemic

Kevin Bardosh

Prologue: The anatomy of a viral birth

The name *Zika* comes from a small forest patch along the shores of Lake Victoria in Uganda, not far from Entebbe International Airport. The word itself means *overgrown* in the local Lugandan language, a descriptor of the tall jungle canopy but also, since 2015, an apt metaphor for a virus that has, like an inconspicuous vine, crossed continents and borders, invaded millions of human bodies, raised political alarm bells and disrupted the intimacy of pregnancy and childbirth. None of this was known, of course, in 1947 when researchers at the Yellow Fever Research Institute, then funded by the Rockefeller Foundation, isolated the new virus from a feverish rhesus monkey (Rhesus 766), caged in the canopy of the Zika forest, and confirmed its transmission by *Aedes* "tiger" mosquitoes (Dick et al., 1952).

In the preceding 60 years, a mere 14 human cases of Zika were recorded, although sero-surveys suggest the virus was widely distributed in much of Africa and Asia (Gubler et al., 2017). Endemic across the tropics, it was likely confused with some of the other 70 *flaviviruses* and *alphaviruses* known to science (yellow fever, Dengue, West Nile, Chikungunya, Japanese encephalitis) or other common infections such as malaria or leptospirosis. It would have been hard, if not impossible, to anticipate the surge in attention that started in northeastern Brazil in 2015. On the other hand, we should not be too surprised. These types of recurring plagues and pestilences (HIV/AIDS, Ebola, Avian Influenza, SARS) often jump the species barrier from animals/insects to humans and do not emerge in a vacuum: certain social, ecological and political conditions help drive, facilitate and maintain their emergence from the virosphere. Before 2015, Zika was a low-ranking member of the more than 500 other anthropod-borne diseases known to science (Higgs, 2016). It was a little known, mild febrile illness – that is, until it caused its first known epidemic and began its journey to the maternity wards of Pernambuco State, Brazil.

This journey began in 2007, when doctors from the tiny Pacific island of Yap, Micronesia, began noticing a spike in illness cases (rash, fatigue, fever, joint pain and conjunctivitis), lasting about a week. Some patients tested positive for Dengue fever, also transmitted by *Aedes* mosquitoes. Despite the similarities, the Yap physicians suspected something different and sent samples to the Centers for Disease Control and Prevention (CDC) in the United States, where Zika was confirmed. The single-stranded RNA virus is exceedingly difficult to find, partially due to its molecular kinship to other arboviruses which has made developing rapid diagnostic tests very challenging. Although scientists later estimated, through antibody testing, that 73% of the 7,000 people on Yap had been infected over a 6-month period, there had been fewer than 200 reported cases (Duffy et al., 2009). The Yap outbreak told us that Zika could cause epidemics and that the virus, in most cases, was mild and asymptomatic (the current conventional wisdom is that 80% of Zika infections do not cause clinical disease): nothing much to worry about.[1]

A second epidemic, this time in Tahiti, hit the main island of French Polynesia in late 2013, some 5,000 miles away from Yap. Over the next six months, there were more than 8,500 reported cases including travellers who returned to the United States and Europe; later studies estimated this to be closer to 30,000, or 12% of the total population. The Polynesian outbreak revealed that Zika could no longer be viewed as a benign disease: Guillain-Barré syndrome (GBS), a debilitating autoimmune disorder and one of the most common neurological emergencies worldwide, was linked to the virus in 42 people. More than a dozen were rushed off to intensive care units (Musso et al., 2017).[2] Zika was added to the list of nearly 100 known causes of GBS, which also includes Dengue and Chikungunya.[3]

The virus then quietly spread throughout the rest of the Pacific until, in early 2015, physicians in northeastern Brazil began noticing a spike in a mild, Dengue-like illness. At first, people described it as an "awful allergy" and treated the telltale rash with antihistamines, which quickly sold out at local drug shops (Diniz, 2017: 23). At the same time, cases of a "paralyzing syndrome" (GBS) began overwhelming emergency departments. Physicians and bootstrap scientists, at first, suspected it might be connected to the recent 2013–2014 Chikungunya virus (CHIKV) epidemic (again spread by *Aedes* mosquitoes) that had just finished sweeping through the Americas for the first time, including northeastern Brazil. But in June 2015, these local scientists, far from the center of Brazilian science and political power, confirmed Zika's presence and linked it to the rise in GBS.[4]

Then, slowly, from September onwards, maternity wards and neurology clinics across Pernambuco, Bahia and Paraiba began filling up with an unusual surge of hundreds and then thousands of crying newborn babies with microcephaly, prone to seizures and with abnormal brain calcifications.[5] In some cases, the brain was almost entirely absent. Their mothers, with dreams of normality now destroyed were disparate and frantic for help. These were predominately young and poor, Afro-Brazilians, the inhabitants of *favelas*, who lacked adequate levels of sanitation or screened windows and stored their irregularly supplied water in buckets and barrels – all perfect breeding sites for a mosquito well-adapted to the urban jungle of tropical towns and cities.

In late 2015, physician waiting rooms became "like death row" as other now fearful pregnant women, at least those who could afford it, waited anxiously for ultrasound test results (Diniz, 2017: 51). A sudden metamorphosis took place; the joys of pregnancy and motherhood transformed into fear, anguish and uncertainty.

Microcephaly can be caused by other infectious diseases like cytomegalovirus and toxoplasmosis, and so it took pieces falling together, in late October and early November, including the isolation of the virus from amniotic fluid, confirming that it could cross the placenta, and testing of the blood and tissue from a dead infant, to finally confirm Zika's most pathological effects. The Ministry of Health (MoH) announced the discovery at the end of November and called a national health emergency; the World Health Organization (WHO) then declared a global Public Health Emergency of International Concern (PHEIC) in February 2016.[6] Zika's most insidious neurotropic manifestations became tragically visible in the physical contortions and cries of innocent children.

Zika dominated the international health news for much of 2016. With most of the region home to the dexterous *Aedes* mosquito, and a checkered vector control history, epidemic pandemonium set in. The US CDC issued travel alerts for whole countries, even if the virus had only been detected in a small area; it was as if the entire southern hemisphere (all of Latin America and the Caribbean) was suddenly hazardous. Brazil declared a new war against the mosquito and deployed military troops onto the streets armed with fumigators, larvicide and information pamphlets in a show of force as the nation prepared for the summer Olympics in Rio de Janeiro; at the same time, a group of 200 international scientists petitioned for the games to be cancelled.[7] Health ministers from Brazil, El Salvador and Jamaica took the unprecedented step of telling women to "not get pregnant until more is known about the virus." Some advised abstaining from child-rearing for two years; the media drew parallels with China's one-child policy, and others contemplated whether the outbreak would cause a demographic birth dip.[8] The tourism industry in the Caribbean took a massive blow. Conspiracy theories and misinformation circulated on Facebook and Twitter. And climate scientists emphasized the severe El Niño year, envisioning a future of recurring mosquito-borne plagues with rapid climate chaos.

Cases then began in Puerto Rico, Florida, Singapore and elsewhere. Protesters took to the streets in downtown Miami to stop the government's anti-mosquito aerial spraying of Naled due to fears about chemical toxicity.[9] Millions of honeybees then turned up dead in South Carolina due to state-led spraying aimed at preventing Zika, compounding existing fears about declining bee populations already under siege from colony collapse disorder.[10] Stories emerged of pregnant women wearing Hazmat suits in trendy Miami neighborhoods as they sealed themselves off in their air-conditioned fortresses.[11] For millions of women in Latin America and the Caribbean, options were much more limited.

To add to all of these anxieties, Zika was confirmed to be the first sexually transmitted disease (STD) spread by mosquitoes, something suggested back in 2008 when a US scientist, who had worked in Senegal, infected his wife with Zika in Colorado after a trip abroad (Foy et al., 2011). With greater evidence, "people visiting infected areas", to say nothing of those who lived there, were now advised to avoid all sexual contact for weeks or even months; one man was found with Zika in his semen 60 days after infection. Health experts wondered aloud how much emphasis they should be placing on condoms and sex education, in addition to labor-intensive vector control activities and calls for repellants and long-sleeved clothing. Over time, blood transfusions, urine, saliva and breast milk as well as other species of mosquitoes, such as the abundant household *culex* mosquito, were also implicated in Zika transmission; the uncertainty about how important these routes were only added to the confusion.

Nothing had been seen like this since the rubella epidemics of the 1960s in Europe or the thalidomide disaster which had left thousands of children with microcephaly, with many more dying in the womb and others born deaf or blind. The prospect of tens of thousands of affected infants was terrifying. Slowly evidence began to emerge that microcephaly was only the tip of a much larger clinical iceberg that could, possibly, take many years to be noticed. A new category was created: Congenital Zika Syndrome (CZS). Some contemplated a whole "Zika generation" affected by various physiological, neurological and behavioral disabilities. These would prove herculean to track, especially as pediatricians wondered if the virus would contribute to rising rates of autism, epilepsy and schizophrenia (McNeil, 2016:86).

Anne Schuchat, the principal deputy director of the US CDC at the time, called Zika "the most difficult" emergency response the agency had ever had. True, it was the first time the agency had to issue an advisory against travel to parts of the continental United States. In the immediate aftermath of the 2014–2015 West African Ebola epidemic, a WHO official was quoted in the *Washington Post* as saying that Zika was "much more insidious, cunning and *evil*" than Ebola.[12] The Zika response took on quasi-theological tones.

But then something happened. Spikes in microcephaly did not emerge in other countries, or indeed other areas of Brazil, in the same way that they had in the northeast. The Olympics passed with very little epidemiological humdrum, except for some new fashionable repellant athletic wear and street protests about government corruption and violence in Latin America's largest, but most unequal, democracy. The WHO's emergency was called off in November 2016, and refocused on a "long-term" strategy to address the care and support needs of affected families, preparedness for future outbreaks and capacity strengthening for vector surveillance, prevention and control.

Like Chikungunya before it, Zika became but one more neglected disease, co-circulating with other malevolent creatures, a forgotten pathogen of forgotten people. However, at the same time, Zika has also challenged our assumptions about mosquito-borne pathogens, generated new investments in arboviral science and vector technology and remained a lingering concern for the tourist industry and women of reproductive age. The virus tested the resilience of global health systems (in the immediate aftermath of the West African Ebola epidemic) and embedded itself within local sociocultural worlds with major implications for environmental, sexual, reproductive and pediatric health. Two years after the PHEIC ended (at the time of writing), uncertainty about the virus remained high; outbreaks were reported in 2018 in several places, including Japan, India and Angola, with evidence of new clusters of CZS. Some governments have been more open than others in reporting Zika, while low capacity for clinic, pediatric and vector surveillance also hampers our collective efforts to track it. Although we have not seen a repetition of the high microcephaly rates in northeastern Brazil in other locations, 26 countries in Latin America and the Caribbean (LAC) reported Zika-related microcephaly between 2015 and 2017.[13] Why the pattern of microcephaly manifested the way it did, and when epidemic Zika will resurface in the Americas (possibly influenced, like yellow fever, by an enzootic cycle in wild primates) are important, unanswered questions, as is the effect of low-grade endemic transmission on health systems and population health.

In this book, a group of engaged social science scholars and public health practitioners working and living across the Americas explore and locate the response to the 2015–2016 Zika epidemic within its broader biosocial and historical context. The book brings together a diverse series of case studies from Brazil, Venezuela, Ecuador, Mexico, Colombia, the United States and Haiti. Through these chapters, we explore how mosquito-borne disease epidemics intersect with social change and health governance and reflect on the ways in which situated knowledge and social science approaches can contribute to more effective health policy and practice for mosquito-borne disease threats. In the remainder of this introductory chapter, I provide some context and general reflection on the state of epidemic preparedness, response and recovery, based on my work on mosquito-borne diseases in Haiti and with international organizations, policymakers and scientists in the United States.[14]

The global health machinery: The governance of epidemics

Evaluating the effectiveness of the response to Zika in the Americas, as a case study in epidemic control, is more difficult than one would first assume. On the positive side, we can point to improvements in risk communication (including travel advisories and efforts by the mainstream media to dispel rumors and misinformation), rapid investments in new diagnostics and clinical vaccine trials, better coordination and data sharing and increases in vector surveillance across the region.[15] However, by any epidemiological measure the response was, on the whole, slow, clumsy, fragmented and inadequate.[16] Battered by criticisms about the delayed response to Ebola in Liberia, Guinea and Sierra Leone, global health players sought to be more assertive in 2016. In some ways, this did take place. But a number of factors conspired to outpace them: the nature of Zika, the abundance of *Aedes* vectors, the geographical scale of the pandemic, long-standing gaps in vector control capacity, deep-seated socio-political pressures and global travel patterns. Few claim anti-mosquito operations had any profound impact, and phylogenetic data from Honduras and Haiti (for example) now shows the virus was circulating in LAC in mid-2014, one-year before it was even noticed in Brazil (Theze et al., 2018; Lednicky et al., 2016). Mosquito-transmission of Zika has now been reported in over 84 countries and dependent territories around the world.[17]

From SARS in 2002–2003, H1N1 in 2009 and Ebola in 2014–2016 (to name a few epidemics), much has been written about the need to reform the global architecture of epidemic preparedness and response (CHRF Commission, 2016). Some have called for a new social movement to "end epidemics" (Quick and Fryer, 2018).[18] The world's richest philanthropist, Bill Gates, has stressed the need for greater investments in technological innovation (Gates, 2018). Experts agree that we are not well prepared for a global pandemic (a recent Gates-funded model simulation showed 33 million people would die in the first 6 months of a 1918-like pandemic influenza). Arguments run both ways about whether we are better preparedness to face a novel high-impact pathogen on the scale of the devastating 1918 Spanish Influenza (estimated to have killed 50–100 million people): social, economic and immunological conditions have improved since the European trenches and we have better pharmaceuticals, global institutions, rapid communication systems and science. On the other hand, the speed and severity of the pandemic would quickly overwhelm us and disrupt the global networks on which we depend, for food and drugs, and we also have larger and more urbanized populations. Political instability and violence, as we now see with a new Ebola outbreak in the eastern Democratic Republic of the Congo (begun in 2018), may bog us down. Rumors and misinformation spread by digital communication and fueled by increasing skepticism about experts and governments may stymie even the most effective medical countermeasures.

The speed and scale of the Zika pandemic – across multiple countries in a matter of a few months – reflects the ability for pathogens to jump our "viral superhighway" (Armelagos, 1998). Some 34 million flights carried nearly 4 billion passengers in 2016 (~10 million per day), not to mention trains, cars and cruise ships; tens of millions traveled between the United States and South America and the Caribbean.[19] There were about 5,500 symptomatic Zika cases reported in the continental United States alone. Although most were acquired abroad, more than 200 were due to local mosquito transmission in Florida (Grubaugh et al., 2017).

During the West African Ebola epidemic, the anthropologist-physician Paul Farmer called for "staff, stuff and systems."[20] With Ebola, infections could be found, monitored and followed within only a few days or weeks of infection. The outbreak could be visibly tracked. A threat that is not easily localized, like Zika, is more like an environmental toxin or chemical pollutant. Diffused, it can seem to be everywhere and nowhere at the same time. Mosquito bites go unnoticed. It can take nine months to witness any birth defects, and potentially much longer for other malformations. Zika reminded us, once again, that our systems move much slower than the invisible microbial worlds that threaten to rain down on us like the plague. In order to move faster organizations, expertise and "stuff" needs to be mobilized not only with greater speed but also agility, which comes from better preparedness and stronger healthcare systems. Here, too, Zika is instructive.

With cases reported in Hawaii, Puerto Rico and the US Virgin Islands, on February 22, 2016, President Barack Obama (who had supported the Global Health Security Agenda [GHSA] in 2014)[21] requested $1.89 billion in supplemental funding from a Republican-controlled Congress that had become increasingly gridlocked along ideological-party lines since 2010.[22] Without any emergency funds available, $510 million (including $295 million from USAID) was redirected in April from "existing Ebola resources" that were intended to strenghten health systems in West Africa to Zika as a stopgap. A cat-and-mouse game began, with multiple efforts to push the bill through the US Congress. But this failed and lawmakers went on summer recess just as mosquito season began in the southern

United States and more domestic Zika cases hit the newspapers. Eventually, $1.1 billion of funding for Zika was passed; yet it took seven months to be approved, signed by Obama on September 29, 2016. By November, when the WHO declared an end to the PHEIC, little US funding had moved out of the treasury. This had repercussions for the newly reformed WHO Health Emergencies Program (the United States is the major donor), which also took nine months to receive most of the funds that it had requested from donors in February 2016.[23] Additional emergency funding came from the World Bank, the Inter-American Development Bank and European agencies and governments.

Some have attributed this delay to xenophobic discrimination among US lawmakers (the framing of Zika as an "immigrant disease" from Latin America), a general neglect for Puerto Rico (an unincorporated territory of the United States that saw 90% of all reported US cases), longstanding conflicts in the use of federal funds for sexual and reproductive health (especially abortion), political tensions concerning Obamacare and the low mortality rate of the virus. All certainly played some role. Importantly, to actually get the bill passed it was bundled with flood relief in Louisiana and the Flint, Michigan water crisis and connected to veteran affairs and military defense spending (which tend to gather significant bi-partisan support).

Too often, this is how health emergencies are funded; US funding for a counter-terrorism operation would have been much more swift. In this case, CDC had to redirect finances from routine vaccination and other activities to address Zika, while the US government's broader post-Ebola funding for preparedness and health system strengthening efforts in West Africa was severely cut. By the time that Congress approved the bulk of its funding, Puerto Rico had already reported 22,358 confirmed Zika cases. From an epidemiological standpoint, a lot of basic science work was also needed to track and understand this new virus. But, as a frustrated senior global health researcher based in the United States told me in an interview at the time:

> No one can get money to do the basic science that needs to get done. Where is Zika? What is it doing outside Brazil? It is a mess. CDC gave some extramural funds it had available, but they don't play with others. So they keep it in-house. You can't really go to NIH, since it will take at least one year. NSF is small money; you can't really do anything significant with it. The EU bureaucracy is terrible. WHO has no money, and PAHO too. It is a joke.

The lack of funds in epidemic response has helped drive a number of innovations in recent years. This includes the World Bank's new global insurance mechanism, the Pandemic Emergency Financing Facility (PEF), used for the first time in the 2018 DRC Ebola outbreak, and the public–private Coalition for Epidemic Preparedness Innovations (CEPI), which aims to mobilize $1 billion over 5 years for vaccine development, including for Chikungunya (Yamay et al., 2017). Although these are welcomed institutional additions to the pandemic response landscape, there are many questions about how effective they will be.

Tied to geopolitics and economic interests, health security moves up and down the corridors of international authority and power. Epidemics disrupt the status quo: flights stop, consumer behavior shifts, people stay indoors and do not go to work or school and they avoid restaurants, hotels and shopping centers. The cascade effects can be huge, especially for tourism, and epidemics also drive surges in other endemic diseases and conditions as they reduce routine health services and capacity. The World Bank projected the short-term economic impacts from Zika in 2016 to be $3.5 billion or 0.06% of GDP in LAC (World Bank, 2016). A separate analysis by IFRC and UNDP (2017) estimated that the pandemic would cost LAC $7–18 billion in the short term and billions more in long-term costs associated with GBS and CZS (UNDP, 2017). By one estimate, each Zika-affected child could cost the US health system $10 million. The long-term effects on Caribbean cruises and other regional tourism remains murky.

Perhaps the most significant, obvious and yet difficult to put into practice lesson from past epidemics has been the importance of robust health systems. Over 57 countries are classified as being in Human Resources for Health (HRH) crises around the world with severe shortages of health care workers, resources and systems, and a health sector highly dependent on international aid, NGOs and a fragmented private sector. Epidemics exasperate these fault lines. They require task shifting, and reveal governance and capacity holes, although they can also be times of learning and reform.[24] Once the US Congress finally approved Zika funding, $230 million of USAID funding was unlocked; however, in the end it took until early to mid-2017 to really get the majority of these international projects off the ground. Most focused on Central America and the Caribbean, and on small geographical areas. USAID health funding to LAC had decreased significantly since Obama took office, which meant there were few International NGOs with established links to USAID desks, especially for vector control.[25] By the time this money actually moved into countries, the epidemic itself was over. The feeling, then, was that these should be arbovirus *preparedness* projects, but project activities and deliverables had been written for an epidemic response to Zika and this limited their scope: what were these projects responding to, exactly (some public health experts asked)? The ability to respond rapidly to epidemics requires that institutional mechanisms be in place well before an emergency, something discussed by Stewart-Ibarra and colleagues in Ecuador in Chapter 6 of this volume.

The Zika epidemic also showed that health communication units across most of the LAC region, at the level of Ministry of Health, were overly technical, hierarchical and under-funded, and in a general state of disrepair. For instance, it was common for local media reports to declare only official confirmed Zika cases; the simultaneous urgent calls-to-action for community prevention seemed out of touch with the scale of the threat, contributing to suspicions, misinformation and rumors. Social media posts related Zika emergence and spread to fertilizers, transgenic mosquitoes, vaccination campaigns, insecticides/agrochemicals, CIA bioweapons, and a global plot to control the population of poor countries by "the Rockefellers." USAID projects aimed to build capacity for health communication and community engagement (RCCE).[26] Social science research shed light on the pitfalls of unrealistic recommendations, like telling women to use repellents and wear long sleeves in humid tropical cities, and to abstain from sex and reproduction. Initial risk communication messages were often broad and somewhat confusing, as public health staff struggled to communicate emerging knowledge

Table 1.1 Behaviors targetted in Zika risk communication in LAC

Household and community vector control	Remove standing water; Scrub water containers (pilas); Cover water containers; Put screens on windows and doors; Participate in community cleanup activities; Close trash bags and bins; Keep doors and windows closed; Change water in pets' bowls at least 3 times/week; Fill holes in the ground with dirt; Keep a lid on garbage cans inside and outside the house; Avoid having trash on your patio; Don't throw trash on the street; Cover containers where you collect water; Change water and scrub water barrels with bleach at least once per week; Eliminate or place a hole in containers that can accumulate water; Control breeding sites; Wash and scrub water container (untadita) once a week; Cover all water containers where you store water; Keep your patio and lot of ground clean, free of weeds and trash; Clean your drainpipe once a week; Eliminate tires, cans, bottles, and lids that can accumulate water; Use small fish to eliminate larvae in pilas and barrels. In this case, don't use bleach or larvicides; Cover water containers with a robust plastic lid and secure it with tape or a rubber band; Change the water in vases and flower pots; Turn over containers, crates, cans, or any container that has standing water; Cover all containers where you store water; Clean rainwater and tap water gutters; Throw away bottles, tires, cans, or pots that you don't use; Store tires under roofs to avoid accumulating water; Plant basil in a pot; Cut the grass and bushes around the house; Keep alert during the morning and evening hours when mosquitoes bite; Use insecticide to eliminate mosquitos inside the house; Pay attention to fumigation campaigns in your community so that you can have your home fumigated; Use hermetic seals for water containers.
Care seeking	Attend prenatal visits; Seek information on family planning from your provider; Rest; Drink water, juices, soups and other; Take acetaminophen; Do not take aspirin; Go to health center to confirm whether you have Zika; Visit the closest health center if you present symptoms; Drink a lot of liquids; Rest; All pregnant women should attend the closest health center for consultations.
Personal protection	Wear repellent containing DEET or picaridin; Use condoms in all sexual relations to prevent sexual transmission of Zika; Always sleep under a mosquito net; Wear long sleeves and long pants; Wear light colored clothing; Use repellent only with doctor's authorization.

Note: These behaviors were taken from ZIKV IEC materials. The list is not comprehensive but is meant to be illustrative of the wide range of behaviors covered by ZIKV risk communication. Provided by Arianna Serino, USAID.

on an emerging virus, especially regarding sexual transmission (see Table 1.1 for a list of behaviors targeted by risk communication teams). A meta-analysis of socio-behavioral data, collected by NGOs and commissioned by UNICEF, found that the elimination of stagnant water, cleaning of water containers, sweeping and cleaning of the house and yard and use of mosquito nets were the most commonly reported community prevention practices undertaken for Zika; however, the last two are not particularly effective for *Aedes* control.[27] Activities focused exclusively on Zika then had to be adapted, in 2017, to communicate risks from Dengue and Chikungunya as USAID projects shifted towards arbovirus preparedness plans more generally. This revealed the tensions between the time-bound nature of "emergency" response and the long-term needs of stronger health systems (Lakoff, 2017), a conflict also made visible in the initial re-appropriation of "Ebola preparedness money" to respond to Zika.

Locating mosquito pandemics in the world

So are we really in an era of mosquito pandemics, as the title of this book suggests? Yes and no. There has been a precipitous decline in infectious disease over the last 50 years, as low- and middle-income countries have narrowed gaps in life expectancy and reduced extreme poverty (Rosling, 2018). Today, unlike in the past, infectious microbes are responsible for less than 10% of global death and disability in most regions of the world, albeit this is higher in South Asia (20%) and sub-Saharan Africa (44%).[28] Thomas Bollyky (2018), in his book *Plagues and the Paradox of Progress*, argues that this has occurred in a categorically different way than it did in Europe and the United States in the 19th and 20th centuries. Here, epidemics linked to their noxious living conditions drove substantial political, cultural and civil action for water and sanitation infrastructure, social and educational reforms and broader changes in government and trade. While this connection between microbes, governance and social change are still occurring, Bollyky argues that the deployment of vaccines, therapeutics and diagnostics today disentangles them from some of the past pressures for social, governance and infrastructure reform.

There are two caveats to this argument. First, while infectious disease may have decreased, their propensity for disruptive epidemics have not. Outbreak events, new spillovers from animals and evolutionary pressures from anthropogenic change continue to increase, as do their health and socioeconomic impact (Bardosh, 2016). Second, arboviruses fit uneasily into this narrative, as we can see with the re-emergence of Dengue, Chikungunya, Rift Valley fever and now Zika. Let's explore this more.

Known as "breakback fever" due to the severe back and muscle pain it causes, Dengue only really emerged on the public health radar in the 1950s in Southeast Asia. There are four distinct serotypes, and multiple viral lineages; while infection with one serotype provides long-term immunity, infection with a different one increases the severity and chance of hemorrhagic infection through antibody-dependent enhancement. Today, Dengue circulates in more than 100 countries, a risk to 30% of the global population. Estimates vary and are difficult to nail down; a recent analysis found 390 million infections every year, with 96 million (67–136 million) developing clinical disease, about half-a-million hospitalizations and 25,000 deaths (Bhatt et al., 2013). Epidemics occur in cycles of 3–10 years, driven by localized climatic, socioeconomic and immunological factors. They are, then, seasonal emergencies.

The global emergence of Chikungunya virus (a *Makonde* word[29] for "to become contorted") has also been remarkable since 2005, through a series of devastating outbreaks linked to genetic shifts that have changed the virus' virulence and vector competence (Schuffenecker et al. 2006). Epidemics in India have been particularly bad. From 2013 to 2015, a game of viral tag occurred in the Pacific as CHIKV passed through Polynesia months after Zika and reached northeastern Brazil in September 2014. Once in the Americas, it caused millions of reported cases, killed about 700 and burdened an estimated 400,000 with the long-term effects of chronic inflammatory rheumatic disease (Morens and Fauci, 2016).

Estimating the true prevalence of arboviruses is difficult, due to the high number of asymptomatic infections, the short and self-limiting nature of many clinical episodes, the lack of diagnostics and therapeutics and gaps in reporting systems. This was all very clear with Zika. The official WHO estimate was that 3–5 million people would be infected during 2016. Data from PAHO/WHO (2015–2017) shows less than one million cases (Table 1.2).[30] With over 650 million people in more than 50 countries and territories, and 13 million births each year,[31] it is clear that the actual number of Zika cases in 2016 in LAC were vastly underreported. A study in Mexico estimated the true prevalence as 30–40 times higher than the reported number of symptomatic infections (Hernandez-Avila et al 2018). Modeling studies suggested that 93–117 million people would actually get infected, including 1.65 million pregnant women during the first wave (Perkins et al. 2016). In Chapter 2 of this book, Henderson and Bardosh discuss the challenges that modelers and their models faced during the epidemic.

Can we really assume that Zika spread throughout the entirety of each of the countries in which it has been reported? Who is still susceptible and when and where will another epidemic occur? Colon-Gonzalez et al. (2017) have projected that, with endemic Zika virus, an average of 12 million Zika cases (0.7–162.3) will continue each year in the Americas. Very few cases have been reported in 2018, most likely due to herd immunity. Evidence from CHIKV and ZIKV seroprevalence studies suggest that upwards of 40–70% of a population is infected during an epidemic wave. Zambrana et al. (2018) found ZIKV antibodies in 36% of a pediatric cohort and 46% in a separate household survey in Managua, Nicaragua. It is likely, however, that climactic factors in 2017 and 2018 have also helped reduced the force of the epidemic. Data from PAHO, for example, shows a significant reduction in Dengue cases, not only Zika, in 2017 and 2018 in the Americas (Table 1.3).

It is not coincidental, then, that Zika was discovered in a yellow fever research station. Entomologists have recorded over 50 resident species of mosquitoes in the Zika forest alone and multiple other viruses including Chikungunya, West Nile and Bwamba, Semliki forest, O'nyong'nyong and Kadam viruses.[33] Scientists are increasingly finding that this viral chatter interacts; for example, co-infection

Table 1.2 Cumulative Zika virus cases reported by country and region in the Americas, 2015–2017

Region	*Autochthonous cases*		*Imported cases*	*Incidence Rate*	*Deaths*	*Confirmed CZS*	*Population (*1,000)*
	Suspected	Confirmed					
North America	0	12,032	5,900	9	0	123	490,275
Central American Isthmus	63,514	7,802	77	154	0	190	46,437
Latin Caribbean	90,187	42,236	205	350	5	145	37,887
Andean Area	173,172	17,078	41	136	0	276	139,615
Brazil	231,725	137,288	0	176	11	2,952	209,553
Southern Cone	1,254	298	76	2	0	7	72,360
Non-Latin Caribbean	23,599	6,743	30	411	4	27	7,382
TOTAL	**583,451**	**223,477**	**6,329**	**80**	**20**	**3,720**	**1,003,509**

Note: PAHO/WHO data, as of Jan 4, 2018.

Table 1.3 Dengue cases reported in the Americas, 2014–2018

Year	*Dengue cases*	*Lab confirmed*	*Severe Dengue*	*Deaths*
2014	1,184,809	366,396	15,982	683
2015	2,416,732	646,103	12,496	1,355
2016	2,174,514	479,148	4,225	913
2017	580,414	117,544	2,065	311
2018	484,111	181,485	2,707	267

Note: PAHO data.[32]

between Dengue, CHIKV and Zika are not uncommon (Singer, 2017). Some postulate that the previous Dengue epidemic in northeastern Brazil contributed to the severity of Zika-related microcephaly in 2015–2016. It is difficult to distinguish between these arboviruses in many standard diagnostic tests. And many of these viruses can also cause neurological and developmental impairments when infections occur in pregnancy, something that has been better appreciated as a by-product of the Zika epidemic and amplified concerns about the maternal-pediatric risk of arboviral infections more generally (Mehta et al. 2018).

These viral diseases also share a common method of transmission: the pesky mosquito or "flying syringe." These insects have had an incalculable influence on human history shaping empires, deciding battles and helping to define and reinforce social and economic relations (McNeill, 2010). Mosquitoes and yellow fever, and a mountainous Haitian landscape, prevented Napoleon's brother from crushing the first successful slave revolt in 1804, for example. There are over 3,000 species worldwide, although only a small fraction (*anopheles*, *Aedes*, *culex*) spread the pathogens that sicken millions and kill 700,000 each year.[34] Global programs for lymphatic filariasis (LF) and malaria have significantly decreased these parasitic infections; however, biomedical tools have proven to be less effective for arboviruses. Part of this has to do with the nature of *Aedes agypti* and *Aedes albopictus* (commonly known as *Asian Tigers*) and their evolutionary past in tropical forests. Both feed largely on human blood, bite during the day, have a local flight distance (100–400m) and are highly invasive. Mimicking their forest niche in tree-holes and plant axils, they now breed predominately in the urban and peri-urban jungles of modern cities, in plastic buckets and jars, discarded tires, water storage containers, flower vases, cemeteries and blocked gutters. In Miami, the Zika epidemic was blamed on the tropical plant – bromeliads – that collects water and larvae on manicured hotel lawns. *Aedes* do not lay all their "eggs in one basket" but spread them out over multiple water containers and enjoy taking blood meals from multiple human hosts, all of which increases their vector efficiency and viral transmissibility. They are also highly invasive, *Aedes albopictus* more so than *Ae agypti*. Shipments of used tires in the 1980s introduced *Aedes albopictus* into the Americas from Asia, and the mosquito is now found as far north as Canada.

The expansion of Dengue, Chikungunya and Zika has followed a similar pattern but, at its core, this expansion has been linked to urbanization, or what

Bollyky (2018) called the emergence of "poor cities" in the tropics. In the period 1950–2014, the world's urban population rose from 746 million to 3.9 billion. Much of this growth was in the tropics; 80% of the populations of Latin America and the Caribbean, for example, now live in urban areas, and most of the world's megacities (of 10 million or more) are now in low- and middle-income countries. Urban scholars have commented on how this new growth of cities, far outpacing the ability of new infrastructure, employment and social policy, may nullify the economic benefits that are typically associated with city living (Bollyky, 2018). Nowhere is this more obvious than in the proliferation of slums and shantytowns, which are expected to grow to be home to 2 billon people by 2030[35] including about 20% of the population of Latin America and the Caribbean.[36] Factors conspire together in these deteriorated urban ecosystems: rural-urban migration, poor planning and infrastructure, colonial histories, social and economic exclusion, an absence of government investment, corruption and economic stagnation. The lack of nutritious food, education and environmental sanitation compromises health. Unemployment and the informal economy are entangled, in some locations, with crime, violence and sexual predation. These areas are also prone to climatic change and natural disasters, and efforts to address them often disadvantage the poor, who lack formal land ownership rights (Figure 1.1).

The slum is a visible manifestation of the social and political pathologies that drive arboviruses, but do these infectious RNA strands really affect the poor

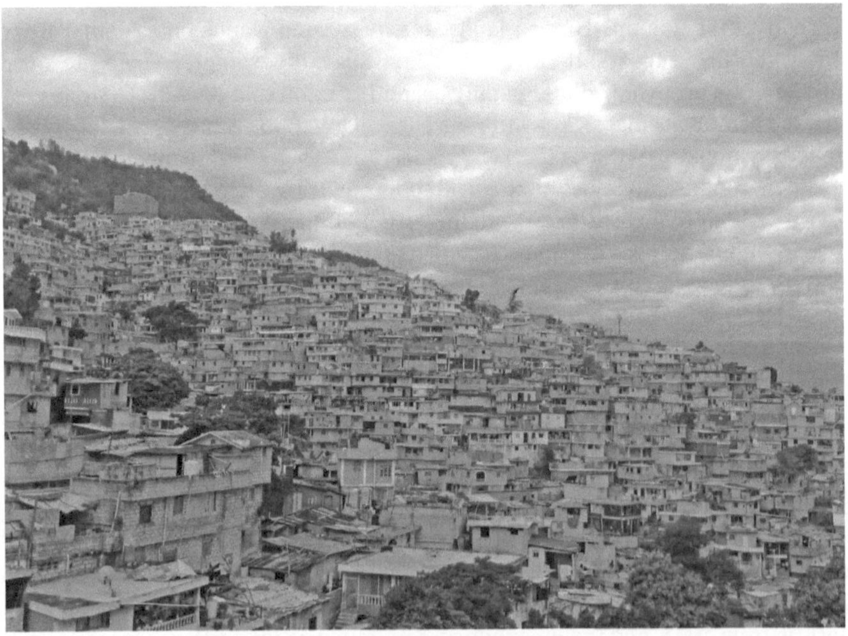

Figure 1.1 Port-au-Prince, home to roughly one-third of Haiti's 11 million people. Photo: author.

disproportionately? The evidence for Dengue is mixed, as mosquitoes breed along the social gradient: in fancy flower vases on a poolside resort, in the storage containers and backyards of middle-income households and in the plastic and metal waste accumulated by some low-income households (Mulligan et al. 2015). In many cases, these socio-ecological realities are within flight-distance.

Social inequalities, however, do shape the lack of access to health care, employment and political leverage that prevent improvements in basic living conditions. Nancy Scheper-Hughes' (1992) classic ethnographic study, *Death Without Weeping: The Violence of Everyday Life in Brazil*, described the ways in which poor Brazilians in Pernambuco State (what became the epicenter of the Zika epidemic) negotiated conditions of sickness, hunger, shantytown violence and child death in the 1980s. Re-reading this classic book, I was struck by the similarities between her poignant descriptions of the *Nordeste* region, with contemporary scars leftover from colonial-era sugar plantations, and Deborah Diniz's (2017: 107) account of the early days of the Zika outbreak:

> We cannot speak of people in terms of ageless, sexless masses; it is young women who are pregnant, or planning to be, who are now terrified by the mere act of living in the land of Zika. Simply because they are poor Northeasterners, ordinary women have been ignored by policies that should respond to suffering in a country as unequal as Brazil's ... women from the elites will find alternative ways to ensure a safe pregnancy despite Zika.

History also has a long shadow in northern Haiti, where I have worked with the Ministry of Health and Population (MSPP) on mosquito control since 2015. While Brazil was the last Western nation to free its slave (1888), Haiti was the first Black Republic (1804). Brazil is one of the most unequal societies on earth; but Haiti, so the saying goes, is the only country with a last name: the poorest country in the Western Hemisphere.[37] I was in Haiti when the Zika wave hit. I noticed more *Aedes* mosquitoes fluttered around homes, shops, decrepit clinics and public health offices. I recall training community health workers as swarms of mosquitoes flew overhead in the humidity. I was bitten more than once. As I watched the news unfold in Brazil, I also saw there was little preparedness planning and, really, no surveillance system. In 2016–2017, I asked people, including a few American missionaries running a variety of orphanages, about infants born with microcephaly and tried to keep track of about a dozen cases. A Haitian friend had a miscarriage: was it Zika? At the time, we anticipated tragedy. But as microcephaly cases did not mount, we all signed some relief.

Declarations of an epidemic are political events. In Haiti, the government did not declare a public health emergency. US news headlines read: "Forget Zika, Haiti has bigger problems – a doctors' strike" and "While Latin America struggles over Zika, Haiti faces epidemic with a shrug." During this time, a contested national election ushered in an uncertain transitional government (one of many since the end of the Duvarier era in 1986), public hospitals were shutdown for months as medical residents (paid $150 a month) went on strike, the infamous cholera epidemic – imported by Nepali UN troops in late 2010 – continued in the face of meager international donations, hurricanes threatened the coast, allegations of massive fraud in billions of loans from Venezuela's PetroCaribe surfaced and the 13-year-old United Nations Stabilization Mission in Haiti (MINUSTAH) began its withdrawal (Figure 1.2).

The NGO-ization of Haiti's health system and the politics of dependence have long been themes in the anthropological and political science literatures. The 2016 presidential election had a 21% turnout rate among a population deeply pessimistic with politics and the hollow rhetoric of change; this disenchantment has emerged alongside the withering of populist democratic hopes that began in the early 1990s. During the Zika epidemic, I was also working on improving mass drug administration (MDA) for lymphatic filariasis (LF) in northern Haiti, and tried to encourage an emergency Zika control program (funded by USAID) to also focus on the street canals, that were infested with *culex* larvae, and to help with the MDA (Bardosh et al. 2017). This town, an important Voodoo pilgrimage site, was a hotspot for LF and had already undergone 14 years of MDA (the WHO says 5 years should eliminate the parasite). I would occasionally see cases of lymphedema and elephantiasis and hear of hydroceles, all untreatable conditions that are immensely painful, debilitating and stigmatizing. There were also lots of mosquitoes. Early successes with the LF program had started the lag; local health staff had become less motivated once an international NGO had taken over and some community members refused to take the medication. It was a simple idea: use staff from the Zika program to help organize more community engagement focused on cleaning-up the canals, give out food with the drug (to help with side effects) and do house-to-house distribution of the MDA drugs rather than at

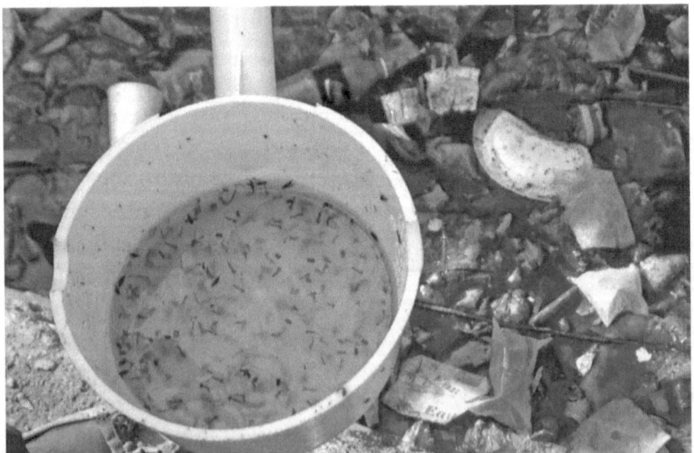

Figure 1.2 A street canal in northern Haiti, clogged with garbage and mosquito larvae. Photo: author.

central points (which is the current standard approach. But the emergency program refused: had to stick with the predefined deliverables. Sorry, I was told, we can only do household vector control – leaving the canals clogged with garbage and mosquito larvae. My Haitian colleagues found this absurd (especially given the absence of Zika) but they laughed it off just as they did with more significant sociopolitical events occurring at the time.

In Haiti, and throughout the region, communities found it hard to understand how a familiar vector was spreading a new disease. Empirical experience mixed with biomedicine and folk beliefs, and people reported different transmission routes that included air, food, climate and vectors (Jansen, 2013). In my fieldwork, no one spoke or seemed to really care about Zika. Others have highlighted that people do not really care about Dengue in the context of multiple other pressures in their lives (Nading, 2014). Nading (2014) discussed Dengue epidemics as temporal or "seasonal emergencies" without a clear beginning or end, blurring ideas of risk and responsibility – that is, until you or a close family member suffers from it. In Haiti, if you spoke about Chikungunya at a community meeting, more than half of the crowd would tell you stories about weeks off work, horrendous back pain and long-term ailments that they attributed to the virus. As you can see from Figure 1.3, local understadings of Chikungunya in Haiti are linked to chronic, non-communicable disease conditions like hypertension. The health director I worked with had long-lasting muscle pain and fatigue, and the epileptic seizures one of my Haitian colleagues had had as a child came back after her Chikungunya infection. CHIKV was a forgotten pandemic, but not so for communities in northern

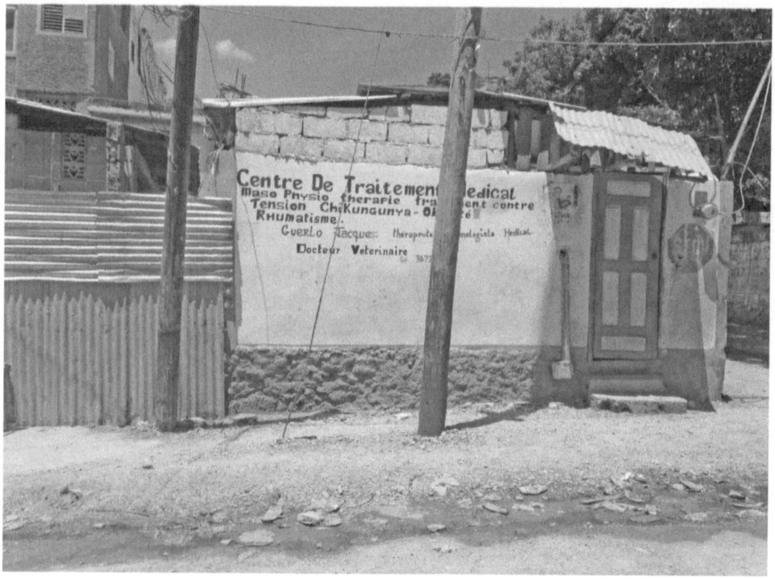

Figure 1.3 An advertisement for a local doctor, showing the local aetiological links between hypertension, obesity and Chikungunya. Cap-Haitien, Haiti. Photo: author.

Haiti. In fact, estimates have shown that upwards of 50% of infected people may develop these long-term ailments (Schilte et al. 2013). Epidemiological studies have begun to explore potential links to kidney disease, heart disease and diabetes (de Almeida Barreto et al. 2018). Arboviruses now seem to exasperate non-communicable disease conditions on top of their maternal-pediatric risks.

Vector wars and state bureaucracy

One of the great lessons from the West African Ebola epidemic was the importance of communities in controlling epidemics. Ebola has a strong social component to infection: caring for the sick, burying the dead, sharing bodily fluids. Paul Richard (2016), based in Sierra Leone, argued in *How a People's Science Helped End an Epidemic* that: "common sense, improvisation, distributed practical knowledge and collective action are invaluable elements in a people's science of infection control." Health interventions are most effective when they support this.

Zika's social dimensions are different, entangled in human–mosquito–ecological relationships. They need to be located in the history of vector control, with roots in the military tactics of the colonial past, and the urban landscapes now increasingly inhabited by female mosquitoes. The general sentiment, for many health experts in 2016, was that vector control would do little to stop the virus. In *Zika: The Emerging Epidemic*, veteran New York Times reporter Donald McNeil (2016) reflected this dismissal:

> I kept asking mosquito experts to name one place I could go where mosquito eradication was demonstrably lowering infections rates. I usually heard long pauses, followed by 'I can't think of one.'

In Haiti, the feeling was mutual. As a senior Ministry of Health and Population official told me in early 2016:

> As far as I am concerned, there is no hope for any public health prevention with Zika. Look around you. The place is rampant with mosquitoes and everyone needs to store water to survive. You cannot control mosquitos. You might reduce them here…but they come back from around the corner … what is my public health policy, you ask? It is to hope that everyone gets infected quickly, that there are few microcephaly cases and that like Chikungunya, the population acquires immunity. … I want people to get the virus, just not pregnant women.

The narrative that *Aedes* are the *cockroaches* of the mosquito world, that they breed in "nothing but" a bottle cap, and thrive where water, sanitation and garbage collection services are lacking, was frequently repeated and furthered the sense of helplessness. I recall a senior WHO official, working on the concurrent yellow fever outbreak in Angola at the time, laughing at me for suggesting that vector control could help. Without a vaccine, McNeil's recommendation, as an emergency measure, was to protect pregnant women during the epidemic wave, allowing the rest of the population to be infected. In this atmosphere, vector control became a show. Large plums of smoke emanating from the gun of the fumigator, symbolism of the state's attempt to assert itself against an enemy that had already won. Spray trucks were mostly for political brownie points; government mobilization an exercise in cosmetics. In some places Zika became a political tool; garbage management could be improved or starved of funds, or garbage deliberately dumped onto the streets, depending on political loyalties. These issues are explored in Chapter 5 of this volume, in the context of the history of vector control before and after the Bolivian revolution and the tragic circumstances of contemporary Venezuela (Figure 1.4).

There have been two major victories in the annals of *Aedes* control. The first was the source reduction campaigns in the early 20th century, led by William Gorgas, the most infamous being in Havana and the Panama Canal. Environmental sanitation mixed with economic interests, US imperialism and military tactics. Yellow fever, which had devastated US cities since the 18th century, was only linked to mosquitoes in 1900 in Cuba. Gorgas's efforts in Havana, managed under US-led martial law during a yellow fever epidemic, centered on various

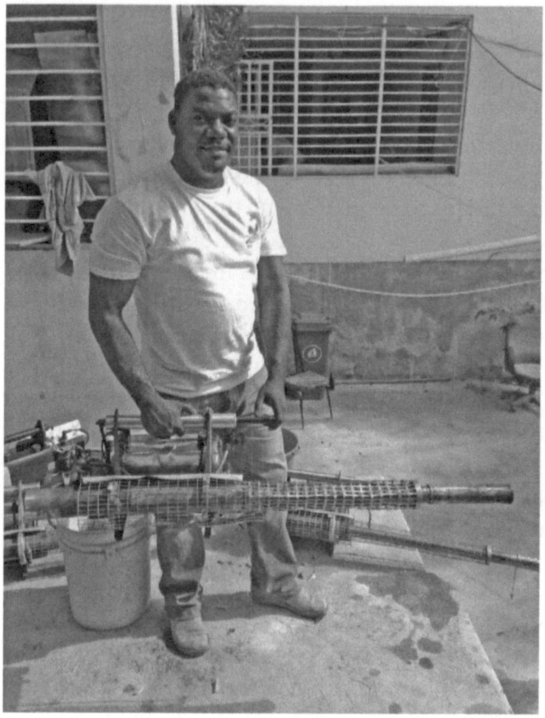

Figure 1.4 A vector control officer in Haiti, with hand-held fumigator, early 2016. Photo: author.

chemicals, fumigation and clean-up techniques, including crude oil and sulphur-based compounds, the closing of bars and cafes and the sealing-off of drinking water tanks and use of special larvae-eating fish (Stepan, 2011: 48). The city was meticulously mapped, each household visited regularly and fines and penalties imposed. Cuba was free from the virus for decades, and the methods were replicated with significant funding from the Rockefeller Foundation in other countries including Brazil and Mexico.

The second victory was the *Aedes agypti* eradication effort run by PAHO, started in 1947 under the direction of Fred Soper, with the goal of "species sanitation": the complete eradication of *Aedes agypti* from the Western hemisphere. This replicated many aspects of the Gorgasian campaigns including its disease-specific focus, detailed mapping and record keeping, general authoritarianism and, of course, the central role of chemicals – in this case DDT (Stepan, 2011). By this time, yellow fever had reduced significantly in the Americas, so the campaign was cast in moral and economic robes and success (and failure) as a problem of political will and organization. It was also often linked with malaria eradication efforts that were being organized in parallel. By 1964, over 18 countries in South and Central America, from Mexico to Argentina, had eradicated the *Aedes* mosquito, and cases (when they did emerge) of yellow fever were predominately found in the interior, away from urban foci and in areas with sylvatic transmission. The United States was a laggard, preferring to focus on the new yellow fever vaccine; areas of Mexico bordering the United States were re-infested because of a lack of US interest. The program ended in the late 1960s; DDT was banned in the United States in 1972; and severe Dengue epidemics then began in LAC in the 1980s.

The demise of *Aedes* eradication efforts, abandoned by PAHO and others, coincided with the rise of the primary health care movement, post-Alma Ata (1978). As Dengue cases rose, interest in community participation and the integration of vector control with other health and government services grew. But at the same time, the hollowing out of malaria control meant that vectors and their viruses received little financial support: labs, insectaries, surveillance systems, basic research and entomological expertise reduced. A review of Dengue programs by Horstick et al. (2010) in four countries presented a dismal assessment: lack of personnel, budgets and expertise, overreliance on insecticides, little community engagement and almost no monitoring and evaluation. As discussed in Chapter 7 of this volume, Villegas-Chim and collegues from Mexico discuss the need for a "socio-political surveillance" of vector control programs to better understand their functioning.

To complicate things further, the evidence on the effectiveness of the current "toolbox" is mixed in terms of arboviral control. A recent meta-analysis on Dengue found only 41 rigorous studies from 1980 to 2015 (Bowman et al. 2016). Some found no statistical significance; there were few randomised control trials (RTCs) or evaluations of insecticide susceptibility. Overall, things like house screening, community-based environmental management and covering water containers reduced Dengue risk, while indoor residual spraying (IRS), skin repellents, insecticide-treated bednets and mosquito coils did not. Study designs and data were noted to be of low quality, especially for outdoor fogging, which is the main response to Dengue (and was widely used for Zika) around the world. Most of the data focused on entomological indexes and not changes in disease transmission.

Approaches such as PAHO's COMBI (Communication for Behavioral Impact) strategy, developed in the late 1990s, aimed to re-orientate *Aedes* control to have a greater focus on environmental management and community-based interventions. Again, here, evidence is mixed (Heintze et al. 2007). A recent RCT, *Camino Verde* (Green Way), piloted in 20,000 households in Mexico and Nicaragua, aimed to test chemical-free community mobilization and was found to have lowered Dengue infection in children by 30% – the first such trial to demonstrate an impact on Dengue infection. But an experimental RCT is very different from a national program. Even in this trial, most households continued to believe that chemicals (*Temephos*) were the best control method (Legorreta-Soberanis et al. 2017). Without piped water, the demand to constantly clean storage containers is hard, repetitive work. Volunteers and health staff can be mobilized to conduct house visits, clean up public areas and do community education. But this type of "evangelical ecology," as Nading (2014: 96) called it, can only go on for so long. Households behind locked gates are not always easily accessible and, in areas of political uncertainty, suspicion of government agents entering homes, like spies, can surface. In Haiti, some would tell me that to control mosquitoes would require that "we change the whole face of the country" (Figure 1.5).

Public health officials cannot assume that, in urban geographies, there is enough social cohesion, shared interest and mutual bonds to carry out this type of anti-mosquito work. Throughout the Zika pandemic, I would hear phrases like "communities are not accustomed to working for the common good." Others would speak about cascade effects: when the state takes care of its citizens, then the citizens will help the state. At the local municipal level, we might suspect that better vector control could translate into brownie points for elected officials. A study in Pernambuco, in northeastern Brazil, however, found that informing citizens about the use of municipal funds to combat Dengue, CHIKV and ZIKV had no effect on the major's reelection bid (Boas and Hidalgo, 2019). There is also an important gender dimension here, a feminization of *Aedes* control. It is females in the household that need to control female mosquitoes, a type of interspecies housekeeping.[38]

Mosquito control, especially environmental sanitation and chemical brigades, has often been a method for the state to show its power, to establish its credentials. In the United States and Europe, mosquito control is funded by municipal taxes, mostly for nuisance mosquitoes. The Cuban Dengue program developed in 1981, after a severe epidemic, is often regarded as one of the most robust in the LAC region. It has included elements of community participation on top of fines, the use of army brigades, decentralized decision-making and traditional chemical vector control. Cuba claimed to have prevented the spread of Zika in 2016 because of this intersectoral approach (Castro et al. 2017). But this requires strong management and funding; for Cuba, this was grounded in one of the best primary healthcare systems in the developing world and a one-party communist state that has remained in power since the 1950s Cuban revolution. Even here

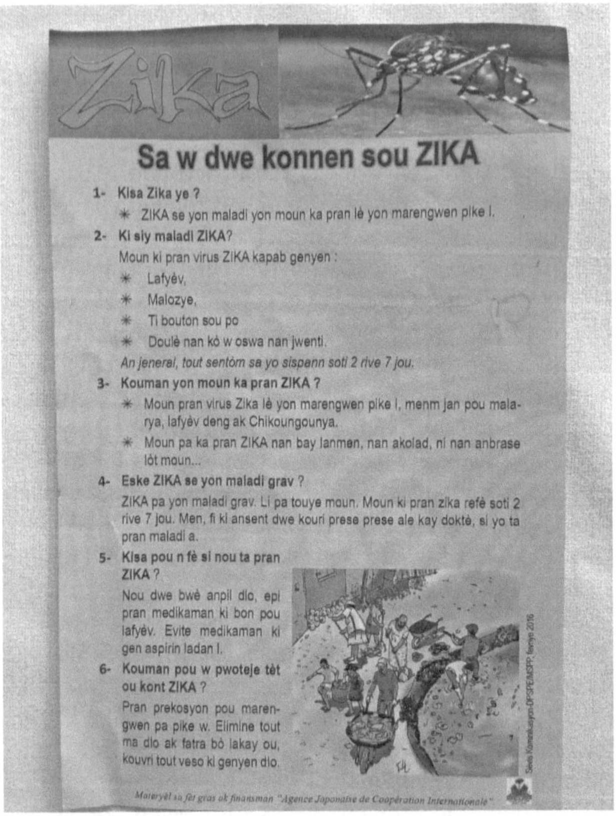

Figure 1.5 A Zika educational flyer, Haiti, emphasizing the need for community clean-up activities.

however, more recent genomic analysis has suggested that these intensive vector control efforts only delayed the virus in Cuba, with a Zika outbreak emerging in 2017.[39]

In the absence of strong tax revenue, militarized anti-mosquito brigades and/or strong health systems, perhaps only a vaccine or genetically modified mosquito can save things? After two decades of work, Sanofi's new Dengvaxia vaccine ran into controversies in the Philippines in 2017 after it was linked to several deaths in children, thought to be due to immunological factors associated with antibody-dependent enhancement. Zika clinical trials have run into the mud because it has been hard to find sero-negative populations. New vector control tools have also been hailed as a welcome addition to the armory: endosymbiotic (Wolbachia) bacteria and dominant lethal genes, such as those developed by the UK-based company, Oxitec. But these too can be problematic. As Bennett discusses in Chapter 9 of this book, experimental technologies such as Oxitec's trial in the

Florida Keys can generate a great deal of controversy and are not the magic bullet some originally assumed.

The state, human rights and the social determinants of health

Zika's social dimensions not only involve mosquitoes but also the more intimate and private spaces of human sexuality and reproduction, as well as the broader social policies and macroeconomic trends that influence people's lives. Framing Zika as a problem of individual behavior change – of cleaning backyards or wearing condoms – ignores the role of the state as a caregiver, of civil society as the glue of social change and of the interlocking of Zika with policies on health care, sexual and reproductive health, social protection, disability rights and the elephant in the room: climate change. During, and after the epidemic, this was articulated by families in northeastern Brazil in their struggle to care for their Zika-affected children, as well as feminist activists in their search for social justice and reproductive rights (see Pimentel and colleagues in Chapter 4 of this book).

As the WHO moves to embrace Universal Health Coverage (UHC), founded on ethical and legal principles of equal access to health care, in some cases even preferential treatment for the poor, major disparities exist across the region and within countries. From Colombia, Cuba and Costa Rica's more developed health and social protection systems to the erratic public-private mix of Haiti, Zika has reflected the challenges and fissures of universalist prescriptions for reform. Puerto Rico, an unincorporated territory of the United States since the 1898 Spanish-American war, was in the gripes of an economic crisis during the epidemic, accelerated since the 2008 global financial meltdown; 46% live below the American poverty line, twice the rate of Mississippi (Gomez et al. 2018). This limited Puerto Rico's resource mobilization in the face of an epidemic, and contributed to over 20% of the population being infected with Zika (85% of all US cases) (Rodríguez-Díaz et al. 2017).

Understanding the state response to Zika requires appreciating various ongoing political and economic struggles across the LAC region, and how these shape the unequal expansion of health policies (see Matta and colleagues' discussion in reference to Brazil in Chapter 3). These include the political and social ramifications of volatile global commodity markets and macroeconomic policies, such as the dramatic effects of the oil and gas industry on Venezuelan society and public life (discussed in Chapter 5). Tensions and conflicts in the social contract between citizens, institutions and elites are linked to the fabric and logics of economic liberalization and democratization itself (Whitehead, Fair and Payne, 2010). Within these struggles for a just and equal society, politics takes different forms with different implications for health: from revolutionary communist rhetoric, populist socialism, liberal democratic sentiment and strongman politics. Political conflict also becomes embodied in physical violence. Latin America holds the unfortunate global distinction of having the most violence cities, with 41 of the top 50 (including 21 in Brazil alone).[40] These locations are home to various forms of vigilantism, drug cartels, police corruption and state-directed human rights violations that coexist with the noxious living conditions of shantytowns and the marginalization of indigenous peoples. Without taxation, social services and universal health care seem a distant fiscal dream – but without trust in the state, who wants to pay taxes?

This is all reflected, in various ways and at different levels, in sexual and reproductive health, albeit interwoven into social and cultural norms, and in the response and recovery to Zika. Modeling studies have shown that sexual transmission, although low in comparison to the significance of mosquitoes, may still be able to sustain endemic transmission (Allard et al. 2017). However Catholic bishops and archbishops condemned the use of condoms as Zika spread. Paternalism and chauvinism (*Machismo*) dominated discussions about the links between Zika and the prevention of sexual transmission, including problems of access and use of contraception and reproductive rights (Guerra-Reyes and Iguiniz-Romero, 2018).[41] An estimated 56% of pregnancies, many from adolescent girls in poor communities, are unplanned in Latin America (Bott et al. 2012). According to some experts, the lack of public health advice for the postponement of pregnancy during the epidemic was "the single greatest travesty" of the Zika response and was "hideously racist hypocrisy … female American tourists were given the best and safest public health advice, while brown Puerto Rican inhabitants were told something else entirely."[42] Data does suggest that Zika had some impact on reproductive health decision-making. Studies have found a ~10–15% drop in hospital births during the epidemic's peak in different Brazilian cities, which may have been due to early miscarriages due to infection, delayed pregnancy and/or increases in abortion (Castro et al. 2018). In 2015, the Guttmacher Institute estimated there were 6.5 million abortions in Latin America and the Caribbean, 95% of which were unsafe.[43] Abortion laws are stricter in some nations (Brazil) than others (Colombia). A lack of access to ultrasound tests run two ways: they can limit a women's decision *for* or *against* an abortion. While much of the discussion has focused on the right to abortion, emerging reports from India in 2018 suggest that pregnant women with Zika infection may also be actively pressured to undergo abortions by the state and medical professionals.[44]

Despite promises, support for families affected by the virus has largely fallen off the political radar and even scientific studies tracking their insidious neurodevelopmental impacts have been under-funded, according to some researchers. Families with Zika-affected children remain in the aftermath, where Zika is a chronic ailment and not a mild virus. As they navigate emotions of apathy, rejection and develop *theologies of hope*, they have formed support groups, finding ways to survive and address stigma and discriminations that their children are "little devils" or the result of sinful sexual transgressions. Most remain "poor northeasterners (de Oliveira et al. 2017), and many are single mothers: the men often have left. This is to say nothing of the less visible pathogenic effects on the "Zika generation." We are left to wonder how many have fallen through the surveillance cracks entirely. In the aftermath, affected families and allied health professionals are left to fight for the rights of the disabled, and to remind the state and society of the threat of doing nothing to address the systemic risks for future arboviral epidemics.

It is, after all, clear that these mosquito-borne epidemics will continue to circulate in the geographies of northeastern Brazil, in the thousands of cities and towns affected by Zika in 2016 and in the urban jungles and "poor cities," around the world, that now define our planet's ecology. As I left Haiti for Florida one day before Hurricane Irma hit in 2017, I was reminded of the impact of climate change: destroyed homes, power outages, evacuation orders, disrupted food supplies and compromised health care. Zika was influenced by a particularly severe 2015–2016 El Niño weather pattern in the eastern equatorial Pacific Ocean that brought multiyear drought to some regions and extreme flooding and humidity to others.[45] Unfortunately, the continued failures of global climate agreements, and of our ability to address unfettered neoliberalism, will remain another factor, among many, in the complex web of arboviral causation.

Notes

1 According to a more recent analysis, this may be much less, from 27% to 50% of cases being symptomatic (Mitchell et al. 2018).
2 GBS causes neurological problems and paralysis of the limbs, and although it often resolves within months, severe complications do occur, especially when it paralyzes the breathing muscles and causes brain inflammation, typically in older people. It requires sophisticated medical care, including intensive care and rehabilitation services. About 20% of people continue to have symptoms throughout their lives and 5% die from it (Yuki and Hartung, 2012).
3 Data showed that the spike in Polynesia was notable; an estimated 1 GBS case for each 4,200 Zika infections, 25 times higher than the "normal" background rate.
4 Much of this early account of the pandemic from Brazil comes from Debora Diniz's (2017) excellent book, *Zika: From the Brazilian Backlands to Global Threat.*
5 By January 2016, over 3,000 cases of microcephaly were under investigation and, by mid-2016, over 8,000 with many more possible cases simply forgotten about or ignored (Diniz, 2017: 99).
6 The WHO's declaration of Zika as a PHEIC was a decision that had broad consequences. However it focused not on Zika infection per say but on its relationship to increasing cases of neonatal microcephaly in northeastern Brazil and, through a retroactive analysis of the 2014 outbreak, in French Polynesia. It also considered the potential for rapid geographical spread, the lack of diagnostics and therapeutics, and the lack of immunity.
7 https://www.theatlantic.com/health/archive/2016/06/rio-de-janeiro-brazil-olympics-zika-risk-postpone-cancel-move/485183/
8 https://www.latimes.com/opinion/op-ed/la-oe-0421-klein-zika-population-drop-20160421-story.html
9 https://www.nytimes.com/2016/09/18/us/outcry-erupts-over-miami-beachs-pesticide-spraying-to-curb-zika.html
10 https://www.theguardian.com/environment/2016/sep/04/zika-mosquito-neurotoxin-kills-bees-livelihoods-beekeepers
11 https://www.miamiherald.com/news/health-care/article109554377.html
12 https://www.washingtonpost.com/national/health-science/mysterious-and-fast-moving-zika-virus-has-worlds-health-leaders-scrambling/2016/02/13/c2aac122-d119-11e5-abc9-ea152f0b9561_story.html?utm_term=.ec2b4f94cf72
13 Studies have shown that CZS rates range from 1–19% of women infected with the virus in their first trimester, and epidemiological studies continue to turn-up new clinical consequences.

14 This includes: fieldwork in Haiti since 2015 (see Bardosh et al., 2017); extensive in-depth interviews I have conducted with scientists, policy-makers, NGOs, funders and public health practitioners in the United States and Europe on Zika, including a month of fieldwork in Washington, DC, in the fall of 2016; and work for UNICEF analyzing social, cultural and behavioral data collected by NGOs during the epidemic (Bardosh et al., 2018).

15 See also https://www.nytimes.com/2017/01/16/health/zika-virus-response.html

16 https://www.nytimes.com/2017/01/16/health/zika-virus-response.html

17 https://www.who.int/emergencies/zika-virus-tmp/en/

18 The Commission on a Global Health Risk Framework for the Future (CGHRF), convened by the US National Academy of Medicine, after the 2014-16 Ebola epidemic estimated that pandemics will cost the global economy some $6 trillion in the 21st century and recommend spending $4.5 billion per year (or 65 cents per person worldwide) on upgrading public health infrastructure, improved governance and financing mechanisms and new pathways for drug, vaccine and product development.

19 https://www.washingtonpost.com/national/health-science/mysterious-and-fast-moving-zika-virus-has-worlds-health-leaders-scrambling/2016/02/13/c2aac122-d119-11e5-abc9-ea152f0b9561_story.html?utm_term=.ec2b4f94cf72

20 https://www.pih.org/article/for-ebola-countries-need-tools-to-treat-patients-in-their-communities

21 https://www.ghsagenda.org

22 This included a request for $1.51 billion for the Department of Health and Human Services, $335 million for USAID and $41 million for the Department of State. See Epstein and Lister (2016).

23 The influence of the United States is significant. Just after confirmation of a Zika-related microcephaly case in Hawaii and a Zika case in the US Virgin Islands, the WHO declared its PHEIC. Hoffman and Silverberg (2018) highlight the political correlation between US disease spread and WHO PHEIC announcements.

24 See Mason (2016) for a discussion of pubic health reform in China after SARS.

25 Other US funding included a Grand Challenges round for vector control innovations and other funds to support vaccine development.

26 This included a Knowledge, Attitudes and Practice (KAP) resource pack and RCCE strategy documents developed by the WHO, PAHO, UNICEF and others. A website on social science and ZIKV was launched by WHO, tracking studies across the region, and a "Zika Communication Network" was established (see www.zikacommunicationnetwork.org).

27 This data was from a meta-analysis of 14 quantitative surveys (n = 41,657 participants) and 8 qualitative studies gathered in 6 countries in 2016–2017: Dominican Republic, El Salvador, Guatemala, Honduras, Nicaragua and Peru.

28 From Bollyky (2018).

29 Makonde is spoken by the Makonde, an ethnic group found between the borders of Tanzania and Mozambique.

30 The majority of reported cases came from Brazil, Colombia, Venezuela, El Salvador, Honduras, Puerto Rico, Martinique and Guadeloupe.

31 https://data.worldbank.org/region/latin-america-and-caribbean

32 http://www.paho.org/data/index.php/en/mnu-topics/indicadores-dengue-en/dengue-nacional-en/252-dengue-pais-ano-en.html?start=1

33 See http://www.uvri.go.ug/index.php/about-uvri/history

34 https://www.who.int/en/news-room/fact-sheets/detail/vector-borne-diseases

35 https://unhabitat.org/pmss/listItemDetails.aspx?publicationID=2917

36 https://data.worldbank.org/topic/poverty?locations=ZJ

37 Nearly 60% live under the national poverty line of $2.40/day.

38 See Chapter 8 of this volume, where García-Betancourt and team explore the theme of belonging in a small Colombian city, in relation to the design of a participatory vector control intervention.

39 https://www.biorxiv.org/content/biorxiv/early/2018/12/14/496901.full.pdf
40 A study in Colombia, with > 6 million IDPs (12% of Colombia's population, second only to Syria) found a strong association between high homicide rates and Dengue infection (Krystosik et al., 2018). See https://www.independent.co.uk/news/world/the-most-violent-cities-in-the-world-latin-america-dominates-list-with-41-countries-in-top-50-a6995186.html
41 Access to birth control methods across LAC vary from an estimated 73% in Colombia to 35% in Haiti, for example. https://www.guttmacher.org/sites/default/files/report_pdf/unmet-need-for-contraception-in-developing-countries-report.pdf
42 https://www.nytimes.com/2017/01/16/health/zika-virus-response.html
43 https://www.guttmacher.org/sites/default/files/factsheet/ib_aww-latin-america.pdf
44 https://www.downtoearth.org.in/news/health/zika-has-unborn-victims-in-madhya-pradesh-62459
45 https://www.who.int/hac/crises/el-nino/22february2016/en/

References

Allard, A., Althouse, B. M., Hébert-Dufresne, L., & Scarpino, S. V. 2017, 'The risk of sustained sexual transmission of Zika is underestimated', *PLoS Pathogens*, vol. 13, no. 9, pp. e1006633.

Armelagos, G. J. 1998. 'The viral superhighway', *The Sciences*, vol. 38, no. 1, pp. 24–29.

Bardosh, K. (ed.) 2016, *One Health: science, politics and zoonotic disease in Africa*. Routledge.

Bardosh, K., Garica, T., Franco, C., Ignuiniz, R., Ormea, V., Amaya, M., Chitnis, K. and Serino, A. 2018, *Risk Communication and Community Engagement in the Zika Response: A Meta-Analysis of Knowledge, Attitude and Practice (KAP) Research Across 6 Latin American and Caribbean Countries*. UNICEF/USAID Technical Report.

Bardosh, K., Jean, L., Beau De Rochars, V. M., Lemoine, J. F., Okech, B., Ryan, S. J., et al. 2017, 'Polisye kont moustik: a culturally competent approach to larval source reduction in the context of lymphatic filariasis and malaria elimination in Haiti', *Tropical Medicine and Infectious Disease*, vol. 2, no. 3, pp. 39.

Bhatt, S., Gething, P. W., Brady, O. J., Messina, J. P., Farlow, A. W., Moyes, C. L., et al. 2013, 'The global distribution and burden of dengue', *Nature*, vol. 496, no. 7446, pp. 504.

Boas, T. C., & Hidalgo, F. D. 2019, 'Electoral incentives to combat mosquito-borne illnesses: experimental evidence from Brazil.' *World Development*, vol. 113, pp. 89–99.

Bollyky, T. J. 2018, *Plagues and the paradox of progress: why the world is getting healthier in worrisome ways*. MIT Press.

Bott S., Guedes A., Goodwin M., Mendoza J. A. 2012, *Violence against women in Latin America and the Caribbean: a comparative analysis of population-based data from 12 countries*. Pan American Health Organization, Washington, DC.

Bowman, L. R., Donegan, S., & McCall, P. J. 2016, 'Is dengue vector control deficient in effectiveness or evidence?: Systematic review and meta-analysis', *PLoS Negl Trop Dis*, vol. 10, no. 3, pp. e0004551. DOI:10.1371/journal.pntd.0004551.

Castro, M. C., Han, Q. C., Carvalho, L. R., Victora, C. G., & França, G. V. 2018, 'Implications of Zika virus and congenital Zika syndrome for the number of live births in Brazil', *Proceedings of the National Academy of Sciences*, 115(24), 6177–6182.

Castro, M., Pérez, D., Guzman, M. G., & Barrington, C. 2017, 'Why did Zika not explode in Cuba? The role of active community participation to sustain control of vector-borne diseases', *The American Journal of Tropical Medicine and Hygiene*, vol. 97, no. 2, pp. 311–312.

CHRF Commission (Commission on a Global Health Risk Framework for the Future). 2016, *The neglected dimension of global security: a framework to counter infectious disease crises*. National Academies Press, Washington, DC.

Colón-González, F. J., Peres, C. A., São Bernardo, C. S., Hunter, P. R., & Lake, I. R. 2017, 'After the epidemic: Zika virus projections for Latin America and the Caribbean', *PLoS Neglected Tropical Diseases*, vol. 11, no. 11, pp. e0006007.

de Almeida Barreto, F. K., Montenegro, R. M., Fernandes, V. O., Oliveira, R., de Araújo Batista, L. A., Hussain, A., et al. 2018, 'Chikungunya and diabetes, what do we know?' *Diabetology & Metabolic Syndrome*, vol. 10, no. 1, pp. 32.

de Oliveira W, et al. 2017, 'Infection-related microcephaly after the 2015 and 2016 Zika virus outbreaks in Brazil: a surveillance-based analysis', *Lancet* vol. 390, pp. 861–870.

Dick, G. W. A., Kitchen, S. F., & Haddow, A. J. 1952, 'Zika virus (I). Isolations and serological specificity', *Transactions of the Royal Society of Tropical Medicine and Hygiene*, vol. 46, no. 5, pp. 509–520.

Diniz, D. 2017, *Zika: from the Brazilian backlands to global threat*. Zed Books.

Duffy, M. R., Chen, T. H., Hancock, W. T., Powers, A. M., Kool, J. L., Lanciotti, R. S., et al. 2009, 'Zika virus outbreak on Yap Island, federated states of Micronesia', *New England Journal of Medicine*, vol. 360, no. 24, pp. 2536–2543.

Epstein, S. and Lister, S. 2016, 'Zika response funding: request and congressional action', *Congressional Research Service*, 7–5700, pp. R44460. <https://fas.org/sgp/crs/misc/R44460.pdf>

Foy, B. D., Kobylinski, K. C., Foy, J. L. C., Blitvich, B. J., da Rosa, A. T., Haddow, A. D., et al. 2011. 'Probable non–vector-borne transmission of Zika virus, Colorado, USA', *Emerging Infectious Diseases*, vol. 17, no. 5, pp. 880.

Gates, B. 2018, 'Innovation for pandemics', *New England Journal of Medicine*, vol. 378, no. 22, pp. 2057–2060.

Grubaugh, N. D., Ladner, J. T., Kraemer, M. U., Dudas, G., Tan, A. L., Gangavarapu, K., et al. 2017, 'Genomic epidemiology reveals multiple introductions of Zika virus into the United States', *Nature*, vol. 546, no. 7658, pp. 401.

Gubler, D. J., Vasilakis, N., & Musso, D. 2017, 'History and emergence of Zika virus', *The Journal of Infectious Diseases*, vol. 216, no. suppl_10, pp. S860–S867.

Guerra-Reyes, L., & Iguiñiz-Romero, R. A. 2018, 'Performing purity: reproductive decision-making and implications for a community under threat of zika in iquitos, Peru', *Culture, Health & Sexuality*, 21(3), 309–322.

Heintze, C., Garrido, M. V., & Kroeger, A. 2007, 'What do community-based dengue control programmes achieve? A systematic review of published evaluations', *Transactions of the Royal Society of Tropical Medicine and Hygiene*, vol. 101, no. 4, pp. 317–325.

Hernández-Ávila, J. E., Palacio-Mejía, L. S., López-Gatell, H., Alpuche-Aranda, C. M., Molina-Vélez, D., González-González, L., & Hernández-Ávila, M. 2018, 'Zika virus infection estimates, Mexico', *Bulletin of the World Health Organization*, vol. 96, no. 5, pp. 306.

Higgs, S. 2016, 'Zika virus: emergence and emergency', *Vector Borne and Zoonotic Diseases*, vol. 16, no. 2, pp. 75.

Hoffman, S. J., & Silverberg, S. L. 2018, 'Delays in global disease outbreak responses: lessons from H1N1, Ebola, and Zika', *American Journal of Public Health*, vol. 108, no. 3, 329–333.

Horstick O., Runge-Ranzinger S., Nathan M. B., Kroeger A. 2010, 'Dengue vector control services: how do they work? A systematic literature review and country case studies',

Transactions of the Royal Society of Tropical Medicine and Hygiene, vol. 104, no. 6, pp. 379–386.

Jansen, K. A. 2013, 'The 2005–2007 Chikungunya epidemic in Reunion: ambiguous etiologies, memories, and meaning-making', *Medical Anthropology*, vol. 32(2), 174–189.

Krystosik, A., Curtis, A., LaBeaud, A., Dávalos, D., Pacheco, R., Buritica, P., et al. 2018, 'Neighborhood violence impacts disease control and surveillance: case study of Cali, Colombia from 2014 to 2016', *International Journal of Environmental Research and Public Health*, vol. 15, no. 10, 2144.

Lakoff, A. 2017, *Unprepared: global health in a time of emergency*. Univ of California Press.

Lednicky, J., De Rochars, V. M. B., El Badry, M., Loeb, J., Telisma, T., Chavannes, S., et al. 2016, 'Zika virus outbreak in Haiti in 2014: molecular and clinical data', *PLoS Neglected Tropical Diseases*, vol. 10, no. 4, pp. e0004687.

Legorreta-Soberanis, J., Paredes-Solís, S., Morales-Pérez, A., Nava-Aguilera, E., Santos, F. R. S., Sánchez-Gervacio, B. M., et al. 2017, 'Coverage and beliefs about temephos application for control of dengue vectors and impact of a community-based prevention intervention: secondary analysis from the Camino Verde trial in Mexico', *BMC Public Health*, vol. 17, no. 1, pp. 426.

Mason, K. 2016, *Infectious change: reinventing Chinese public health after an epidemic*. Stanford University Press.

McNeill, J. R. 2010, *Mosquito empires: ecology and war in the Greater Caribbean*, 1620–1914. Cambridge University Press.

McNeil, D. G. 2016, *Zika: the emerging epidemic*. WW Norton & Company.

Mehta, R., Gerardin, P., de Brito, C. A. A., Soares, C. N., Ferreira, M. L. B., & Solomon, T. 2018, 'The neurological complications of chikungunya virus: a systematic review', *Reviews in Medical Virology*, vol. 28, no. 3, pp. e1978.

Mitchell, P. K., Mier-y-Teran-Romero, L., Biggerstaff, B. J., Delorey, M. J., Aubry, M., Cao-Lormeau, V. M., et al. 2018, 'Reassessing serosurvey-based estimates of the symptomatic proportion of Zika virus infections', *American Journal of Epidemiology*, 188(1) 206–213.

Morens, D. M., & Fauci, A. S. 2016, 'Meeting the challenge of epidemic chikungunya', *The Journal of Infectious Diseases*, vol. 214, no. suppl_5, pp. S434–S435.

Mulligan, K., Dixon, J., Joanna Sinn, C. L., & Elliott, S. J. 2015, 'Is dengue a disease of poverty? A systematic review', *Pathogens and Global Health*, vol. 109, no. 1, pp. 10–18.

Musso, D., Bossin, H., Mallet, H. P., Besnard, M., Broult, J., Baudouin, L., et al. 2017, 'Zika virus in French Polynesia 2013–14: anatomy of a completed outbreak', *The Lancet Infectious Diseases*, 18(5) 172–182.

Nading, A. M. 2014, *Mosquito trails: ecology, health, and the politics of entanglement*. Univ of California Press.

Perkins, T. A., Siraj, A. S., Ruktanonchai, C. W., Kraemer, M. U., & Tatem, A. J. 2016, 'Model-based projections of Zika virus infections in childbearing women in the Americas', *Nature Microbiology*, vol. 1, no. 9, pp. 16126.

Quick, J. D., & Fryer, B. 2018, *The end of epidemics: the looming threat to humanity and how to stop it*. St. Martin's Press.

Richards, P. 2016, *Ebola: how a people's science helped end an epidemic*. Zed Books Ltd.

Rodríguez-Díaz, C. E., Garriga-López, A., Malavé-Rivera, S. M., & Vargas-Molina, R. L. 2017, 'Zika virus epidemic in Puerto Rico: health justice too long delayed', *International Journal of Infectious Diseases*, vol. 65, pp. 144–147.

Rosling, H. 2018, *Factfulness: ten reasons we're wrong about the world--and why things are better than you think.* Flatiron Books.
Scheper-Hughes, N. 1992, *Death without weeping.* University of California Press.
Schilte C, Staikovsky F, Couderc T, Madec Y, Carpentier F, Kassab S, et al. 2013, 'Chikungunya virus-associated long-term arthralgia: a 36-month prospective longitudinal study', *PLOS Neglected Tropical Diseases*, vol. 7, no. 3, pp. e2137. DOI:10.1371/journal.pntd.0002137.
Schuffenecker, I., Iteman, I., Michault, A., Murri, S., Frangeul, L., Vaney, M. C., et al. 2006, 'Genome microevolution of chikungunya viruses causing the Indian Ocean outbreak', *PLoS Medicine*, vol. 3, no. 7, pp. e263.
Singer, M. 2017, 'The spread of Zika and the potential for global arbovirus syndemics', *Global Public Health*, vol. 12, no. 1, pp. 1–18.
Stepan, N. L. 2011, *Eradication: ridding the world of diseases forever?* Reaktion Books.
Thézé, J., Li, T., du Plessis, L., Bouquet, J., Kraemer, M. U., Somasekar, S., et al. 2018, 'Genomic epidemiology reconstructs the introduction and spread of Zika virus in Central America and Mexico', *Cell Host & Microbe*, 23(6) 855–864.
UNDP, 2017, *A socio-economic impact assessment of the Zika virus in Latin America and the Caribbean: with a focus on Brazil, Colombia and Suriname.* UNDP press.
Whitehead, N. L., Fair, J. E., & Payne, L. A. 2010, *Violent democracies in Latin America.* Duke University Press.
World Bank 2016, *The short-term economic costs of Zika in Latin America and the Caribbean (LCR).* World Bank Group, Washington, DC.
Yamey, G., Schäferhoff, M., Aars, O. K., Bloom, B., Carroll, D., Chawla, M., et al. 2017, 'Financing of international collective action for epidemic and pandemic preparedness', *The Lancet Global Health*, vol 5, no. 8, pp. e742–e744.
Yuki, N., & Hartung, H. P. 2012, 'Guillain–Barré syndrome', *New England Journal of Medicine*, vol. 366, no. 24, pp. 2294–2304.
Zambrana, J. V., Carrillo, F. B., Burger-Calderon, R., Collado, D., Sanchez, N., Ojeda, S., et al. 2018, 'Seroprevalence, risk factor, and spatial analyses of Zika virus infection after the 2016 epidemic in Managua, Nicaragua' *Proceedings of the National Academy of Sciences*, vol. 115, no. 37, pp. 9294–9299.

2 Counting Zika

Insidious uncertainties and elusive epidemic facts

Rebecca Rose Henderson and Kevin Bardosh

Introduction

In early 2016, the WHO, CDC and other global public health agencies announced that Zika virus transmission was widespread in all of Central America, much of South America, and many countries in the Caribbean, and that these countries should be avoided "until more is known about the virus."[1] Fearful that the consequences of Zika infection, first seen in northeastern Brazil in 2015, were now emerging at a larger scale across the continent, disease modelers and their models painted a worrisome picture of the future of Zika and of the risks to pregnant women and their unborn babies. In a 2016 press briefing, the WHO predicted that 3 to 4 million Zika cases were expected in the Americas,[2] and an early article in the *New England Journal of Medicine* described the disease as "explosive" (Fauci and Morens, 2016). Early estimates of the risk of congenital malformation from Zika infection during pregnancy were thought to be 14% or higher, frequently compared to congenital rubella syndrome (Nishiura et al., 2016). Entomological maps depicted moderate-to-high abundance of *Aedes aegypti* throughout US cities (including New York, Philadelphia and Washington, DC), suggesting that the summer of 2016 would bring with it a new mosquito-borne disease (Monaghan et al., 2016). The conversation quickly evolved to emphasize other potential ways for Zika to spread, including the distribution of *Aedes albopictus* (a mosquito found as far north as the Canadian border), sexual transmission, blood transfusions and breast milk.

Two years later, however, the epidemic has largely faded from public view. Catastrophic predictions of skyrocketing rates of microcephaly around the region have not been realized, at least thus far. About half-a-million suspected cases of Zika, and nearly 4,000 cases of congenital Zika syndrome (CZS), have been officially reported to the Pan American Health Organization (PAHO).[3] The reasons for this discrepancy are now open to intense scientific debate and public health reflection. A more measured, incremental and endemic image of Zika has emerged.

Maps and models of disease, and their corresponding epidemiological predictions, have important influences on the political conversation and public anxieties, and play an increasingly important role in emerging disease epidemics. In fact, predictive models have come to define a central task of epidemic response, where epidemiologists and disease modelers (among others) interact, and through their scientific logics and techniques create our collective social knowledge of disease spread, reduction and containment (Morse et al., 2012). Demographic data, disease trends, the life cycles of insects and animals, geospatial analysis, sophisticated mathematical algorithms and super-computers increasingly intermix to produce statistics, causal inferences and public policy.

Yet in tracking diseases epidemiologically, scientists exhibit fundamental assumptions about *what counts* and *how it should be counted.* In reality, "good numbers" – numbers that are representative of lived (microbial, animal and human) experience, and account for complexity, divergence and contingencies – are hard to find. Instead, these data are sometimes created, at least in part (Adams, 2016). Imperfect numbers are seen through prisms of available assumptions, theoretical models, tools and methodologies. During epidemics of new emerging infectious pathogens, producing such epidemiological knowledge is also shaped by ideas about the ontological status of disease and socio-scientific ideas about how disease is experienced, detected and combatted. But as scientific data grows, our ideas about disease also change. With each new epidemic, assumptions can be made more visible. Crises and outbreaks generate opportunities to question accepted scientific norms and concepts.

In this chapter, we are concerned with tracing the emerging science of Zika as it manifested itself, both in the scientific and political world, between 2016 (a time of "epidemic Zika") and 2018 (a time of "endemic Zika"). To do so requires exploring some of the initial epidemiological predictions, scientific logics and modeling approaches that emerged during the early stages of the epidemic, and following how epidemiology assembled particular framings of "Zika" based on limited knowledge, various assumptions, best guesses, contingencies and the pull of public anxiety. Following scholars of science and technology studies (Adams, 2016; Latour, 1987), we are concerned here with how scientists, in the context of uncertainty and partiality, make choices about how to treat their data, and the implications of these choices on unfolding policy and epidemic response.

Locating Zika: Tracking invisibilities and partialities in the world

One central task in tracking an emerging disease epidemic, like Zika, is to be able to reliably identify human cases. To do so, epidemiologists first need to decide what "counts" as a disease case. Here, the task is simplified when Rapid Diagnostic Tests (RDTs) are available. RDTs have done wonders for the epidemiological surveillance of malaria, for example, but many emerging viral pathogens cannot be counted through a simple finger-prick or even standard microscopy. Rather, counting Zika depends on serological and molecular testing, often located only in sophisticated laboratories, found mostly in capital cities and regional hubs (Charrel et al. 2016). In the typical clinic, then, where testing is unavailable, Zika is counted by presumptive diagnosis, based both on potential exposure history and clinical picture. In areas where Zika is known to be circulating, diagnosis revolves around presumption, based on clinical criteria and case definition.

Case definition is a standardization tool by which a complex clinical picture is transformed into epidemiological statistics. These case definitions are typically formulated by government agencies for the purpose of tracking disease, and, as mentioned earlier are used wherever possible in conjunction with exposure history and confirmatory testing. For example, Rabe et al.'s (2016) case definition for Zika includes the criteria summarized in Table 2.1.

As mentioned earlier, counting Zika has relied on a hierarchy of evidence and related terminology. In countries where exposure is presumed and laboratory testing is unavailable, case definition criteria suffice to count a "suspected" case. During the 2014–2016 epidemic, confirmatory testing was only available in a few countries, and even in these the logistics of transporting samples from the clinic to the lab further mediated the act of confirmation. For example, as of January 2018, the PAHO/WHO has reported only five confirmed cases of Zika in Haiti, not because the disease was through to be rare but due to the lack of availability of confirmatory testing.[5] These difficulties were especially acute during the height of the epidemic in Brazil, for example, when LACEN (Laboratório Central de Saúde Pública) reported a wait time of at least nine months for laboratory confirmation (Faria et al., 2016). Even in the United States, delays with a median wait of 42 days were reported during the first month of local transmission in 2016 (Shiu et al., 2018). Instead of waiting for test results, epidemiologists relied on counting "suspected" or "probable" cases.

The use of the case definition, however, obscures as much as it reveals. First, the virus' circulation in human bodies is predominantly invisible: up to 80% of Zika cases are thought to be asymptomatic. While some data suggests this number is an overestimate, it is likely that at least half of all patients are asymptomatic (Moghadas et al., 2017).

Even in cases where Zika shows symptoms, the use of a clinical profile has its own particular challenges. Symptoms are nonspecific and mild; they are easy to

Table 2.1 Typical case definition for Zika Virus infection[4]

Zika is defined as:
A person with one or more of the following not explained by another etiology:

1. Clinically compatible illness that includes:
   - Acute onset of fever (measured or reported), **OR**
   - maculopapular rash, **OR**
   - arthralgia, **OR**
   - conjunctivitis
2. Complication of pregnancy:
   - fetal loss; **OR**
   - fetus or neonate with congenital microcephaly, congenital intracranial calcifications, other structural brain or eye abnormalities, or other congenital central nervous system-related abnormalities including defects such as clubfoot or multiple joint contractures
3. Guillain-Barré syndrome or other neurologic manifestations

miss and ignore. This is particularly true in the context of poverty, where health resources are limited and reserved for cases of serious illness or emergency. In order for diseases to be *counted* through the use of a case definition, individual patients have to go to the doctor (and not elsewhere for their health care, such as a traditional healer or pharmacist) and this doctor has to be sufficiently *connected* to a surveillance system to make the case visible, which depends on physical and cognitive infrastructures to support epidemiological accounting.

These requirements mean that Zika counting as manifested in official disease reports are necessarily partial and incomplete. With a lack of health insurance, disposable income or confidence in health providers, impoverished individuals are much less likely to seek medical care in general (Peters et al., 2008) especially for mild illnesses that resolve spontaneously within a matter of days. Fevers reported by patients with Zika are rarely high; patients normally do not require hospitalization. Symptoms such as conjunctivitis (red eyes), arthralgia (muscle aches) and maculopapular (red bumpy) rash could further be due to many other causes. An agricultural laborer, for example, who comes home with a low fever, red, irritated eyes, a red bumpy rash and muscle aches could easily attribute these mild symptoms to working outside among plant and insect irritants, as well as to exposure to sun and pesticides. In any case, they may lack time or money to go to the doctor, and within a few days would recover and, generally speaking, be back to normal. Surely, many such cases of Zika did not make their way into epidemiological reports.

To further complicate things, consider a second example: a pregnant woman with the same symptoms, who is acutely aware of the details of Zika virus infection. Such a woman, more concerned about her symptoms and more likely to go to a doctor, would also be more likely to be "counted," as reported by Lozier et al. (2017) in Puerto Rico. Furthermore, when cases of congenital fetal malformations are suspected or confirmed, Zika counting frequently depends on the mother's memory. Mild symptoms manifested many months previously need to be disentangled from other physiological changes during pregnancy, in the emotional context of caring for a newborn baby with congenital malformations and the newly discovered reality of its life-long impact (Diniz, 2017). Similar to the maternal health statistics explored by Wendland (2016), these statistics are reflections of both visible and invisible disease temporalities that are dependent on expert interpretation and acts of translation. These hidden realities are further complicated by the unpredictable behavior of infected mosquitoes and human bodies.

Although Zika, as depicted by its case definition, can look like many different things, it most closely resembles its viral cousins: Chikungunya and the four accepted Dengue serotypes. Both are carried by the same vector (*Aedes aegypti*) and are endemic in precisely the same geographical areas as Zika. All three viruses are positive, single-stranded RNA enveloped Arboviruses with an icosahedral shape. While Chikungunya is an Alphavirus, Dengue and Zika are both members of the genus Flavivirus (Lycke & Norrby, 2014; Faye et al., 2014) (Table 2.2).

Table 2.2 Case definitions of Dengue, Chikungunya and Zika[6]

Dengue (without warning signs)	*Chikungunya or other non-neuroinvasive arbovirus*	*Zika (non-congenital)*

• Fever
• Two of the following:
  • Nausea, vomiting
  • Rash
  • Aches and pains
  • Leukopenia
	• Fever (chills) as reported by the patient or a health-care provider, **AND**
	• Absence of neuroinvasive disease, **AND**
	• Absence of a more likely clinical explanation.
	• Other clinically compatible symptoms of (arbovirus disease headache, myalgia, rash, arthralgia, vertigo, vomiting, paresis and/or nuchal rigidity)
		• Acute onset of fever (measured or reported), **OR**
		• maculopapular rash, **OR**
		• arthralgia, **OR**
		• conjunctivitis

Where diseases look similar, the use of case definition to categorize them becomes even more problematic, and is increasingly reliant on prevailing public health discourse. In a setting where everyone is looking for Zika, but there are simultaneously co-occurring epidemics of Dengue (DEN-1 to DEN-4) and Chikungunya (not to mention, other many other viruses),[7] physicians are more likely to label these vague symptoms "Zika." By worrying about Zika, we may become more likely to find it.

Interestingly, although statistics on the prevalence of Zika in most places rely almost exclusively on case definition, most governments have not tested the efficacy of this approach. In Brazil, Braga et al. (2017) evaluated several clinical case definitions used to identify Zika in the context of simultaneous Dengue and Chikungunya circulation. They found that case definitions offered by WHO, ECDC, PAHO, and Brazilian Ministry of Health each had very low specificities, and that the case definitions used by the Brazilian Ministry of Health and PAHO misclassified 48% of Zika cases as Dengue (Braga et al., 2017).

In government reports, statistics published about the number of "suspected" cases are depicted on maps and in graphs in ways that, to the untrained eye, may hide these uncertainties and approximations. For example, country-level data from WHO/PAHO case reports are based on case definition criteria alone. In El Salvador, to take just one example, we find higher incidence rates for infants and young adults, which likely mirrors the issues discussed above regarding clinical care; parents are more likely to take children to the doctor than they are to go themselves. Looking at these authoritative representations, we may be easily forgiven for mistaking these numbers for exact counts, and conclude that Zika is more likely to occur in children.

Although "suspected" case numbers may be unreliable, it is likewise dangerous for governments without access to diagnostic testing to rely only on "confirmed" cases. Early risk communication efforts in Jamaica, for example, led by the Ministry of Health, only reported the few confirmed cases while simultaneously emphasizing to the public that Zika was a public health emergency and that communities needed to take action (Bardosh, personal communication, Jamaica, September 2016). This is a recipe for confusion, rumours and even social resistance (Briggs and Nichter, 2009). Choices about how to communicate Zika count to the public, then, and have practical consequences for interventions at community-level. These interventions have tended (after some initial emphasis on confirmed cases) to have evolved to focus on suspected cases, as well as incantations that everyone is at risk.

Unlike in most of the Americas, however, public pronouncements in the United States followed officially confirmed laboratory cases and test results. This presented a different set of ambiguities. Currently, the CDC recommends RNA NAT (Nucleic Acid Testing) or RT-PCR (Reverse Transcription Polymerase Chain Reaction) for symptomatic pregnant women who may have been exposed to Zika (CDC, 2018). Molecular and serological tests, such as Enzyme-Linked Immunoabsorbant Assays (ELISA) and plaque reduction neutralization tests (PRNT) locate antibodies; testing for these antibodies is a common and relatively low-cost method of tracking infection. However, like clinical presentations and case definitions, recent studies have demonstrated that Zika virus antibodies cross-react with other flaviviruses, especially Dengue but also Japanese Encephalitis, Saint Louis Encephalitis, West Nile and Yellow Fever (Vorou, 2016). These closely related viruses co-circulate in many of the areas in which Zika was emerging, impacting the reliability of tests involving antibodies. While rates of sensitivity (true positive rate) and specificity (true negative rate) vary by commercial test, cross-reactivity means that Zika antibody tests will sometimes be falsely positive, particularly in the case of Dengue (Dejnirattisai et al., 2016). As antibodies persist in the body, cross-reactivity may not be time-specific; it can occur based on flavivirus infections decades earlier. In areas where Dengue infection rates are high, this creates a major problem for diagnostic confirmation. A retrospective study in Miami, where laboratory conditions are at their best, suggested a false positive rate of 25% for women tested for IgM antibodies (Curry et al., 2017).

Testing problems, and the challenges of disentangling multiple arboviruses at the molecular level, do not stop here. For example, although the Plaque Reduction Neutralization Test (PRNT) is the reference standard for the detection of neutralizing antibodies to flaviviruses, it requires live viral cultures, takes days to weeks to perform and is a more difficult and expensive test compared to immunoassay (Theel and Hata, 2018). As a result, this test was not widely available for clinical care during the Zika epidemic (Granger et al., 2017). Cross-reactivity is also a problem with PRNT, at least in secondary infections, which works both ways – patients who really have Zika will test falsely positive for Dengue and vice versa (Felix et al., 2017; Granger et al., 2017). Due to the expense of PRNT and other factors, ELISA continues to be used due to its relative cheapness, speed and accessibility. But again, cross-reactivity complicates the work of epidemiology.

One study found that combining ZIKV-NS1 IgM and IgG ELISAs could detect Zika with a specificity of only ~67%; cross-reactivity from secondary Dengue infection ranged from 28% to 67% (Tsia et al., 2017).

These diagnostic difficulties were briefly made publically visible in 2016 when a whistle-blower at the CDC went public with the information that the agency-recommended Tripolex RT-PCR test, which tested simultaneously for Zika, Chikungunya and Dengue, reduced the sensitivities of the individual tests to the point that up to 40% of Zika cases were missed (Sun, 2016).

Due to the problems of immunoassay, the only way to tell if a patient *definitively* has Zika is to test their serum for viral RNA using RT-PCR. This gold standard runs into the hundreds of dollars per test. Even if national labs, like LACEN in Brazil, can carry out the test, many cannot manage high-test volumes during an actual epidemic. Samples for RT-PCR must be taken, packaged, shipped and stored carefully to prevent degradation of RNA samples and inaccurate test results (CDC, 2017); remote districts and bad roads stand in the way. Even in the United States (where RT-PCR is used to confirm ELISA positive tests), bottlenecks and long delays occurred during the epidemic.

But perhaps a bigger difficulty is that finding and counting Zika RNA is a precarious process. Once the active virus has been cleared from the patient's blood (a maximum of 14 days after symptoms), viral RNA is untraceable. The virus has left. It is gone. This means that if a patient faces delays in testing or fails to go to the doctor while they have symptoms or has no symptoms at all, a positive RT-PCR test is impossible. Counting a "confirmed case" requires that an expensive and largely unavailable test be performed within a specific 14-day window.

In light of the multiple difficulties in testing for Zika, the CDC's guide to Zika testing is convoluted and difficult to follow (see CDC, 2017). Definitive testing for Zika, even in the best laboratory conditions in the world, remains difficult and fraught with uncertainty. Poorly-defined symptoms, inadequate testing resources and imperfect tests are just some of the problems epidemiologists faced as they attempted to measure Zika's presence in the world during the 2016 global health emergency.

Zika models: Imperfect predictions and the art of forecasting

The invisibilities and partialities inherent to counting Zika in the world, socially and scientifically, have also influenced the burgeoning field of Zika modeling, albeit in different ways and with different results. A quick PubMed search shows more than 500 papers published in 2017 with the word "Zika" in the title. Due to the nature of Zika transmission, ecological modeling approaches (that predict disease movement based on the environmental factors that determine mosquito presence and abundance) were central to early scientific efforts to predict the course of the epidemic. However, a review paper by Carlson et al. (2017), based on data from the United States, concluded that methodological conflicts hindered the development of appropriate predictions, and that most models had unacceptable margins of uncertainty that "could misrepresent the risk faced by millions of people in the United States within a single year." Keegan et al.'s (2017) review of quantitative Zika models was not less critical:

> In Europe and the United States, for example, areas predicted to have seasonal or year-round transmission risk were extensive and varied across models. However, through March 2017 no vector-borne transmission had been documented in Europe and just over 200 locally acquired mosquito-transmitted cases reported in the United States occurred in small regions of southern Florida and Texas.

While Zika science has blossomed, the predictions made by many models have failed to come to pass. Why is this? As Carlson et al. (2017) and Keegan et al. (2017) point out, both mechanistic and ecological models predicted radically different scenarios, and few seem to have been even remotely accurate.

One major problem is that it is very challenging to compare the predictions of different types of modelers, who produce widely different-looking products. Ecological modelers often produce maps depicting the possibility of transmission in various regions, and at different scales taking into account a multitude of parameters such as host density, environmental conditions like temperature, elevation and humidity and geographical barriers (Escobar and Craft, 2016). Quantitative modelers, in turn, focus on understanding pathogen spread. This is focused on generation of an accurate "reproductive number," R_0, which represents the number of individuals infected by a single infected person in an immunologically naive population. After estimating R_0 for a given disease, quantitative modelers then plug these epidemiological parameters into mathematical equations and statistically depict the speed at which a disease will spread through a population.

Within these modeling subfields, a great deal of uncertainty and disagreement exists. Both Keegan et al. (2017) and Carlson et al. (2017) attempt to compare the results of various predictive Zika models, and to graphically demonstrate the variability inherent in these predictions. They found that R_0 has ranged from 1 to 10, a huge variability, leading to widely divergent forecasts of the epidemic's size. R_0 is thought to be different for each disease and each epidemic. As a comparison, the R_0 in the 2014–2016 West African Ebola epidemic has been estimated at between 1.5 and 2.5 (Althaus, 2014).

Essentially, the challenges with counting clinical cases of Zika meant that modelers were forced to estimate disease parameters at multiple levels, embedding uncertainties within these products. In order to justify these guesses, modelers frequently cite other models, entangling together different estimates, assumptions and shaky epidemiological data. There is a tendency to employ an "empiricist repertoire" that rhetorically portrays results as belonging to the realm of accepted, socially neutral scientific fact instead of adequately and fully communicating uncertainty (Mulkay and Gilbert, 1984). Furthermore, as different researchers and policy-makers use each other's data, the amount of uncertainty increases while simultaneously becoming more obscured.

One example of the problematic assumptions embedded in disease models involves the key variable of "attack rate," which describes the speed by which a disease spreads. In order to model the spread of Zika, disease modelers were forced to construct an estimate of this important variable. Many of these estimates were based on the well-documented Zika outbreak on Yap Island in 2007. However, the attack rate in Brazil is generally thought to have been much lower than in Yap, where it was documented to be 14.6 infected individuals per 1,000 people. In Brazil, it was estimated to be 4.4/1,000 at the height of the epidemic in Bahia State, for example (MacDonald and Holden, 2018). If this rate is correct (and it may not be, for reasons discussed earlier), the Yap outbreak models would have wildly overestimated the extent of Zika infection and spread in Latin America and the Caribbean in 2016. Practically speaking, the models that informed early policy-orientated discussions about how Zika was spreading would, then, have been widely inaccurate.

This also demonstrates a problematic assumption at the heart of disease models: that there are fundamental aspects of disease that work the same ways in very different times and places. But, in reality, data drawn from different places yields different predictions and parameters. Examples of variables assumed to be the same across multiple sites include the transmissibility of Zika, the bite rate of mosquitoes, the period of infectivity and the rate of microcephaly caused by Zika. By discovering, or at least closely estimating, these disease parameters on the basis of known data, models attempt to extend these parameters to make predictions about how diseases will work in other times and places. While this assumption is taken for granted within disease modeling, in many ways it flies in the face of our knowledge about how viruses work. Even given equal exposure, everyone does not get sick equally. If I am exposed to a disease, the chances that I will get sick depend on the health of my immune system and my nutritional status, to name just a few factors. Furthermore, the rates at which individuals are exposed to disease are never equal. Disease models often assume a homogenously mixing population, in which every person is equally at risk, an assumption that is clearly not only incorrect but also obscures important social inequalities and sociocultural practices that remain at the heart of why certain people get sick and others do not.

Microcephaly: Vanishing consequences, unexplained biosocial puzzles

The long-term consequences of Zika infection are in many ways no less amorphous and difficult to track and scientifically explain than the virus and vector. Early in the Brazilian epidemic (mid-2015), cases of febrile rash were linked to a 20-fold increase in neonatal microcephaly in northeastern Brazil (Oliveira Melo et al., 2016). However, the magnitude of risk posed during pregnancy remains elusive. This link has also been expanded to include a range of other insidious neurological and developmental disorders that may take months, or possibly years, to notice after birth (Kapogiannis et al., 2017): these include mental retardation, motor disabilities and visual and auditory impairments (Table 2.3). In effect,

Table 2.3 The clinical spectrum of congenital Zika syndrome[10]

Classic findings	• Severe microcephaly (often >3 SD below the mean for gestational age and sex) • Brain abnormalities (subcortical calcifications, ventriculomegaly, cortical thinning, gyral pattern anomalies, hypoplasia of the cerebellum, or corpus callosum anomalies) • Occular findings • Congenital contractures • Neurologic impairment
Other possible findings	• Severe spinal cord injury • Facial dysmorphia • Clubfoot • Hearing loss • Congenital cardiac disease • Unilateral diaphragm paralysis
Chronic effects	• Seizures, tremors, posturing, hypertonia with spasticity, severe irritability, dysphagia, postnatal hydrocephalus • Motor and cognitive disabilities, impairment in vision and hearing • Postnatal microcephaly due to decreasing rate of head circumference growth

microcephaly is now considered to be the tip of a much larger, more nuanced and chronic clinical iceberg, or spectrum, termed Congenital Zika Syndrome or CZS (Oliveira Melo et al., 2016).[8] CZS is a complex and shifting set of symptoms that may occur together or apart, with varying degrees of severity.[9]

It is perhaps unsurprising that rates of CZS have been calculated differently at different times and places during the course of the epidemic, although most studies confirm a much higher risk when women are exposed during the first trimester and early second trimester of pregnancy (Moore et al., 2017). Coelho et al. (2017) summarized various studies that found rates from 1% to 17% of pregnancies in women with ZIKV infection, and in a systemic review and meta-analysis of eight cohort studies, Coelho and Crovella (2017) estimated the average rate of microcephaly due to Zika infection in the first trimester to be 2.3%. Alternatively, a study of women testing positive and negative for Zika in Rio de Janeiro estimated the risk of microcephaly at 3.4% but noted a broad spectrum of neonatal consequences beyond microcephaly. A study based on 442 completed pregnancies registered with the US Zika Pregnancy Registry found a 6% overall Zika-related birth defect rate and 11% rate when the women had been infected during the first trimester (Honein et al. 2017).

Clearly, understanding the full extent and occurrence of CZS will require longitudinal studies in different countries and population groups. A recent review in *The Lancet Infectious Disease* commented:

> Reports regarding the prevalence of microcephaly and adverse birth outcomes found that these ranged from 3–4% in Rio de Janeiro and 5–42% in the USA.

> A 2017 study in São Paulo, Brazil, found adverse outcomes in 15 (28%) of 54 infants (95% CI 17–41) of pregnant women infected with Zika virus, but these outcomes appeared to be substantially milder than those observed in the Rio de Janeiro study, causing speculation of possible variation in risk across regions. However, case-control, prospective cohort, and enhanced surveillance investigations have not yet yielded insights on why a small fraction of fetuses of infected mothers develop microcephaly and severe sequelae.

Before Zika moved into Brazil and invaded Recife and neighboring cities it was not documented to cause microcephaly. The potential for maternal-fetal transmission was suspected during the 2013–2014 epidemic in French Polynesia but not confirmed; subsequent retrospective studies suggest a strong association between microcephaly and Zika.[11] Rather, Zika had a rather lackluster and low-profile history, since it was first "counted" in a rhesus monkey by Rockefeller Foundation program staff investigating the sylvatic cycle of Yellow Fever in the canopy of the Zika Forest in Uganda. There remains some controversy about when the first human cases were found, with a report from Nigeria in 1954 and others in Uganda in 1962–1963 competing for the title (Gubler et al. 2017). None of these early reports or subsequent identifications in Asia (1977 Central Java) and elsewhere suggested anything more than mild febrile illness. Epidemics of Zika were never recorded, and fewer than 20 human cases were reported, although the data suggests silent infection was occurring between humans, animals and mosquitoes for over 70 years in Africa and Asia (Gubler et al. 2017). But, then again, perhaps this was because no one was looking, a question that some epidemiologists have been interested in, attempting to locate clusters of possible Zika-related microcephaly; Majumder et al. (2018) hypothesized that seasonal birth defects in a West African hospital may be explained by Zika.

At the center of this story is genetic mutation – a deadly shift of viral RNA nucleotides, emerging from the sea of random transcription errors and/or selective pressures in host-cell machinery. There are three accepted phylogenetic lineages of Zika virus: the African, Asian and American lineage, with distinct characteristics. Gubler et al. (2017) hypothesized that the Asian lineage may have adapted to generate higher viremia levels in humans, which would have facilitated more efficient mosquito spread and enhance transplacental transmission. But none of this is confirmed, and remains speculative.

What is not speculative is that Zika-related cases of microcephaly are not evenly distributed (see Figure 2.1). As noted earlier, it is impossible to tell the extent to which this skewed distribution reflects not only the distribution of cases but also the ability to count confirmed cases of the congenital effects of Zika infection. Researchers at the Latin American Collaborative Study of Congenital Malformations warned as early as 2016 that a surge in microcephaly diagnosis could be at least in part due to increased vigilance for Zika (Butler, 2016). Vigilance, in this sense, is mediated by public health surveillance systems and their methods of counting, crosschecking and confirming. However, many studies of CZS, particularly in low-resource countries and districts, have struggled in linking the congenital syndrome with the virus. In January 2016, for example,

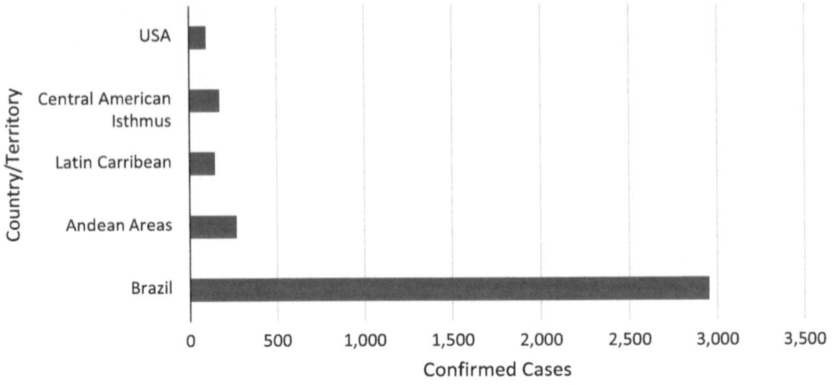

Figure 2.1 Confirmed cases of congenital syndrome associated with Zika infection through 2015–2018.

the Brazilian government reported that of 4,180 suspected cases of microcephaly recorded since October, it had rejected 462 as false diagnosis and confirmed only 270 (Butler, 2016). Cases are frequently classified based on the amount of information available and reported per case, which is often incomplete and inadequate to distinguish CZS from other congenital syndromes (França et al., 2016), and the ranking of cases according to degrees of certainty reveals the extent to which congenital Zika syndrome is an uncertain, shifting category.

As of 2018, around 3,000 cases of Zika-related microcephaly have been reported from 29 countries since its initial appearance in Brazil. As shown in Figure 2.1, the vast majority of these cases (n = 2,366) have been reported from Brazil, and most (> 80%) only from the Northeastern region (de Araújo et al., 2016). While Zika raised global health security alarm bells, it would appear that the virus' most insidious effects (on neonates – we should not forget GBS)[12] have been markedly localized to a particular corner of Brazil – what Diniz (2017) has called the "backlands" of northeastern Brazil. Why is this? A mutation does not account for why Zika should appear so profoundly important to microcephaly in northeastern Brazil, but not seem to have had the same effect elsewhere in Latin America and the Caribbean.

First, it is important to acknowledge that measures of microcephaly are dependent on clinician knowledge, situated within the state's medical bureaucracy and accepted surveillance norms and protocols. As Quintó et al. (2017) describes, a diagnosis of microcephaly requires accurate knowledge of gestational age, or the estimated age of the pregnancy, a value used to calculate the baby's maturity or prematurity at birth. Premature babies are small and thus have naturally smaller heads; microcephaly is often measured as an absolute value (head circumference) rather than as a ratio of body-to-head. An inaccurate estimate of gestational age would lead small, premature babies to be misclassified as having microcephaly, in this case clinically termed "relative microcephaly" (deSilva et al., 2017).

Gestational age is particularly difficult to calculate in the context of poor maternal health care, as it requires knowledge of the mother's last menstrual period and is often correlated with ultrasound measurements. Without this knowledge, newborn gestational age exams are, like clinical case definitions, open to different degrees of interpretation. One frequently used estimate, the Ballard exam, was demonstrated to overestimate gestational age, misclassifying 80% of premature neonates as full term; this would lead researchers attempting to classify cases of microcephaly to believe that infants had unusually small heads when in fact they were simply small due to prematurity (Quintó et al., 2017). Among cohorts of infants in Mozambique, Guatemala, Brazil, and Colombia, Quintó et al. (2017) compared the calculated prevalence of microcephaly using different systems of rating gestational age. Using one set of guidelines, the rate of microcephaly was calculated to be 1.7%; using the other, it was calculated at 4.1%.

Notably, before February 2016, the Brazilian Ministry of Health adopted a 30-cm head circumference limit, which was later increased to 33 cm. This value was a very sensitive measure (meaning that it potentially captured more cases of microcephaly) but was not necessarily scientifically validated (Osorio-de-Castro et al., 2017). In fact, in a recent clinical review of the case definition for microcephaly, de Silva et al. (2017) described four different levels of diagnostic certainty with which one can diagnose a case of zika-related microcephaly. Each of these four levels requires different amounts, and kinds, of evidence.

For this reason, multiple studies since the Zika epidemic have pointed out that "background" rates of microcephaly prior to Zika, which were largely unknown across the region, presented a second problem. Estimates of pre-Zika microcephaly prevalence rates have varied widely based on the definition used, region, methods and populations studied, and have been found to range from 0.6 to 9 per 10,000 live births (Dufort & White, 2018), Furthermore, small head circumferences are not always the result of congenital infection with Zika but can be caused by a variety of other exposures (deSilva et al., 2017); for example, many teratogens, such as alcohol, radiation, tobacco, marijuana, cocaine and toluene place neonates at risk for microcephaly. Maternal health conditions, such as maternal hypothyroidism, folate deficiency and placental insufficiency, can also cause this effect. There are also a variety of infectious diseases, such as toxoplasma, rubella, measles, cytomegalovirus (CMV), herpes, HIV and syphilis. A 2016 retrospective review of microcephaly in northeastern Brazil, for example, showed previously undetected seasonal peaks of microcephaly dating back to at least 2012, and becoming more severe as time went on (de Araújo et al., 2016). Finally, a common cause of microcephaly appears to be related to a combination of stress, malnutrition, socioeconomic status and intrauterine growth retardation (delayed growth in the womb) (Alvarado-Socarras et al., 2016). One study in Brazil noted that rates of microcephaly (prior to Zika) were correlated with maternal schooling, marital status, smoking during pregnancy, primiparity (first time birth), vaginal delivery and intrauterine growth restriction (Silva et al., 2018). De Souza et al. (2018) have shown that microcephaly in Recife, the epicenter of the Zika epidemic, were correlated with precarious living conditions and poverty. And in other impoverished places in Latin America, such as rural Guatemala, Zika has forced the realization that so-called "background" rates of microcephaly are much higher than was previously thought (Rick et al., 2017).

Campos et al. (2018) note that in tracing out the causes of heightened rates of microcephaly in Northeast Brazil, it is important to simultaneously unpack several co-occurring factors. They note that Northeast Brazil has the highest rate of poverty and the poorest environmental management, providing ideal conditions for *Aedes* mosquitoes. Furthermore, while Zika and Dengue were widespread throughout Brazil, Chikungunya rates were highest in the northeast, where peak rates of microcephaly occurred. It is difficult to disentangle these interlinked epidemiological, biological and social worlds and the multiple forces working in them. Microcephaly can be caused by multiple factors interacting simultaneously, or be caused by a single factor; thus, attempting to link microcephaly and Zika as if these two conditions could be tracked, measured and related in a vacuum risks both inaccurate measurement and erasure of the ways that microcephaly may be socially mediated.

Many of these biosocial factors, however, are not unique to Northeastern Brazil. Several possible explanations have been provided, then, for why rates of Zika were so much higher in the "backlands" of Northeastern Brazil (Diniz, 2017). An earlier study, Parens et al. (2017), argued that it was possible that Zika itself was not responsible for these cases, but that microcephaly spikes could be caused by the pesticide pyriproxyfen, which was being used in drinking water to control *Aedes* mosquitoes. This generated significant media attention in the early stages of the epidemic. However, other studies have shown that the distribution of cases of microcephaly does not map on to the distribution of pyriproxyfen use (Albuqueque et al., 2016), and an influential case-control study in *The Lancet Infectious Diseases* concluded there was no association between pyriproxyfen exposure and cases of microcephaly, while these cases were strongly associated with Zika infection (de Araújo et al., 2018). Possibilities for alternative explanations, however, become more attractive as rates of microcephaly comparable to Northern Brazil do not materialize elsewhere.

Other explanations for this gap exist. Some are located in co-circulating epidemics. For example, Northeastern Brazil has faced critical shortages of the antibiotic used to treat syphilis, and had recently suffered from both a Chikungunya and measles epidemic only a few years before (Garcia Serpa Osorio-de-Castro, et al., 2017). The pathogenesis of Zika has been shown to be enhanced by preexisting infection to other flaviviruses, notably Dengue serotypes but also, so some postulate, Chikungunya (Bardina et al., 2017).

Additional explanations have to do with the virus itself and how the threat of Zika may have increased risk mitigation behaviors in high-risk areas outside of the epicenter. The most severe congenital effects of Zika, for example, are thought to result in pregnancy loss, particularly in the very early stages of pregnancy – something that would be even harder to track and account for around the world. Coelho et al. (2017) noted that there was a 15% drop in live births in Rio de Janeiro between September and December 2016, which may have been due to early miscarriages due to ZIKV infection or delayed pregnancy due to fears about microcephaly. Marteleto et al. (2017) found a 10% drop in live births one year after the ZIKV epidemic began in Pernambuco, Brazil. A study using data from the 36 largest Brazilian cities (8.2 million births) found a live birth rate reduction of 8% in the second half of 2016, rising to 11% in cities with the highest microcephaly rates (Diaz-Quijano et al. 2018).

On the other hand, it has been proposed that some infants who were exposed to Zika in utero had less profound effects, and may not have met criteria for microcephaly (Oliveira Melo et al., 2016). These infants may still show developmental, emotional or behavioral problems, and may even regress to microcephaly if their heads fail to grow as they age (Kapogiannis et al., 2017). These consequences of Zika may only become visible after months or even years. A final possibility is related to abortion requests, which increased across some areas of Latin America during the epidemic (Aiken et al., 2016). However, while it is possible that this had some influence on reducing congenital malformation rates, the absence of ultrasound tests, required to confirm microcephaly, are not available equally to everyone.

Discussion and conclusions

This chapter has retraced the path of Zika's emergence, the ways in which scientific challenges and epidemiological uncertainty made it appear simultaneously visible and invisible, certain and uncertain, everywhere and nowhere. The corresponding partialities involved in the act of locating and counting Zika in the world operated at several levels. Zika is often asymptomatic, and when it is visible usually manifests as a mild illness with an often-undramatic clinical course, unlikely to be noticed outside of a context of epidemiological alarm. It is a virus co-circulating with a number of similar viruses carried by the same vector, with similar symptoms and similar distributions, that often cannot be told apart even by clinicians in the absence of good diagnostic testing. And even diagnostic testing may obscure as much as it clarifies: almost all tests embed profound problems, either in sensitivity, specificity, temporality or all three. And, in any case, access and availability to these tests remain very low.

These problems are not methodological flaws; they are problems inherent to the art of tracking disease, the limits of our measurement techniques and the delays inherent to generating new scientific knowledge. Some kinds of facts, like *real* Zika case numbers, simply remain fuzzy and insidiously unknowable – approachable only through approximations.

Yet epidemiologists are required to count disease; some quantification is necessary in order to provide useful science to governments, policy-makers, clinicians and an often-anxious public. Numbers of suspected and confirmed cases emerge from this mire of shifting uncertainty and are depicted in graphs and charts. And from these, they guide resources and shape policy. Health statistics in part made Zika real: these numbers pointed to it, as a real thing, existing in patients in the world. Yet what were they pointing to? At least in part, to poverty, to low access to health care and to a set of very similar endemic illnesses, co-circulating in ways that made them inextricable. And yet many within the sciences continued to treat Zika as if it was occurring in a vacuum, and treated the syndrome as a discrete biological entity rather than as a product of multiple interacting diseases and factors.

As Zika fears grew and clinicians became attuned to a public health discourse that cast Zika as an emerging critical public health threat, it is likely that this sense of needing to look for microcephaly all but guaranteed it would be found. Disease entities, like microcephaly, are often presumed to be discrete biological categories that are universal and self-evident, easily tracked and measured statistically. At every level, however, these categories fall apart, and are instead held together by guidelines, socially created and socially mediated, which allow them to be counted. Microcephaly, like many other disease phenomenon, is more easily measured and counted in contexts where access to health resources are high. In places where resources are scarce, there is increased reliance on case definitions and clinical guidelines, which can under-estimate or over-estimate. Furthermore, microcephaly, like many other disease phenomena, exists in a biological, social and economic context; microcephaly may be caused by one thing, or by a multitude of intersecting factors, such as poverty, lack of access to basic health care and other infectious diseases and environmental factors. By focusing on, and counting, microcephaly as a direct consequence of Zika, we run the risk of making these other factors invisible.

In the context of fundamental uncertainty about how a new disease works, the norms of scientific publication are inadequate to make explicit the degree to which findings are certain, or simply best guesses. It is perhaps no surprise, then, that predictions based on the subjective choices of estimates and assumptions were in many cases inconsistent from each other, and often radically departed from the reality of the unfolding Zika epidemic. They were approximations and estimates of facts. But this does not make the scientific world of epidemiology and disease modeling benign! The imperfections of scientific models have important ramifications for the real world (Morgan, 2012). Even when scientists appreciate the complexities and partialities of their work, the medium of communicating science (as Marshall McLuhan famously stated, *the medium is the message*) helps to generate illusions of certainty. Let us follow a particular example, and follow the social life of Zika modeling, to better illustrate our point.

In a 2016 article in the *New England Journal of Medicine*, Johansson et al. (2016) attempted to estimate a crucial unknown – the risk of microcephaly after first-trimester infection with Zika. Acknowledging that this value is extremely uncertain, the authors estimated the rate for Bahia, Brazil, an early epicenter of Zika and microcephaly. In attempting to model this risk, Johansson et al. (2016) first acknowledged the inherent uncertainty of tracking Zika prevalence, as described earlier, and noted that as infection rates in Bahia cannot be reliably inferred, they would use a wide range – an infection rate of between 10% and 80% of the population. The authors also attempted to account for potential over-reporting, and the unknown baseline of microcephaly in the region. After a thorough acknowledgement and attempt to account for this uncertainty, the risk of microcephaly was estimated at 0.88%, if the authors assumed an 80% Zika infection rate, and 13.2%, assuming a 10% infection rate. The authors compared their findings to data from the outbreak in French Polynesia, which estimated the risk of microcephaly in first-trimester infection to be 0.95%, based on 8 affected pregnancies in a population of 270,000. The authors noted that the lower end of their estimated range is consistent with both the numbers from French Polynesia and the absence of cases seen on Yap, which has a small enough population that at this low rate no cases would be expected.

The predictions of Johansson et al. (2016) were then mobilized, as data, by other Zika modelers. Ellington et al. (2016) attempted to estimate the number of pregnant women who may become infected with Zika virus in Puerto Rico, and to use this number to project the number of expected infants with microcephaly. In estimating the rate of microcephaly, they used the wide range produced by Johansson et al. (2016), assuming that rates of microcephaly in Puerto Rico would be similar to those in Brazil. While retaining the wide range of values projected by the uncertain predictions of Johansson et al. (2016), Ellington et al. (2016) offered no discussion of the source of these estimates, or the multiple sources of uncertainty inherent in the original paper. At the same time, new sources of uncertainty are embedded; for example, the authors are once again forced to estimate the infection rate of Zika, this time in Puerto Rico, as well as to project the rate of pregnancy during this period. They also, notably, estimate the risk of birth defects caused by Zika infection during the second and third trimesters, despite the fact that neither of the two papers cited contain any attempt to measure this risk – these are pure estimates. Using Johansson et al. (2016) as well as these estimates, the authors predicted 110 to 290 microcephaly cases occurring between mid-2016 and mid-2017.

In January, Li et al. (2017) used the predictions of Ellington et al. (2016) in another modeling paper, this time attempting to model the cost-effectiveness of increasing the availability of access to contraception during a Zika epidemic in Puerto Rico. Once again, in using Ellington et al.'s (2016) prediction for the number of microcephaly cases, the authors failed to convey the uncertainty inherent in this metric, and the potentially problematic nature of Johansson et al.'s (2016) original use of data from Brazil, which was, by this time, beginning to be recognized as having had anomalously high rates of microcephaly. Once again, the paper embeds its own uncertainty, including, notably, assumptions, unsupported by data, about the number of women who would utilize contraceptives if they were provided. In using these high projected numbers of microcephaly cases, and assuming, for example, that more than 50% of women would visit a doctor, and 50% of these would switch contraceptive measures, Li et al. (2017) found that the estimated costs of an intervention to introduce additional contraceptive resources in Puerto Rico would be about half of the amount needed to care for the infants estimated to be born with congenital Zika syndrome.

Other researchers used Li et al. (2017) to justify the need for US government interventions and investments (Ahrens et al, 2017; Darney et al., 2017; Fitzpatrick et al., 2017; Vermund, 2017). In particular, many of the authors of Li et al.

(2017) were researchers affiliated with the CDC, which in May 2016 launched Z-CAN, the Zika Contraception Action Network, through the CDC Foundation, which helps to provide women in Puerto Rico with contraceptive options (CDC Foundation, 2017). Notably, there was a significant overlap in authorship between Li et al. (2017), who published a cost justification for an intervention much like this program, and Lathrop et al. (2018), who published a description of the program. The program functioned between March 2016 and August 2017, serving > 2,100 women. As of August 2017, the Puerto Rican Department of Health had confirmed only 29 cases in which a baby born, or a fetus lost, had Zika-related birth defects – in contrast to the 110 to 290 microcephaly cases that had been predicted by Ellington et al. (2016).

What are we to make of this example? Should we interpret this chain of events as a sign of positive, science-driven policy? Epidemiological data, while uncertain (Johansson et al., 2016), was used to create predictive models (Ellington et al., 2016), which, while likewise uncertain, was used to create cost estimates (Li et al., 2017) that helped to justify and measure an intervention (Lathrop et al., 2018). On the one hand, it is possible that Z-CAN (and other related programs) is at least in part responsible for the low rates of microcephaly reported in Puerto Rico; certainly, it helped in providing affordable access to contraceptives to a few thousand women. On the other hand, in each of these publications, the authors admit significant uncertainty, not only about the rate of microcephaly caused by Zika but also about rates of infection, rates of pregnancy, uptake of contraceptives and costs of care, to name just a few. While each article acknowledges its own significant uncertainties, each also reports the results of preceding papers without a discussion of where these results come from, and the uncertainties they contain. Uncertainties within these papers are not simply additive; they increase exponentially until predictions become a series of best guesses, easily influenced by the choice of model parameters. These can drive policy. In our example, cost justification was published in January 2017 for an intervention that had already been planned by the CDC Foundation since May 2016. In what direction does the arrow of causality go: was policy driving research, research driving policy, or both?

As almost any scientist attempting to influence policy will point out, getting governments to respond to science is easier said than done. Furthermore, while the uncertainty and inherent assumptions of epidemiological predictions may cause inaccuracies in predictive models, in the face of a new disease, epidemic uncertainty is in many important ways unavoidable. In pointing out a lack of consensus between disease models, Carlson et al. (2017) worried that "the lack of a consensus among different models renders the literature less credible to policymakers." We can ask, rather provocatively: is it better to bury, rather than highlight, uncertainty in order to fight against a policy climate that increasingly has no use for science (is even "anti-science")? As Villa (2016) has pointed out, in the case of uncertainty surrounding Zika, public health agencies are in a lose-lose situation; either they are accused of raising alarm unnecessarily and wasting health resources, or of acting too slowly and remaining passive while a crisis unfolds.

Conversely, epidemiologists and disease modelers are not always advocates for policy change; disease modeling papers, in particular, are frequently abstract and geared towards a scientific audience. In this way, they reflect the need for modelers to produce science, and the appearance of certainty, cohesion and sophistication, to maintain their research funding, prestige and position. Perhaps these publications were never intended to guide policy, but to produce approximations and further develop the field? It is important to acknowledge, however, that whether they intend it or not, science is picked up by the policy world. Academic publications are frequently used and reused (even by other scientists) in ways that do not acknowledge the serious uncertainties that were obvious to those who created them.

It is possible (but unlikely) that disease predictions of the rapid and widespread transmission of Zika in LAC in 2015–2016 resulted in policies and programs that prevented the worst of predictions from fully coming to pass through public health interventions and population-level behavior change. However, it is also possible that these had negative, unintended consequences. As Carlson et al. (2017) noted, over-predictions of Zika spread almost certainly resulted in increased use of pesticides, which resulted in the killing of millions of honeybees in the United States alone. Policy could also have simply have resulted in wasted money. For example, while access to contraception in August 2017 was of benefit to preventing pregnancy, that funding could have been of greater use to physicians in Puerto Rico in September 2017 when the island was slammed by devastating hurricanes. Furthermore, we are now aware that predictions have overestimated the potential harm of Zika for pregnant women and babies across the Americas. However, the power of hindsight runs the risk of obscuring an even greater danger for epidemiology: underestimating and underpreparing for an epidemic that exceeds predictions and overwhelms human lives.

Notes

1 https://wwwnc.cdc.gov/travel/notices
2 https://www.bbc.com/news/health-35427493
3 https://www.paho.org/hq/index.php?option=com_content&view=article&id=12390&Itemid=42090&lang=en
4 https://wwwn.cdc.gov/nndss/conditions/zika/case-definition/2016/06/
5 https://www.paho.org/hq/index.php?option=com_content&view=article&id=12390&Itemid=42090&lang=en
6 See: https://wwwn.cdc.gov/nndss/conditions/zika/case-definition/2016/06/
https://wwwn.cdc.gov/nndss/conditions/dengue-virus-infections/case-definition/2015/
https://wwwn.cdc.gov/nndss/conditions/chikungunya-virus-disease/
7 Such as Japanese Encephalitis, Saint Louis Encephalitis, West Nile and Yellow Fever, among others.
8 In a recent US-based study, CDC researchers identified n = 2,962 infants/fetuses with birth defects that they believed were likely due to Zika infection: 49% with microcephaly/brain abnormalities, 20% with early brain malformations, 9% with eye abnormalities only and 22% with other CNS dysfunctions (Delany et al., 2018).
9 Some are under way; see the EU-funded project Zikaction: http://zikaction.org
10 See the work of Adachi and Nielsen (2018) and Moore et al. (2017).

11 An estimated 66% of the population of French Polynesia (roughly 280,000) are thought to have been infected during 2013–2014, with over 30,000 suspected cases, some with neurological complications. With an estimated baseline prevalence of 2 microcephaly cases per 10,000 neonates, a retrospective study found that Zika virus infection increased this to 95 cases per 10,000 women infected with Zika in the first trimester (Cauchemez et al. 2016).

12 In this chapter, we focus predominately on microcephaly. However, Zika has also been demonstrated to cause Guillain-Barré Syndrome (GBS), a rare autoimmune attack on the nervous system caused by viral infection. While estimates for the rate by which Zika causes microcephaly are uncertainty, due to its low frequency, the rates at which it causes GBS are even more difficult to estimate. Estimates range from between 1 and 8 cases per 10,000 (see Keegan, Lessler, & Johansson, 2017).

References

Adachi, K., & Nielsen-Saines, K. 2018, 'Zika clinical updates: implications for pediatrics', *Current Opinion in Pediatrics*, vol. 30, no. 1, pp. 105–116.

Adams, V. 2016, *Metrics: what counts in global health*. Duke University Press.

Ahrens, K. A., Hutcheon, J. A., Gavin, L., & Moskosky, S. 2017, 'Reducing unintended pregnancies as a strategy to avert zika-related microcephaly births in the United States: a simulation study', *Maternal and Child Health Journal*, vol. 21, no. 5, pp. 982–987.

Aiken, A. R., Scott, J. G., Gomperts, R., Trussell, J., Worrell, M., & Aiken, C. E. 2016, 'Requests for abortion in Latin America related to concern about Zika virus exposure', *New England Journal of Medicine*, vol. 375, no. 4, pp. 396–398.

Albuquerque, M. D. F. P. M., de Souza, W. V., Mendes, A. D. C. G., Lyra, T. M., Ximenes, R. A., Araújo, T. V., et al. 2016, 'Pyriproxyfen and the microcephaly epidemic in Brazil-an ecological approach to explore the hypothesis of their association', *Memórias do Instituto Oswaldo Cruz*, vol. 111, no. 12, pp. 774–776.

Althaus, C. L. 2014, 'Estimating the reproduction number of Ebola virus (EBOV) during the 2014 outbreak in West Africa', *PLoS Current,* vol. 6.

Alvarado-Socarras, J. L., Ocampo-González, M., Vargas-Soler, J. A., Rodriguez-Morales, A. J., & Franco-Paredes, C. 2016, 'Congenital and neonatal chikungunya in Colombia'. *Journal of the Pediatric Infectious Diseases Society*, vol. 5. no. 3, pp. e17–e20.

Bardina, S. V., Bunduc, P., Tripathi, S., Duehr, J., Frere, J. J., Brown, J. A., et al. 2017, 'Enhancement of Zika virus pathogenesis by preexisting antiflavivirus immunity', *Science*, vol. 356, no. 6334, pp. 175–180.

Braga, J. U., Bressan, C., Dalvi, A. P. R., Calvet, G. A., Daumas, R. P., Rodrigues, N., et al. 2017, 'Accuracy of Zika virus disease case definition during simultaneous Dengue and Chikungunya epidemics', *PloS One*, vol. 12, no. 6, pp. e0179725.

Briggs, C. L., & Nichter, M. 2009, 'Biocommunicability and the biopolitics of pandemic threats', *Medical Anthropology*, vol. 28, no. 3, pp. 189–198.

Butler, D. 2016, 'Zika virus: Brazil's surge in small-headed babies questioned by report', *Nature News*, vol. 530, no. 7588, pp. 13–14.

Campos, M. C., Dombrowski, J. G., Phelan, J., Marinho, C. R.F., Hibberd, M., Clark, T. G., et al. 2018, 'Zika might not be acting alone: using an ecological study approach to investigate potential co-acting risk factors for an unusual pattern of microcephaly in Brazil', *PloS One*, vol. 13, no. 8, pp. e0201452.

Carlson, C. J., Dougherty, E., Boots, M., Getz, W., & Ryan, S. 2017, 'Consensus and conflict among ecological forecasts of Zika Virus Outbreaks in the United States,' *Scientific Reports* 8(1) 4921.

Cauchemez, S., Besnard, M., Bompard, P., Dub, T., Guillemette-Artur, P., Eyrolle-Guignot, D., et al. 2016, 'Association between Zika virus and microcephaly in French Polynesia, 2013–15: a retrospective study.' *The Lancet*, vol. 387, no. 10033, pp. 2125–2132.

CDC Foundation 2017, 'Zika contraception access network', <https://www.cdcfoundation.org/sites/default/files/upload/pdf/CDCFoundation-ZCAN-FactSheet.pdf>

Centers for Disease Control and Prevention 2017, 'Trioplex real-time RT-PCR Assay', <https://www.cdc.gov/zika/pdfs/trioplex-real-time-rt-pcr-assay-instructions-for-use.pdf>

Centers for Disease Control 2018, *Types of Zika Tests*. <https://www.cdc.gov/zika/laboratories/types-of-tests.html>

Charrel, R. N., Leparc-Goffart, I., Pas, S., de Lamballerie, X., Koopmans, M., Reusken, C.. 2016, 'Background review for diagnostic test development for Zika virus infection', *Bulletin of the World Health Organization*, vol. 94, no. 8, pp. 574.

Coelho, A. V. C., & Crovella, S. 2017, 'Microcephaly prevalence in infants born to Zika virus-infected women: a systematic review and meta-analysis', *International Journal of Molecular Sciences*, vol. 18, no. 8, pp. 1714.

Curry, C. L., Kwal, J., Bartlett, M., Crane, A., Greissman, S., Gunaratne, N., et al. 2017, 'Challenges in universal testing for zika in the setting of local mosquito-borne transmission', *American Journal of Obstetrics and Gynecology*, vol. 217, no. 6, pp. 726.

Darney, B. G., Aiken, A. R., & Küng, S. 2017, 'Access to contraception in the context of zika: health system challenges and responses', *Obstetrics and Gynecology*, vol. 129, no. 4, pp. 638–642.

de Araújo, J. S. S., Regis, C. T., Gomes, R. G. S., Tavares, T. R., dos Santos, C. R., Assunção, P.M., et al. 2016, 'Microcephaly in north-east Brazil: a retrospective study on neonates born between 2012 and 2015', *Bulletin of the World Health Organization*, vol. 94, no. 11, 835–840.

Dejnirattisai, W., Supasa, P., Wongwiwat, W., Rouvinski, A., Barba-Spaeth, G., Duangchinda, T., et al. 2016, 'Dengue virus sero-cross-reactivity drives antibody-dependent enhancement of infection with zika virus', *Nature Immunology*, vol. 17, no. 9, 1102.

de Silva, M., Munoz, F. M., Sell, E., Marshall, H., Kawai, A. T., Kachikis, A., et al. (2017). 'Congenital microcephaly: case definition & guidelines for data collection, analysis, and presentation of safety data after maternal immunisation', *Vaccine*, vol. 35, no. 48, pp. 6472–6482.

Diaz-Quijano, F. A., Pelissari, D. M., & Chiavegatto Filho, A. D. P. 2018, 'Zika- associated microcephaly epidemic and birth rate reduction in Brazilian cities', *American Journal of Public Health*, vol. 108, no. 4, pp. 514–516.

Diniz, D. 2017, *Zika: from the Brazilian backlands to global threat*. Zed Books.

Dufort, E., & White, J. 2018, 'Pre-Zika microcephaly in Brazil: closer to the elusive baseline and new questions raised', *Pediatrics* 141(2): e20173811.

Ellington, S. R., Devine, O., Bertolli, J., Quiñones, A. M., Shapiro-Mendoza, C. K., Perez-Padilla, J., et al. 2016, 'Estimating the number of pregnant women infected with Zika virus and expected infants with microcephaly following the Zika virus outbreak in Puerto Rico, 2016', *JAMA Pediatrics*, vol. 170, no. 10, pp. 940–945.

Escobar, L.E., & Craft, M.E., 2016. 'Advances and limitations of disease biogeography using ecological niche modeling', *Frontiers in Microbiology*,vol. 7, no. 1174.

Faria, N. R., Sabino, E. C., Nunes, M. R., Alcantara, L. C. J., Loman, N. J., & Pybus, O. G. 2016, 'Mobile real-time surveillance of Zika virus in Brazil', *Genome Medicine*, vol. 8, no. 1, pp. 97.

Fauci, A. S., & Morens, D. M. 2016, 'Zika virus in the Americas—yet another arbovirus threat', *New England Journal of Medicine*, vol. 374, no. 7, pp. 601–604.
Faye, O., Freire, C. C., Iamarino, A., Faye, O., de Oliveira, J. V. C., Diallo, M., et al. 2014, 'Molecular evolution of Zika virus during its emergence in the 20th century', *PLoS Neglected Tropical Diseases*, vol. 8, no. 1, pp. e2636.
Felix, A. C., Souza, N. C. S., Figueiredo, W. M., Costa, A. A., Inenami, M., da Silva, R. M., et al. 2017, 'Cross reactivity of commercial anti-dengue immunoassays in patients with acute Zika virus infection', *Journal of medical virology*, vol. 89, no. 8, pp. 1477–1479.
Fitzpatrick, M. C., Singer, B. H., Hotez, P. J., & Galvani, A. P. 2017, 'Saving lives efficiently across sectors: the need for a Congressional cost-effectiveness committee', *The Lancet*, vol. 390, no. 10110, pp. 2410–2412.
França, G. V., Schuler-Faccini, L., Oliveira, W. K., Henriques, C. M., Carmo, E. H., Pedi, V. D., et al. 2016, 'Congenital Zika virus syndrome in Brazil: a case series of the first 1501 livebirths with complete investigation', *The Lancet*, vol. 388, no. 10047, pp. 891–897.
Granger, D., Hilgart, H., Misner, L., Christensen, J., Bistodeau, S., Palm, J., et al. 2017, 'Serologic testing for Zika virus: comparison of three Zika virus IgM-screening enzyme-linked immunosorbent assays and initial laboratory experiences', *Journal of Clinical Microbiology*, vol. 55, no. 7, pp. 2127–2136.
Gubler, D. J., Vasilakis, N., & Musso, D. 2017, 'History and emergence of Zika virus', *The Journal of Infectious Diseases*, vol. 216, no. suppl_10, pp. S860–S867.
Honein, M. A., Dawson, A. L., Petersen, E. E., Jones, A. M., Lee, E. H., Yazdy, M. M., et al. 2017, 'Birth defects among fetuses and infants of US women with evidence of possible Zika virus infection during pregnancy', *Jama*, vol. 317, no. 1, pp. 59–68.
Johansson, M. A., Mier-y-Teran-Romero, L., Reefhuis, J., Gilboa, S. M., & Hills, S. L. 2016, 'Zika and the risk of microcephaly', *New England Journal of Medicine*, vol. 375, no. 1, pp. 1–4.
Kapogiannis, B. G., Chakhtoura, N., Hazra, R., & Spong, C. Y. 2017, 'Bridging knowledge gaps to understand how Zika virus exposure and infection affect child development', *JAMA Pediatrics*, vol. 171, no. 5, vol. 478–485.
Keegan, L. T., Lessler, J., & Johansson, M. A. 2017, 'Quantifying Zika: advancing the epidemiology of Zika with quantitative models', *The Journal of Infectious Diseases*, vol. 216, no. suppl_10, pp. S884–S890.
Lathrop, E., Romero, L., Hurst, S., Bracero, N., Zapata, L. B., Frey, M. T., et al. 2018, 'The Zika contraception access network: a feasibility programme to increase access to contraception in Puerto Rico during the 2016–17 Zika virus outbreak', *The Lancet Public Health*, vol. 3, no. 2, pp. e91–e99.
Latour, B. 1987, *Science in action: how to follow scientists and engineers through society*. Harvard University Press.
Li, R., Simmons, K. B., Bertolli, J., Rivera-Garcia, B., Cox, S., Romero, L.,et al. 2017, 'Cost-effectiveness of increasing access to contraception during the Zika virus outbreak, Puerto Rico, 2016', *Emerging Infectious Diseases*, vol. 23, no. 1, pp. 74.
Lozier, M. J., Burke, R. M., Lopez, J., Acevedo, V., Amador, M., Read, J. S., et al. 2017, 'Differences in prevalence of symptomatic Zika virus infection by age and sex—Puerto Rico, 2016', *The Journal of Infectious Diseases* 217(11) 1678–1689.
Lycke, E., & Norrby, E. (eds.) 2014, *Textbook of medical virology*. Butterworth-Heinemann, London, UK.
MacDonald, P. D., & Holden, E. W. 2018, 'Zika and Public Health: understanding the Epidemiology and Information Environment', *Pediatrics*, vol. 141, no. Supplement 2, pp. S137–S145.

Majumder, M. S., Hess, R., Ross, R., & Piontkivska, H. 2018, 'Seasonality of birth defects in West Africa: could congenital Zika syndrome be to blame?' *F1000Research*, vol. 7, no. 1, pp. 159.

Marteleto, L. J., Weitzman, A., Coutinho, R. Z., & Valongueiro Alves, S. 2017, 'Women's reproductive intentions and behaviors during the Zika Epidemic in Brazil',. *Population and Development Review*, vol. 43, no. 2, pp. 199–227.

Moghadas, S. M., Shoukat, A., Espindola, A. L., Pereira, R. S., Abdirizak, F., Laskowski, M., et al. 2017, 'Asymptomatic transmission and the dynamics of Zika infection', *Scientific Reports*, vol. 7, no. 1, pp. 5829.

Monaghan, A. J., Morin, C. W., Steinhoff, D. F., Wilhelmi, O., Hayden, M., Quattrochi, D. A., et al. 2016, 'On the seasonal occurrence and abundance of the Zika virus vector mosquito Aedes aegypti in the contiguous United States', *PLoS Currents*, vol. 8.

Moore, C. A., Staples, J. E., Dobyns, W. B., Pessoa, A., Ventura, C. V., Da Fonseca, E. B., et al. 2017, 'Characterizing the pattern of anomalies in congenital Zika syndrome for pediatric clinicians', *JAMA Pediatrics*, vol. 171, no. 3, pp. 288–295.

Morgan, M. S. 2012, *The world in the model: how economists work and think.* Cambridge University Press.

Morse, S. S., Mazet, J. A., Woolhouse, M., Parrish, C. R., Carroll, D., Karesh, W.B., et al. 2012, 'Prediction and prevention of the next pandemic zoonosis', *The Lancet*, vol. 380, no. 9857, pp. 1956–1965.

Mulkay, M., & Gilbert, G. N. 1984, *Opening Pandora's box.* Cambridge University, Cambridge.

Nishiura, H., Mizumoto, K., Rock, K. S., Yasuda, Y., Kinoshita, R., Miyamatsu, Y., et al. 2016, 'A theoretical estimate of the risk of microcephaly during pregnancy with Zika virus infection', *Epidemics*, vol. 15, pp. 66–70.

Oliveira Melo, A. S., Malinger, G., Ximenes, R., Szejnfeld, P. O., Alves Sampaio, S., & Bispo de Filippis, A. M. 2016, 'Zika virus intrauterine infection causes fetal brain abnormality and microcephaly: tip of the iceberg?' *Ultrasound in Obstetrics & Gynecology*, vol. 47, no. 1, pp. 6–7.

Osorio-de-Castro, C., Silva Miranda, E., Machado de Freitas, C., Rochel de Camargo Jr, K., & Cranmer, H. H. 2017, 'The Zika virus outbreak in Brazil: knowledge gaps and challenges for risk reduction', *American Journal of Public Health*, vol. 107, no. 6, pp. 960–965.

Pan American Health Organization / World Health Organization. (2017). *Zika - epidemiological report El Salvador*. PAHO/WHO, Washington, DC.

Parens, R., Nijhout, H. F., Morales, A., Costa, F. X., & Bar-Yam, Y. 2017, 'A possible link between pyriproxyfen and microcephaly', *PLoS Currents, 9.*

Peters, D. H., Garg, A., Bloom, G., Walker, D. G., Brieger, W. R., Hafizur Rahman, M., 2008, 'Poverty and access to health care in developing countries', *Annals of the New York Academy of Sciences*, vol. 1136, no. 1, pp. 161–171.

Quintó, L., García-Basteiro, A. L., Bardají, A., González, R., Padilla, N., Martinez-Espinosa, F. E., et al. 2017, 'The challenge of assessing microcephaly in the context of the Zika virus epidemic', *Journal of Tropical Pediatrics*, vol. 63, no. 6, pp. 495–498.

Rabe, I.B., Staples, J.E., Villanueva, J., Hummel, K.B., Johnson, J.A., Rose, L., et al. 2016, 'Interim guidance for interpretation of Zika virus antibody test results', *Morbidity and Mortality Weekly Report*, vol. 65(21).

Rick, A. M., Domek, G., Cunningham, M., Olson, D., Lamb, M. M., Jimenez-Zambrano, A., et al. 2017, 'High background congenital microcephaly in rural guatemala: implications for neonatal congenital Zika virus infection screening', *Global Health: Science and Practice*, vol. 5, no. 4, pp. 686–696.

Shiu, C., Starker, R., Kwal, J., Bartlett, M., Crane, A., Greissman, S., et al. 2018, 'Zika virus testing and outcomes during pregnancy, Florida, USA, 2016', *Emerging Infectious Diseases*, vol. 24, no. 1, pp. 1–8.

Silva, A. A., Barbieri, M. A., Alves, M. T., Carvalho, C. A., Batista, R. F., Ribeiro, M. R., et al. 2018, 'Prevalence and risk factors for microcephaly at birth in Brazil in 2010', *Pediatrics* 141(2) pp. e20170589.

Sun, L. 2016, 'CDC whistleblower claims agency has been using wrong Zika test', *The Washington Post.* https://www.washingtonpost.com/news/to-your-health/wp/2016/09/27/cdc-whistleblower-claims-agency-has-been-using- wrong-zika-test/?utm_term=.45414c21c9d5

Theel, E. S., & Hata, D. J. 2018, 'Diagnostic testing for Zika virus: a post-outbreak update', *Journal of Clinical Microbiology*, 56(4) e01972-17.

Tsai, W. Y., Youn, H. H., Brites, C., Tsai, J. J., Tyson, J., Pedroso, C., et al. 2017, 'Distinguishing secondary dengue virus infection from Zika virus infection with previous dengue by a combination of 3 simple serological tests', *Clinical Infectious Diseases*, vol. 65, no. 11, pp. 1829–1836.

Vermund, S. H. 2017, 'The vital case for global health investments by the US government', *Clinical Infectious Diseases*, vol. 64, no. 6, pp. 707–710.

Villa, R. 2016, 'Zika, or the burden of uncertainty', *La Clinica terapeutica*, vol. 167, no. 1, pp. 7–9.

Vorou, R. 2016, 'Letter to the editor: diagnostic challenges to be considered regarding Zika virus in the context of the presence of the vector Aedes albopictus in Europe', *Eurosurveillance*, vol. 21, no. 10: 30161.

Wendland, C. 2016, 'Estimating death: a close reading of maternal mortality metrics in Malawi', in Adams, V., Biehl, J (ed.), *Metrics: what counts in global health.* Duke University Press, pp. 57–82.

3 A literary history of Zika

Following Brazilian state responses through documents of emergency

Gustavo Corrêa Matta, Carolina de Oliveira Nogueira and Lenir da Silva Nascimento

Introduction

In November 2015, the Brazilian Health Ministry declared a Public Health Emergency of National Concern (known as an ESPIN) because of a rapid increase in unexpected, and unexplained, cases of microcephaly in newborn babies in the northeastern region. The ESPIN announcement was issued by the Health Ministry and published as a *portaria* (an ordinance) (2015a). The Brazilian Health Ministry issued a series of such bureaucratic directives during the Zika epidemic, and these documents can shed light on state-directed form of governance by tracing what Veena Das (2006) has called the *literacy of the state*: the series of everyday performances in documents and signatures that act as forms of governance, created by technologies of writing and their corresponding power.

Due to the outbreak in French Polynesia in 2013–2014, and just as Brazil was preparing to host the 2014 FIFA World Cup and 2016 Summer Olympics, Zika was highlighted in a 2014 Epidemiological Bulletin by the Health Ministry (Secretaria de Vigilância em Saúde) as a possible risk to the country. Two issues seemed to be highlighted in this early document: the government's experience in organising mass events and on following the International Health Regulations (IHRs). The document also shows the official state concern with the economic importance of these two events. As Zika emerged, and became known to the global public, some health scholars, such as Attaran (2016), alluded to the potential global health threat that these mass events, especially the Olympic Summer Games, could create as tourists and athletes returned to their countries, many of which also have high *Aedes agypti* populations.

In this chapter,[1] we follow Das's (2006) example and explore the social lives of written documents and what these documents reflect, reveal and omit about the Brazilian government response to the outbreak. Government institutions and mechanisms played important convening roles during the Zika epidemic in Brazil. One central actor was the *Centro de Operações de Emergências em Sáude Pública* (Public Health Emergency Operation Centre or COES) which was formed in 2014 in the aftermath of the West African Ebola epidemic. Thus, its existence as a mechanism of state literacy preceded Zika and is in line with growing international bioinsecurity. A core document of the COES is the *National Plan of Health*

Emergencies Protocol, which divides events according to four levels of alertness. COES provide technical guidance on resource allocation, such as increasing health staff and expanding infrastructure and services, and is also charged with providing information and communication to the public. COES becomes active when an ESPIN is declared, and during the ZIKV epidemic the institution operated on the highest level of alert, as it also did during the yellow fever outbreak in 2017. As an emergency operational unit, COES is connected to the Sanitary Vigilance Department and, during the Zika epidemic, worked alongside municipal, state and federal agencies to strengthen surveillance, disease prevention, care and support to affected families.

On February 2016, following the Brazilian emergency declaration, the World Health Organization (WHO) announced a Public Health Emergency of International Concern (PHEIC), given the suspected correlation between Zika infection and the rise of microcephaly cases in Brazil. This global alert lasted nine months, until November 2016, whereas it took the Brazilian state until July 2017 to officially end the ESPIN and close the *Centro de Operações de Emergências em Saúde Pública* (COES).

Between this time, diverse actions and responses were set into motion by the Health Ministry apparatus. Both of these announcements (the global PHEIC and national ESPIN) directly affected the Brazilian state as it dealt with a series of scientific uncertainties and political and social challenges permeated by a sense of urgency, fear and the demand for rapid action, all with domestic and foreign pressures. Understanding how this process unfolded in 2015–2017 is especially important given the fact that support for the thousands of children and their families affected by the virus, and preparedness planning for future arboviral epidemics, hangs in a cloudy balance in 2018.

The epidemic in Brazil was framed as a *war* – a war of both people against mosquito and women against microcephaly. Ribeiro et al. (2018: 138) pointed out that the Brazilian state "played a fundamental role in defining the terms of the debate" through a "war frame" that was focused on individualised disease prevention, particularly placed on women. This war spectacle masked social and gender inequalities, extending the negligence of poverty and regional inequality.[2]

The Health Ministry has been historically responsible for the creation of the country's public health policies and scientific knowledge. In this sense, the state's authority can be viewed, as proposed by the work of Veena Das (2006), as emanating from a set of temporal documents that inscribe policies and actions. Understanding the state, therefore, demands thinking in terms of literacy. This intensive production of documents and decrees, and the styles of reasoning and *seeing* that emerge from it, shapes the process of scientific knowledge and discourse stabilisation, both of which have consequences for the construing of official narratives. Such documents create temporalities, produce attention and silences, leave trails and inscribe some sense of official history. In this chapter, we explore these issues, using discourse and document analysis to investigate how the Health Ministry responded to the Zika epidemic. As a way to understand how official narratives are constructed, we selected a series of crucial government and scientific documents in order to shed light on the complex relationships among policies, guidelines and actions during an unfolding health emergency. We approach this corpus of documents as a lens to inspect the relationships between, on the one hand, the Brazilian political response to Zika and, on the other, the scientific response to this emergent viral pathogen. In so doing, we aim to write a literary history of ZIKV in Brazil, one that pays special attention to how official documents navigated uncertainty, within the demands of expediency and the sphere of urgency.

In the first part of the chapter, we briefly describe some crucial details about Brazil's public health landscape and the early history of the epidemic. We then turn our attention to how the state came to understand and frame the epidemic itself, as it responded to public anxieties and questions. We do so by exploring the literacy of the Brazilian state, and how its ordinances, protocols and manuals aimed at guiding health professionals produced temporalities.[3] Lastly, we adjust our lens to explore the government response to children and families affected by the virus. By analysing official microcephaly epidemiological bulletins (MEB) and their corresponding epidemiological reports (ER), we question how visible these children became given the biomedical emphasis on performing formal technical solutions disconnected from embodied suffering and affliction.

The birth of Zika: From pathogen to Brazilian politics

In 1988, health as a human right was enshrined in the Brazilian Constitution, ensuring that the state takes appropriate responsibility and action in offering policies and services to all Brazilian citizens. The constitution was created at the end of a 20-year military dictatorship and, in this sense, was representative of newly felt democratic expectations. As stated in the 1988 Constitution:

> Health is the right of everyone and the duty of the State, guaranteed through social and economic policies aimed at reducing the risk of disease and other diseases and universal and equal access to actions and services for their promotion, protection and recovery.

Before 1988, Brazil had a health system founded on meritocratic principles, offering health services for formal employees in a social security model. Other citizens should need to buy health delivery from the private sector, for things such as chronic diseases, child and maternal care and traffic accidents. The health system was centralized and fragmented, and it excluded most informal workers as well as much of the rural population. The authoritarian regime created an unequal, but also highly inefficient, system.

Things changed with the birth of democracy in 1988, when the Brazilian Health System, officially named Unified Health System (Sístema Único de Saúde, or SUS), was scripted into the constitution, with a few at the time radical principles, that continue to structure health policies, services and actions across the country. This includes: (1) *universality*: that every Brazilian citizen has the right to health services for free, guaranteed through state financing and policies; (2) *comprehensive care*: that the state should provide preventive, promotive and curative care, control policies on pharmaceuticals, biological inputs, the quality of food, water and other products for human consumption, and also epidemiological surveillance; (3) *equity*: that the state should pay attention to the health needs of diverse individuals and groups including the social, cultural and economic determinants of health; (4) *decentralization*: that the health system should be managed through a balance of federal, state and municipal control. According to the decentralised system, federal fundings concerning health care are destined to the state and municipal level. Each of the three federal levels are supposed to destined a specific amount of their budget to health care system. Constitutionally, the Ministry of Health (MoH) is also responsible for supporting and funding states and municipalities in case of health emergencies and disasters; and (5) *social participation*: that institutional arrangements should be created and supported to guarantee social participation in health delivery and also the policy-making process. These principles have helped to facilitate many significant advances on health access, primary health care coverage, the involvement in local municipalities in health (including specialized services, such as AIDS treatment, organ transplants and oncological services) and the expansion of the health workforce, to name a few achievements.

In spite of these great efforts to develop the right to health in Brazil, SUS still has serious problems. As with many health systems, this includes inequitable access, regulatory constraints among health care levels, the co-existence of public and private systems, challenges with social participation, federal government centralization and financing, difficulties in organizing local regional management, unequal health worker distribution, intersectoral policies to reduce the social determinants of health and the unequal burden of disease. These challenges can also be seen through the lens of basic health statistics, shown in Table 3.1. Whereas the overarching aim of SUS is to ensure health access to all, in reality, four epidemiological situations put considerable strain on existing resources and capacities: an increasingly ageing population, greater chronic diseases, a continued (and newly emerging) infectious disease burden and violence, both physical and psychosocial.

Table 3.1 Brazilian economic and health statistics

Total population (2016)	*207 million*
Gross national income per capita (2016)	$8,650
Life expectancy at birth, m/f (years, 2016)	71/79
Probability of dying under five (per 1,000 live births, 2008)	21
Total expenditure on health per capita (2014)	$1,318
Total of expenditure on health (public and private) as % of GDP (2014)	8.3%
Estimated population coverage of primary heath care (2017)	64.5%

Sources: WHO, Brazilian Ministry of Health and World Bank

Infectious diseases are still relevant in contemporary Brazil. One of the most notorious is Dengue, an arbovirus responsible for an estimated one million cases and 500 deaths per year in Brazil (Fares et al., 2015). A concerted control program nearly eliminated the *Aedes aegypti* mosquito between the 1950s and 1970s. After a few decades of relative silence, Dengue returned to the country during the 1980s as successive waves of Dengue serotypes spread from Southeast Asia to the Americas, facilitated by modern transport networks and urbanisation. All four Dengue serotypes are now endemic in Brazil.

Dengue is not the only emerging mosquito-borne disease in the country. In 2014, the American Chikungunya (CHIK) outbreak spread rapidly in Brazil. More than 250,000 cases have since been registered with the MoH surveillance system, including 159 reported deaths in 2016 alone (Ministério da Saúde, 2017a), although the virus has certainly infected many more people. To make matters worse, Brazil has been battling resurgent yellow fever epidemics since the end of 2017. The sylvatic (jungle) yellow fever (YF) transmission cycle is endemic in monkey populations. In response, massive vaccination campaigns have been organised in 2017 and 2018.

It was on the tail-end of CHIK, and resurgent Dengue and YF, that Zika emerged in 2015. Brazil has an excellent and well-distributed national health surveillance system and at the very beginning of Zika circulating in the country, the Minister of Health, Arthur Chioro, made a statement to the nation:

> It was confirmed 8 cases in Camaçari-Bahia. The Zika virus does not worry us. It is a benign disease that has a good prognostic. The fever is low, and the biggest annoyance is itching, red spots. It requires very little patient access to emergency room and medical services. All our concern is with dengue because dengue kills.[4]

Brazilian health authorities had identified Zika but dismissed it, believing it to be an insignificant pathogen, a "weak" Dengue-like disease of little consequence. Before the emergence of microcephaly clusters in and around Recife in late 2015, this was the standard scientific view. Before the 2007 epidemic on the isolated islands of Yap, Federated States of Micronesia, in the Western Pacific, there had been fewer than 20 human ZIKV infections reported over a 70-year period following its discovery in Uganda in the late 1940s (Gubler et al. 2017).[5] The link between ZIKV and microcephaly was yet to be suspected: it took the Brazilian scientific establishment, and the world, by surprise.

From the beginning, Zika in Brazil was inseparable from two substantial political events that shaped the discourse and actions of the state towards this new viral disease (see Figure 3.1). On the one hand, there was the embattled presidency of Dilma Rousseff, involved in a lengthy impeachment process, and the political instability related to this. On the other hand, there was the planned Olympic Games in Rio de Janeiro in 2016, which was to host national delegations from 208 countries.

Rousseff's mandate was under attack in parliament. During the lefist Lula and Rousseff governments, from 2003 to 2016, Brazil lived under steady economic

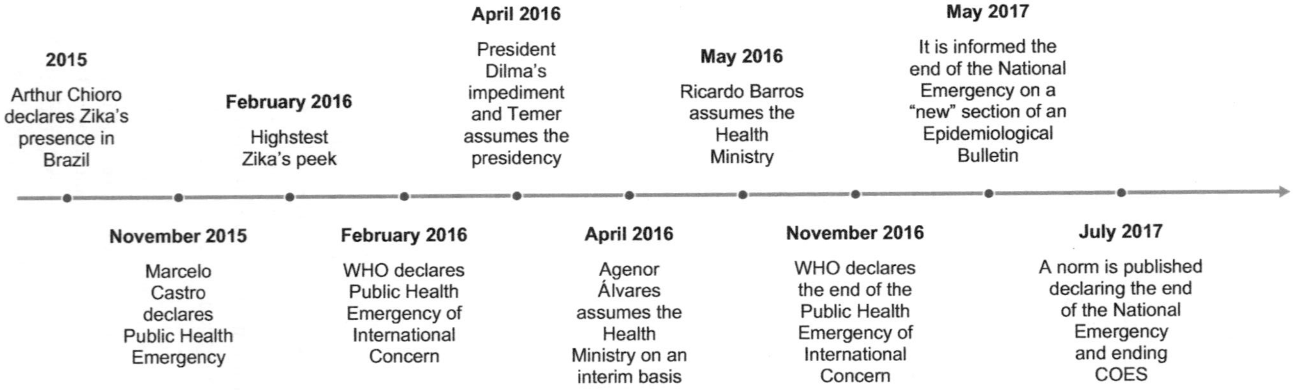

Figure 3.1 A timeline of Zika and political events in Brazil.

growth which helped support major investments in public social policies including support to the lower social classes in access to education, health, essential goods and living conditions. However, conservative undercurrents in politics and the higher classes disagreed with increasing state expenditures. Brazil had entered into a remarkable political and democratic crisis that stayed on throughout the entire Zika epidemic period.[6] On October 2015, in one of several political strategies to maintain power and escape from the impeachment process, Rousseff reshuffled the Minister of Health, widely considered the best-resourced social ministry, removing a member of the Labour Party (PT) with a representative of the Brazilian Democratic Movement Party (PMDB). Marcelo Castro, a psychiatrist and congressman with no actual public health experience, became a crucial actor in the epidemic.

It was this new health minister who found himself having to declare a ESPIN after primary health care physicians in northeastern Brazil began raising the alarm about the rising cases of microcephaly (Diniz, 2017), which were confirmed in November 2015. Marcelo Castro supported his decision by relying on renowned scientific institutions, especially the Oswaldo Cruz Foundation (FIOCRUZ), and on a technical body from the Ministry of Health, specifically the Health Surveillance Secretary.[7] Although there was certainly a great deal of uncertainty at this early stage, Castro and many other key actors from the government as well as scientists were scared. To galvinize support and convey the scope of the potential threat, the focus quickly turned to an on old and traditional narrative: a "war" against the vector:

> About 30 years ago the mosquito has been transmitting diseases to our population and since then we have fought it, but we are losing the war against Aedes aegypti. We are living in a real epidemic. We need Brazilian society to be mobilized in the prevention of these diseases.
>
> (*O Globo* newspaper, Rio de Janeiro, Jan, 2016)

Launching a National Public Health Emergency is both a political and bureacractic exercise. Through administrative mechanisms, it allows financial resources to be mobilized and targetted towards scientific studies, disease control interventions and efforts to fast-track biomedical countermeasures, like new diagnostics and vaccines. A sense of urgency and purpose floated over the actions and debates of those involved. In Brazil, primary care physicians, pediatricians and local epidemiologists in the northeastern region played important roles in unraveling early epidemiological details and raising the alarm. An area known for its history of sugarcane plantations, slavery and poverty, ZIKV hit what Diniz (2017) has called "a forgotten, anonymous region." This meant that physicians and scientists from the periphery of Brazilian science, most unknown figures, made many of the key discoveries. These actors built rapid response networks and knowledge sharing platforms on the go, working with scientists from other regions of the country, in what became known among them as the "Whatsapp Epidemic." These networks were organized organically, and the use of modern technologies (Whatsapp messages, cellphone texting, Skype video and iPhone photos) meant that the epidemic played out in real time, almost instantaneously, with important consequences for the organization of scientific research and political decision making. Of course, this also meant that rumors and misinformation about this mysterious new disease could spread just as quickly as facts and data. Images of microcephalic babies and concerned mothers intermixed with scientific hypothesis, fake news and the ongoing Brazilian political crisis, especially in social media and internet news.

President Dilma Rousseff understood the threat of ZIKV to population health but also to the significance and symbolism of the epidemic to public trust in her presidency and to the Brazilian state. Zika became a priority issue, discussed side-by-side her political fight against the impeachment process taking shape in congress. From October 2015 to April 2016, she had been talking daily with scientists and epidemiologists regarding the epidemic and solutions to control it. In 2015, after the declaration of the ESPIN, the Ministry of Health invested millions of dollars in case-control studies, vaccine and diagnostic tests, community education material and vector control innovation studies, which included genetically modified mosquitoes.

Following in the footsteps of Oswaldo Cruz's sanitation campaigns of the early 20th century, the army went to the people to distribute information guides, to spread insecticides and to inspect houses and streets in search of mosquito breeding sites. In a patriotic show of hands and feet, more than 200,000 military troops and staff were called by the Ministry of Health to assist with vector control activities:

> Armed forces, military police, firefighters, community agents, mayors, state secretaries, are all mobilized against Brazil's number one enemy today, which is the mosquito *Aedes aegypti*, the famous dengue mosquito.
>
> (Minister of Health – February 2016)

Through a public health historical perspective during the 20th century, we see that Rio de Janeiro's landscape, for instance, seems to be a complex meshwork that involved mosquito combat through sanitization attempts, urban planning as well as violent state-induced dislocation of bodies and entire communities under the political discourse of "sanitation" (Hochman 1998; Nogueira 2016).

In April 2016, the impeachment of Dilma Rousseff reached its finish line in the National Congress. Michel Temer, her vice president, assumed the presidency of Brazil and a conservative turn began as Temer cut funding to social services (including health), science and technology policies by more than 20% and deregulated labour laws. The new Ministry of Health, under Ricardo Barros, proposed that new private health plans should be promoted for the lower social classes, threatening the National Health System and the right to health in Brazil. At that moment, Zika started to decrease. The new Ministry of Health chief declared that the mosquito was undisciplined:

> 'If the mosquito committed to biting, only those who live in the house were easy, but unfortunately he is not disciplined,' he said. The new minister

> defended punishments for those who resist the entrance of public agents for house inspections. 'This is the Brazilian culture. People have to be burdened.'
> (Journal Bahia, 2016)

At the same time, President Temer and his government approved a constitutional amendment to impose limits on federal, state and municipal funding for public services and policies. Health, education and science were more affected by this law.

As this quick, and cursory, introduction to Brazilian politics show, the Zika outbreak coincided with a very complex political moment in Brazil, one that is ongoing. Ordinances, policies and health responses to Zika were immersed in these scientific, political, economic and historic contexts. The biopolitics of Zika made visible and invisible selected actors, groups and phenomena.

Paper trails: Official documents and unofficial silences

The war frame – man against mosquito – reinforced what Krieger (2014), in her analysis of 21st-century epidemiology, called the normalization of biomedical reductionism and this perspective reigned in the Brazilian response. A broader social epidemiological approach to the epidemic, that would have brought greater attention to poverty, sanitation, life conditions, social inequalities, reproductive health, climate change, urban planning and local governance did not enter into the conversation of the state nor, really, the scientific agenda (Ribeiro et al. 2018). *Aedes aegypti*-related diseases are widely endemic in the north and northeast regions, as well as in the big cities of Rio de Janeiro, Belo Horizonte, São Paulo and Recife. Oliveira et al. (2018) showed, for Ceará, over 190,000 reported cases of Dengue between 2001 and 2012, with higher peaks during the years of 2001, 2006, 2008 and 2012, with different strains of DENV circulating at the same time. In the city of Rio de Janeiro, Coelho et al. (2016) showed that in 2002 there were over 140,000 reported cases and in 2015 over 55,000 cases of different strains of DENV.

In many ways, ZIKV is a vector-borne disease causing only mild symptoms, one of many infectious diseases that now compose the epidemiological landscape of Brazil, like Dengue, Chikungunya or the seasonal flu (H1N1). But this was not the way ZIKV was framed during the epidemic. The consequences of neurological impairments for newborn babies turned ZIKV into what Veena Das (2006) has called a "critical event." This unprecedented event disrupted a previous narrative and set it apart from other vector-borne diseases. In some ways, this conjunction of a dangerous pathogen with the state response highlighted what seemed to be a threat to the nation and its future. During an interview with *O Globo* newspaper, on January 2016, the Health Ministry expressed its concern and fears regarding the possibility of an entire generation affected by microcephaly, and the implications of this on the social and economic fabric of the country.

Human bodies, in an unequal world, are not subjected to the same effects, access and resources (Lock and Nguyen, 2010). Different neighborhoods and social groups are not provided with the same resources, capacities, interventions and care from the state. People move along urban ecosystems in different ways, traveling along different axes and encountering mosquitoes differently. As Nading (2014) argued in reference to Dengue in urban Nicaragua, vector-borne disease control is not only about mosquitoes and their breeding sites but also about the embedded and complex human-to-human relationships that also need to come under the microscope and into public surveillance. This includes the ways in which different actors invoke the language of "emergencies" and "crises," with their corresponding emotions of fear and urgency. Nading (2014:178) argues that overlapping geographical and political event inform the urban city, often in a continual process of "emergency" and constitute a "political trope".

We want to explore this "political trope" in a slightly different way: instead of looking and thinking about the city, we want to think about the "documents of emergency" that evolved during the Zika epidemic itself, and how these paper trails produced the literacy of the state response.[8] We are concerned with a set of official documents that were created and disseminated through institutionalized channels, such as ordinances, technical notes and protocols. There are two aspects of these documents: historical and institutional. The former create specific temporalities by declaring, in this case, start and end dates to the Public Health National Emergency in 2015 and 2017. The latter include the various ordinances created during the epidemic as well as operational instructions, protocols and epidemiological bulletins. These documents produce guidelines and ordinances on how to do public health in times of epidemic emergency, documents with an institutional power, produced within the Ministry of Health, by technicians and experts, with the purpose of guiding and structuring a set of actions.

Over two years, the ministry issued over 17 ordinances, 6 technical notes, 4 protocols on ZIKV and 4 on microcephaly, and 60 weekly reports monitoring, specifically, cases of microcephaly. These are the main bureaucratic forms that produced and communicated decisions and policies in the health ministry, the health secretaries at both state and municipality levels and to health care professionals. In our analysis of this corpus of documents we have found three broad categories: (1) surveillance protocols; (2) documents concerning non-vector Zika transmission; and (3) documents that outline institutional arrangements between different ministries.

Surveillance protocols

By the end of 2015, and all through 2016, national epidemiological bulletins were announcing the appearance and distribution of new microcephaly cases in different states of the country. Alongside Pernambuco, Bahia and Recife in the north-east, Rio de Janeiro also began showing substantial increases. As cases and public interest in the new emergency increased, important surveillance gaps needed to be quickly filled. In response, during the last month of 2015, two main documents were issued. The first, *Protocol for Implementing Health Sentinel Sites*, stressed the need to better understand viral spread, improve laboratory diagnostics and coordinate the flow of surveillance information. This short and concise document (of only seven pages) settled, among other things, approaches for surveillance of the new virus including how to turn diagnostic laboratories into sentinel sites to trace Zika's movement.

The health ministry, following tenets of decentralized policy-making, decided that every capital city, in each of the 26 federal states, should have at least 1 sentinel laboratory and that some medium-sized cities should also have this capacity, in order to track cases from smaller cities located nearby. These labs, situated in the northeast, were supposed to send 10 samples per week to the federal referral laboratory Instituto Evandro Chagas (located at Pará state in the north of the country). This system only lasted a couple of months. By mid-2015, the referral lab was receiving far more than 10 samples per week, and the health ministry had to find other laboratory facilities to act as referral sites, such as Fiocruz-Pernambuco, in order to respond faster to the outbreak.

The second document, the *National Plan to Combat Microcephaly*, was the first protocol issued after the state officially confirmed the correlation between Zika virus and microcephaly. It is geared towards health professionals and administrators, and is a handy book detailing not only how to deal, medically, with ZIKV (such as on diagnostic issues) but also delves into planning and bureaucratic problems, including how the state should generate, share and store information. Along with providing parameters to classify suspected and confirmed ZIKV infection and microcephaly (in both pregnant women and newborns), it urges health professionals to inform suspected cases of the results of diagnostic tests and assessments as soon as possible. Information should also flow upwards, from the health professional (preferably a doctor) to the municipality, the state and then the national federal entity, the health ministry – a fairly standard notification process. However, it took until early February 2016 for ZIKV virus and ZIKV virus infection among pregnant women to be classified as a reportable disease, to be notified to local health authorities within 24 hours, which meant that passive surveillance was no longer to be solely based on eligible sentinel sites.

This document enunciates some certainties: the geographical dispersation of Zika cases and the fact that the virus can be found in the amniotic fluid of pregnant women whose babies were born with congenital malformation, such as microcephaly. Nevertheless, the document points out some scientific uncertainties: available data could not ascertain the risk to women of having a fetus with congenital malformations if they were infected when pregnant. The document clearly states the necessity of further studies. Other possible forms of virus transmission seemed less important, as the document only mentions the possible presence of the virus in breastmilk, semen, urine and saliva but discards its potential transmissibility, focusing on human-animal relations (mosquitoes).

Negotiating transmission uncertainties

In late December 2015, just three days before Christmas, a technical note was produced by the National Coordination Body on Blood and Blood Products

(Ministério da Saúde, Agência Nacional de Vigilância Sanitária, 2015), which stated:

> The main mode of Zika virus transmission is through mosquitos bites such as *A. aegypti*. However some evidences suggest that the virus can also be sexually transmitted among humans, as well as by blood transfusion.

In light of the other official pronouncements cited earlier, such a declaration reveals the fragmentation within the corpus of "documents of emergency" and inside the Health Ministry. The document addressed blood transfusions protocols, alerting health professionals to be more careful in screening for possible ZIKV-infected blood donors. This work followed a history of monitoring hospital and public blood banks, going back to the 1970s and 1980s, when contamination cases, mainly from Chagas disease and Hepatitis B, were widely known and problematic. Once HIV/AIDS became a global threat, the Brazilian social movement was highly effective at demanding changes on blood transfusion policies, through federal surveillance and reinforced screening policies. While more scientific studies are needed on the risks that blood transfussions pose for the spread of Zika, the coordinating body followed other international institutions (like the US CDC) and altered blood transfusion protocols. A decision had to be made, and scientific uncertainties, as Callon et al. (2009) put it, constitute the everyday lives of policy-makers and political institutions.[9]

Another technical note was issued in March 2016 concerning semen donation. This forbade the donation of sperm in the case of positive or inconclusive blood tests for Zika virus infection. By March 2016, the National Epidemiological Vigilance Agency (ANVISA) issued a technical note altering the protocol for the utilization of both national and imported semen or oocytes for reproductive uses. It is important to highlight that these technical notes were not ordinances, and so did not exert much tangible bureaucratic power, although at the time some inside the MoH were emphasizing the possibility that Zika could be sexually transmitted, although there were no warnings to the general public.

In a recent interview conducted by our research group, a technical member of the health ministry involved in the epidemic outbreak response affirmed that given the amount of vector-borne transmission cases and the uncertainties surrounding sexual transmission, such as the duration of the virus' incubation and its viremia, the health ministry decided to focus on vector control alerts and campaigns. This official statement seems to be in agreement with the epidemiological bulletin (no. 46, published on 2015), affirming the existence of other forms of transmissibility but also downplaying it.

Institutionals arrangements

A little over a month after the ESPIN declaration, a presidential decree was signed by Dilma Rousseff, Marcelo Castro, from the health ministry and Gilberto Ochi, from the national integration ministry. This latter ministry is involved in many national development programs, such as irrigation and drought prevention, but it also has a role in protection and civil defence. This decree combined efforts from these ministries to create the *Sala Nacional de Coordenação e Controle para o Enfrentamento da Dengue, do vírus Chikungunya e Zika vírus* (National Unit of Coordination and Control for Dengue, Chikungunya and Zika viruses). This centralized unit's role was to coordinate and integrate efforts from both the Health Ministry and the Ministry of Social Development, putting together both ministries' efforts into the National Integration Ministry's administrative units.

This decree did not invalidate the ESPIN declaration; rather, it reinforced national concerns by creating a specific institutional device that not only combined forces from different ministries but also transformed, what at first glance could seem like a more regionally localized microcephaly outbreak into a national one, deploying a set of combined institutional efforts. During the ESPIN, the flow of surveillance data becomes particularly important, and is watched very closely and COES issued weekly reports to inform decision makers.

Until this moment, the Health Ministry was the main state institution involved in producing "documents of emergency" – protocols, ordinance, guides and general public communications. One of the presidential decree's effects was to create better coordinated actions between the ministry of health and ministry of social development. Here, there seems to be another governmental entry point into Zika's timeline as the ministry of social development is brought to the political stage to socially and financially address the needs of children and families touched by congenital malformation. Three interministerial ordinances were then issued, in addition to two "combined operational instructions." These five documents dated from early February until late October 2016, and they are analyzed here together as a way to perceive subtle changes and some continutities.

Throughout these documents, there is a sense of emergency regarding the diagnostic accuracy and confirmation of microcephaly. In the first document produced by this interministerial group, there are still doubts concerning the correlation between the high rates of microcephaly and the Zika epidemic. The document points to "unexpected situations" and "possibly associated with Zika virus." Nevertheless, the health ministry and social development ministry created actions aimed to strenghten prevention and care and social protection to pregnant women and women of reproductive age.

As far as prevention activities go, there is a clear focus on individual care and responsibility, as well as vigilance and control at the household level. As Nading (2014) shows in Nicaragua, Dengue and vector control are often seen through the prism of individual vigilance and action, where motivational social and educational programs and campaigns are the main vehicle for state intervention. Engaging the community to fight the mosquito, to create a housing environment that is unfit for the mosquito, as well as being vigilant about the hygiene and personal attitudes of your neighbours, are the main tasks. What is missing from this rhetoric, however, are state actions concerned with public goods and public spaces, such as sewer systems, garbage disposal and better housing – all of which remained largely absent from state documents and campaigns during the Zika crisis. Infrastructural efforts that would indeed make concrete changes in people's lives are, and have been for many years, a political and economic issue that remain, time and again, unaddressed by local and federal policymakers. As scholars of Brazilian anthropology have shown, these infrastructural issues become, at each election, merely a rhetoric slogan for political campaigns, with very little progress made in-between the ballot box (Heredia and Palmeira, 2006; Kuschnir, 2000).

The next three documents, issued between March and October 2016, no longer had any doubts concerning the correlation between high rates of microcephaly and ZIKV. In a detailed epidemiological survey at the time, every state of the country, expect Amapá, had suspected or confirmed cases of microcephaly. Rio de Janeiro was ranked 6th among 26 states; the first 5 were all located in the northeast of the county and each of those 26 states received additional national funding. The amount of the funding was calculated based on the number of confirmed cases of microcephaly, as established by these ordinances.

Another point that is not addressed in any of the documents is the possibility of pregnancy terminations. Abortion in Brazil is only legal when a woman's life is at risk or in rape cases. Sexual and reproductive rights in these five documents concerned only a social and educational approach about contraceptive methods (and its dispensation) and "medical counseling to inform and better evaluate women's decisions on wanting to get pregnant." In a touching documentary film, produced by Debora Diniz, terms as "we will see"; "we will wait and see"; and "it is hard, I know, but have faith, you are strong" are deployed by medical staff when attending to pregnant women whose fetuses had been diagnosed, via ultrasound, with microcephaly. In a country where abortion in those cases is illegal, and when pregnant women are faced with a new challenging reality, it begs the question: what else is there to be said?

In an epidemiological bulletin issued in 2017, the health ministry described the women most touched by Zika's terrible effects. It depicts mostly Afro-Brazilian women, poor and living in neglected urban areas or in the poor countryside. These are the women making routine use of the Unified Health System (SUS), who have no financial resources at their disposal to use private health care. For these women, abortion is not only illegal but also completedly inaccessible.[10] It becomes apparent, through this depictions and many others like it, that Zika's worst and most devastating effects were not only gendered but also embodied in racial and class differences.[11]

Throughout the epidemic, a national campaign slogan could be seen spread across the country: "*Um mosquito não é mais forte do que uma nação inteira*" (a mosquito is not stronger that a whole nation). Obviously, this is a piece of propaganda designed to reinforce a sense of community in a collective effort to combat the mosquito threat. It was used to focus the collective psyche on individual responsibility, on the need to follow environmental sanitation procedures at the household level, and to accept government fumigation and house-to-house vigilance by municipal staff called *agentes de combate de endemias* (combat agents of endemic disease).

However, this slogan did more than this. It reinforced the military idiom that pervaded these campaigns throughout the 19th and 20th centuries (Hochman, 1998), which viewed the mosquito as the enemy and created an impossible battle to be fought in a deeply unequal society. What "nation" is being addressed by this campaign slogan? What "nation" will have its houses inspected on a daily basis by state agents? And on whose shoulders does the weight of this campaign fall? By July 2017, the health ministry published a norm declaring the end to the national emergency, leading each state, in its own way, to continue with the medical and epidemiological follow-up.

Brazilian responses to microcephaly: Caring and forgetting children affected by Zika

Babies affected by ZIKV started to appear in the Brazilian and international press in 2015 in ways that revealed certain things and kept others hidden. Indeed, ZIKV has become a political event in Brazil and a global health problem through the fear and uncertainty surrounding microcephaly, and its related health risks, bodily damage and burden. The disease has a temporal dimension, with its impact dragged from an infected present to a chronically burdened future for those families that are, unfortunately, affected. Nevertheless, it is worth asking: have affected children and families become as perceptible as the virus itself? How has the Brazilian government responded to their plight and suffering, and long-term care needs?

Microcephalic infants were visual centerpieces of the epidemic, but addressing their caregiving needs, and the psychosocial realities of their mothers and families, were not the first priorities of the Brazilian government when they declared the ESPIN in November 2015. Rather, the aim was to obtain continuous and timely knowledge about the disease by strengthening epidemiological surveillance and to prevent more cases by mobilizing long-known strategies to combat the *Aedes aegypti* mosquito (Ministério da Saúde, 2015b).

The fact that ZIKV was already known to science complicated things. A known disease suddenly became unknown, and epidemiologists and public health experts needed to quickly map and evaluate the available data. The unprecedented nature of ZIKV consequences and the rapid increase in the number of cases posed difficulties in reorganizing the Brazilian health system to respond promptly and adequately to these new demands.

The corpus of microcephaly epidemiological bulletins (MEB) (Boletins Epidemiológicos de monitoramento de microcefalia) and their corresponding epidemiological reports (ER), produced by the Health Ministry as tools of monitoring ZIKV and affected children, were important parts of the repertoire of "documents of emergency." The epidemiological bulletin (EB) and the epidemiological report, published online, provided the Sanitary Vigilance Department with a platform to rapidly disseminate results on disease-specific information and investigations, and to orientate public health action.

At the end of 2015, when there were many scientific uncertainties and no guarantees of significant and immediate health system support, mostly because of the troubled political landscape, the official discussions centered on knowing and controlling the disease right away. Regrettably, Dengue has shown us that simply knowing about a disease is not enough to control it.

If the Brazilian state provided medical care in full accordance with its constitutional laws, focused on comprehensive care for example, then all babies with Congenital Zika Syndrome (CZS) ought to get specific pediatric primary care, professional early stimulation and follow up by different specialists, according to the national "Protocol for Surveillance and Response" published in 2015 by the Brazilian Health Ministry (Ministério da Saúde, 2015b). As reported by the Sanitary Vigilance Department (Secretaria de Vigilância em Saúde, 2017), among the 2,681 confirmed CZS cases that remained alive from November 2015 to February 2018, 72% had some kind of care, 31% had all three kinds and 23% had both pediatric and specialist care. According to same document, there were 3,087 confirmed cases of CZS by February 2018. Although life expectancy for these children is considered exceptionally low, 2,681 of them were still alive in 2018. In addition, 12,393 notified cases were still under investigation, or were considered probable, discarded, excluded or inconclusive, for various reasons (Secretaria de Vigilância em Saúde, 2017).

In our analysis, we found three significant moments that shifted the management of the epidemic in Brazil. The first included the government's integrated approach between the Ministries of Health and Social Development, in early 2016, to combat the sanitary emergency (Ministério da Saúde, Ministério do Desenvolvimento Social do Brasil, 2016a,b,c). The second included, in early 2017, the effort to better integrate epidemiological data into the management of the epidemic through surveillance and healthcare data, protocols and guidelines (Secretaria de Vigilância em Saúde, 2017). The final and third shift was seen in the second half of 2017, when the United Nations International Children's Emergency Fund (UNICEF) entered the scene. Although prevention and care of children and families affected by Zika were discussed in official documents, until mid-2017 most actions focused on risk communication in vector control and on individual microcephaly diagnosis.

In the Brazilian health system, diagnostic practices are important, even necessary, vehicles for accessing social service provisions. For children with CZS, a medical report was needed to plan individual care routines and to access the *Benefício de Provisão Continuada* (BPC), a financial security program for low-income families with a victim of Zika-related microcephaly (Congresso Nacional do Brasil, 2016). Benefits in this program, however, seem calculated to an early death; the maximum benefit period is only three years. The BPC has political implications. Social support tied to microcephaly babies is set apart from the greater disability advocacy community and may compromise efforts in strengthening the general health care and social protection of other children and families. In addition, the arrangement between the ministries, affecting health system and social assistance, focused on promoting early stimulation interventions through family involvement, instead of creating conditions to provide pediatric primary care, professional early stimulation and follow up by different specialists, such as neurologists, ophthalmologists and orthopedists.

The aim to better integrate epidemiological data into practices of caring for mothers and children affected by Zika, stated in the 2017 MEBs, promoted the integrated monitoring of changes in growth and development. Nevertheless, in everyday practices the discourse on microcephaly continued to frame biomedical surveillance and health interventions. This situation conflicted with what we know about CZS, or came to know in 2016, that CZS constitutes a range or spectrum of disorders and can occur without microcephaly and can appear after birth (Mota et al., 2016).

The term "CZS," therefore, implies that children exposed to Zika during pregnancy may have multiple development disorders, even though they are considered "normal" at birth. Lowe et al. (2018:9) called these babies the "Zika generation." The microcephaly spectacle blurs their visibility, also because there remain substantial diagnostic difficulties that complicate tracking these more insidious and hidden affects. This threatens a large segment of children born during the Zika epidemic, the "Zika generation," with unknown health, social and economic implications as well as social and state neglect and disregard, which is well known to the wider Brazilian handicapped population (Nações Unidas no Brazil, 2018). The existence of a large segment of "Zika generation," their life conditions and requirements are, therefore, in dispute and remain unaccounted for.

The health apparatus, in the second half of 2017 and in cooperation with UNICEF, created three documents to better address the needs of children affected by Zika (United Nations Children's Fund, 2017a,b,c): (1) guidelines for families and caregivers of children with developmental disorders (*Orientações às famílias e aos cuidadores de crianças com alterações no desenvolvimento*); (2) school and home stimulation of children with developmental disorders: qualification course for health, education and social assistance professionals (*Metodologia para Multiplicadores. Estimulação de crianças com alterações no desenvolvimento no ambiente domiciliar e escolar: Curso para qualificação de profissionais de saúde, educação e assistência social*); and (3) ensuring the rights of families and children with CZS and other disabilities (*Projeto Redes de Inclusão. Garantindo direitos das famílias e das crianças com Síndrome Congênita do Zika vírus e outras deficiências*). These documents drew heavily on the "early childhood development" (ECD) concept that has guided UNICEF's strategies since the 2000s (UNICEF, 2001). Practices established from the ECD approach place strong emphasis on brain enhancement and optimal brain development, as well as the promotion of a child's cognitive, physical, emotional and social potential (UNICEF, 2001). In reality, however, the majority of efforts under the ECD umbrella tend to focus most on cognitive and physical issues, and less so for emotional and social ones (Silva, 2016).

In an atmosphere of limited resources and the need to optimize investments, the collaboration between the Ministry of Health and UNICEF focused on the first three years of life, regarded as the most significant period for structural brain development, although according to the United Nations Committee on the Rights of the Child (2005), early childhood may last up to eight years of age. They also focused largely on early non-professional stimulation, often to be carried out by the families of the affected children. Like mosquito control, the onus of responsibility is on the individual and the household, charged with conducting and maintaining most child development interventions (Silva, 2016). This may sideline the demands of poor families for comprehensive professional care and state intervention.

Discussion and conclusions

This work highlighted some critical nodes in Brazilian health policies in relation to the ZIKV outbreak. Political contexts, scientific uncertainties and state trajectories enact complexities and produce different meanings and actions on Zika. The rapid response of the Brazilian Ministry of Health helped to increase epidemiological surveillance, diagnostic resources, improve financing to research and implement vector control initiatives. This was efficient in some ways and less so in other, but overall followed well-established historical patterns of other medical emergencies, such as outbreaks of H1N1 influenza, Dengue and measles. In a climate of unstable national politics, the Brazilian state response to Zika was predominately biomedical and reactionary, with limited regard for the deep-seated structural issues in the public health system and the social inequities that, in many ways, explain the virus' particular epidemiology. The "war framing" of Zika (Ribeiro et al. 2018), and with it the large, periodic campaigns on vector control, remain the main course of action, regardless of the social determinants of health, structural problems in the health system and other forms of transmission, such as through sex.

The "documents of emergency" we have reviewed and analyzed in this chapter reveal, first and foremost, a policy approach that repeats time-restricted and epidemiological monitoring patterns of previous responses. In the beginning of 2017, the Brazilian government announced the development of a "process of integrated surveillance and health care monitoring in cases of changes in the growth and development of Zika virus infections and other infectious etiologies," but, in February 2018, this processes was still unfinished. If, on the one hand, science learned to know Zika better, then, on the other hand, data from the improvement of epidemiological surveillance did not result in enhanced integration between the surveillance system and health care network planning, much less in guaranteeing access to much needed expanded health care assistance to all babies effected by ZIKV.

In January 2016, a former health minister, Marcelo Castro, declared that women should postpone their pregnancies and that he "hoped" women would get infected early in their lives, before they reached their fertile period.[12] The minister's underlying assumption seems to have revolved around a sort of "permanent immunization" established by a one-time infection with the virus. However, there seems to be no scientific evidence confirming this statement, just as there is no certainty about how the immune system responds to ZIKV and its transmissibility. Individual responsibility here appears entangled in a complex meshwork evolving gender biases, ideas of nation building and an assumption that herd immunity would "naturally" resolve an epidemic that, in many ways, was driven by dominant social, economic and political phenomena.

In this chapter, we situated Zika within a broader landscape of Brazilian politics and health systems. By exploring the literacy of the Brazilian state, and its ordinances, protocols and manuals aimed at guiding health professionals, we provided some reflects on how the state came to understand and frame the epidemic itself. With regard to the official responses to microcephaly, we found three significant moments that shifted the management of the epidemic in Brazil: the government's integrated approach between the Ministries of Health and Social Development, in early 2016, to combat the sanitary emergency; the attempt to integrate epidemiological surveillance data with health care planning; and the shift (in the second half of 2017) in care and support to affected families, where UNICEF played an important convening role.

From a local epidemic to a global threat, from the state's response seen through what we called "documents of emergency" to children and family care, we have attempted to explore, following Nunes and Nacif (2016), how and why certain subjects, issues and groups became visible during the epidemic and its aftermath, while others largely remained hidden and invisible. Through each set of documents analyzed here, such as ordinances, protocols, technical notes and microcephaly epidemiological bulletins, not only do we see differences among the Health Ministry's departments and hierarchies but, most importantly, in each of these set of documents a slightly different ZIKV is put forward, and "enacted" (Mol, 2002).

A Zika construed solely by mosquitoes and their human-animal relations leaves absent other forms of transmission, including sexual transmission, and constitutes a series of silences and erasures of scientific data; a Zika construed by its correlation only to microcephaly constitutes another series of silences, this time concerning an entire "Zika generation" that falls outside the more visible effects of microcephaly; and a Zika with which a considerable number of families, especially women and mothers, are expected to provide early life stimulation hides the need for professional state services and access to specialists.

Scientists now affirm that Zika is here to stay and, just as Dengue and Chikungunya, has become endemic to Brazil and most other countries in the Americas. It will in time reappear in epidemic form once herd immunity wanes. But Zika's transmission, effects and repercussions are embedded in a set of uncertainties. Zika is not the same as other arbovirus diseases. In January 2016, the former health minister (cited earlier) also declared that the fight against Zika was a fight against the need to avoid a "damaged generation" for Brazil. Nowadays, in the aftermath, it is possible to see that the children affected by the Zika virus have been framed and treated, to a large degree, as yet another segment of a neglected population group, inscribing further iniquities in Brazil's genealogy. Some aspects are highly visible, just as microcephaly is highly visible, and yet many aspects are equally silenced and unseen, just as many of Zika's biological effects are also unseen and invisible.

Notes

1 This work was partially supported by the European Union's Horizon 2020 Research and Innovation Program under ZIKAlliance Grant Agreement no. 734548. We would also like to acknowledge the Newton Fund Institute and the British Council for their support. Special thanks to our colleagues at the Zika Social Science Network and at FIOCRUZ.

2 As Hochman suggested (1998), the emphasis on large environmental sanitation campaigns in Brazil reflects a certain history of how the state has dealt with vector control over the years, in fragmented actions carried out for some months during peak epidemics and mainly concerned with individual and household responsibility and the use of chemical fumigation. In this approach, none of the infrastructural issues that surround mosquito breeding are addressed.

3 We use the term "temporalities" here in the terms used by Veena Das (2007) and Alex Nading (2014). Both authors, in different contexts, speak about a state that makes itself present only sporadically in the lives of its citizens, in lacunar actions.

4 See http://www.jb.com.br/ciencia-e-tecnologia/noticias/2015/05/15/especialista-minimiza-riscos-de-zika-no-pais/

5 It is now believed that Zika was likely introduced into Brazil from various soccer and canoe race competitions, between 2013 and 2014, that brought athletes from the South Pacific, as the virus was circulating there (see Gubler et al. 2017).

6 After the Brazilian presidental electrions in 2014, an economic crisis started which supported the political crisis against President Dilma Rousseff and the Labour Party. A conservative wave grew all over the country among high and middle social classes. From 2015 until the time of writing (mid-2018), Brazil was immersed in a polarized battle between democratic and conservative politics.

7 FIOCRUZ is a major public health research institution in Brazil, established in 1900, when it originally worked on sanitation campaigns for smallpox, yellow fever and plague. It has a current workforce of over 7,500 people, with a main office in Rio de Janeiro.

8 In a classic paper on bureaucracy, Weber (2006:50) establishes an articulation between written papers (the archives) and the professionals who work in the administration, and suggests that it is not possible to analyze bureaucratic practices without paying due attention to these papers and their role in structuring and ordering the administrative apparatus. Bourdieu (2014: 113), in a similar sense, emphasizes the "situation of authority" that produces the legitimacy of an "appointment or attestation," making them official acts, endowed with bureaucratic meanings and, in a certain way, creative powers, orders and realities.

9 Such a decision, at least the way it was implemented, has since been questioned in the United States. Saá et al. (2018) showed the high cost of screening each individual donor (which cost over $42 million over a period of 15 months) was likely an unnecessarily sensitive (and expensive) process given the risks involved.

10 It is important to note here that the argument that abortion is a public health issue had been strengthened in 2007 when a former health minister, Mr. Temporão, openly defended revisions to the country's abortion laws, supported by former president Lula. However the two following elections changed this legislative effort (Nogueira and Baptists, 2007).

11 For an ethnographic study on the entanglements produced by official documents construing everyday life in primary health care facilities in Rio de Janeiro, especially concerning prenatal care and HPV screening prevention, see Nogueira (2016).

12 See: http://g1.globo.com/bom-dia-brasil/noticia/2016/01/ministro-da-saude-comete-gafe-ao-falar-sobre-vacina-contra-zika-virus.html.

References

Attaran, A. 2016, 'Zika virus and the 2016 Olympic games', *The Lancet Infectious Diseases*, vol. 16, pp. 619–619. DOI:10.1016/ S1473-3099(16)30069-X.

Bourdieu, P. 2014, *Sobre o Estado*. Companhia das Letras, São Paulo, SP.

Callon, M., Lascoumes, P., Barthe, Y. 2009, *Acting in an uncertain world: an essay on technical democracy*. The MIT Press, Cambridge, MA.

Coelho, J., de Oliveira, M., and Paiva, C. 2016. 30 anos de dengue no Rio de Janeiro: Sua epidemiologia. <http://observatoriodasauderj.com.br/30-anos-de-dengue-no-rio-de-janeiro-sua-epidemiologia/>.

Congresso Nacional do Brasil 2016, *Lei que dispõe sobre a adoção de medidas de vigilância em saúde quando verificada situação de iminente perigo à saúde pública pela presença do mosquito transmissor do vírus da dengue, do vírus chikungunya e do vírus da zika* (Law No. 13.301). <http://pesquisa.in.gov.br/imprensa/jsp/visualiza/index.jsp?data=28/06/2016&jornal=1&pagina=1>.

Das, V. 2006, *Life and words: violence and the descent into the ordinary*. University of California Press, Oakland, CA.

Diniz, D. 2017, *Zika: from the Brazilian backlands to global threat*. Zed Books Ltd, Chicago.

Fares, R. C., Souza, K. P., Añez, G., & Rios, M. 2015, 'Epidemiological scenario of dengue in Brazil', *BioMed Research International*, 2015(5), 1–13.

Gubler, D. J., Vasilakis, N., & Musso, D. 2017, 'History and emergence of Zika virus', *The Journal of Infectious Diseases*, vol. 216(10), S860–S867.

Heredia, B., Palmeira, M. 2006, 'O voto como adesão', *Teoria e Cultura,* vol. 1, no. 1, pp. 35–58.

Hochman, G. 1998, *A era do saneamento: as bases da política de saúde pública no Brasil*. Editora Hucitec, São Paulo, SP.

Krieger, N. 2014, 'Discrimination and health inequities', *International Journal of Health Service*, vol. 44, no. 4, pp. 643–710. DOI:10.2190/HS.44.4.b.

Kuschnir, K. 2000, *O cotidiano da política*. Jorge Zahar, Rio de Janeiro, RJ.

Lock, M., Nguyen, V.K. 2010, *An anthropology of biomedicine*. Wiley-Blackwell, Indianapolis, IN.

Lowe, R., Barcellos, C., Brasil, P., Cruz, O., Honório, N., Kuper, H., et al. 2018, 'The Zika virus epidemic in Brazil: from discovery to future implications', *International Journal of Environmental Research and Public Health*, vol. 15, no. 1, pp. 1–18. DOI:10.3390/ijerph15010096.

Ministério da Saúde 2015a, *Portaria declara Emergência em Saúde Pública de importância Nacional (ESPIN) por alteração do padrão de ocorrência de microcefalias no Brasil* (Ordinance No. 1.813). <http://pesquisa.in.gov.br/imprensa/jsp/visualiza/index.jsp?data=12/11/2015&jornal=1&pagina=51&totalArquivos=120>.

Ministério da Saúde 2015b, *Protocolo de atenção à saúde e resposta à ocorrência de microcefalia relacionada à infecção pelo vírus Zi Protocolo de atenção à saúde e resposta à ocorrência de microcefalia relacionada à infecção pelo vírus Zika. Plano* Nacional de Enfrentamento à *Microcefalia*. ka. *Plano* Nacional de Enfrentamento à *Microcefalia*. <http://www.sbp.com.br/fileadmin/user_upload/2015/12/PROTOCOLO-SAS-MICROCEFALIA-ZIKA-dez-15.pdf.>

Ministério da Saúde, Agência Nacional de Vigilância Sanitária 2015, *Nota Técnica sobre Critérios técnicos para gerenciamento do risco sanitário no uso de hemocomponentes em procedimentos transfusionais frente à situação de Emergência em Saúde Pública de Importância Nacional por casos de infecção por Vírus Zika no Brasil* (Publication No. 001).

Ministério da Saúde, Ministério do Desenvolvimento Social do Brasil 2016a, *Portaria institui, no âmbito do Sistema Único de Saúde (SUS) e do Sistema Único de Assistência Social (SUAS), a Estratégia de Ação Rápida para o Fortalecimento da Atenção à Saúde e da Proteção Social de Crianças com Microcefalia.* (Ordinance No. 405). <http://pesquisa.in.gov.br/imprensa/jsp/visualiza/index.jsp?data=16/03/2016&jornal=1&pagina=27&totalArquivos=68>.

Ministério da Saúde, Ministério do Desenvolvimento Social do Brasil 2016b, *Instrução Operacional Conjunta* (Publication No. 01). <https://www.jusbrasil.com.br/diarios/112900537/dou-secao-1-11-04-2016-pg-61>.

Ministério da Saúde, Ministério do Desenvolvimento Social do Brasil 2016c, *Instrução Operacional Conjunta* (Publication No. 02). <https://www.jusbrasil.com.br/diarios/112900537/dou-secao-1-11-04-2016-pg-61>.

Ministério da Saúde, Secretaria de Vigilância em Saúde 2017, 'Monitoramento dos casos de dengue, febre chikungunya e febre pelo vírus Zika até a Semana Epidemiológica 19, 2017,' *Bol Epidemiológico*, vol. 48, no. 16, pp. 1–10. <http://portalarquivos.saude.gov.br/images/pdf/2017/maio/25/Monitoramento-dos-casos-de-dengue-febre-de-chikungunya-e-febre-pelo-virus-Zika-ate-a-Semana-Epidemiologica.pdf>

Mol, A. 2002, *The body Multiple: ontology in medical practice*. Duke University, Durham, NC.

van der Linden V, Pessoa A, Dobyns W, et al. 2016. Description of 13 Infants Born During October 2015–January 2016 With Congenital Zika Virus Infection Without Microcephaly at Birth — Brazil. MMWR Morb Mortal Wkly Rep 2016;65:1343–1348.

Nações Unidas no Brazil 2018, 'Documentos Temáticos. Objetivos de Desenvolvimento Sustentável 6 – 7 – 11 – 12 -15,' <http://www.br.undp.org/content/dam/brazil/docs/ODS/Documentos%20Tem%C3%A1ticos%20-%20ODS%206,%20ODS%207,%20ODS%2011,%20ODS%2012%20e%20ODS%2015.pdf>.

Nading, A. 2014, *Mosquito trails. Ecology, health, and the politics of entanglement.* University of California Press, Oakland, CA.

Nogueira, C. 2016, *"Dá licença, posso entrar?" Uma etnografia em uma Clínica da Família,* Master's thesis, Universidade Federal do Rio de Janeiro, Rio de Janeiro, Brazil. <http://objdig.ufrj.br/72/teses/844735.pdf>.

Nogueira, C., Baptista, T. 2007, 'Interrupção voluntária de gravidez: panorama do debate político do projeto de lei 1135/91', *Saúde em Debate*, vol. 31, no. 75, pp. 60–75.

Nunes, J., Nacif, D. 2016, 'The Zika epidemic and the limits of global health,' *Lua Nova*, vol. 98, pp. 21–46.

Oliveira, R. D. M. A. B., Araújo, F. M. D. C., & Cavalcanti, L. P. D. G. 2018, Aspectos entomológicos e epidemiológicos das epidemias de dengue em Fortaleza, Ceará, 2001–2012. *Epidemiologia e Serviços de Saúde*, 27, e201704414.

Ribeiro, B., Hartley, S., Nerlich, B., & Jaspal, R. 2018, Media coverage of the Zika crisis in Brazil: The construction of a 'war' frame that masked social and gender inequalities. *Social Science & Medicine*, 200 137–144.

Secretaria de Vigilância em Saúde 2017, 'Monitoramento integrado de alterações no crescimento e desenvolvimento relacionadas à infecção pelo vírus Zika e outras etiologias infecciosas, da Semana Epidemiológica 45/2015 até a Semana Epidemiológica 02/2017,' *Boletim Epidemiológico*, vol. 48, no. 6, pp. 1–18. <http://portalarquivos2.saude.gov.br/images/pdf/2017/fevereiro/27/2017_003.pdf>.

Secretaria de Vigilância em Saúde 2018, 'Monitoramento integrado de alterações no crescimento e desenvolvimento relacionadas à infecção pelo vírus Zika e outras etiologias infecciosas, até a Semana Epidemiológica 05 de 2018,' *Boletim Epidemiológico*, vol. 49, no. 19, pp. 1–8. <http://portalarquivos2.saude.gov.br/images/pdf/2018/maio/04/2018-016.pdf>.

Silva, L. 2016, *A invenção da primeira infância e a constituição contemporânea das práticas de governamentalidade*, Master's thesis, Universidade Estadual do Rio de Janeiro, Rio de Janeiro, Brazil. <http://ppfh.com.br/wp-content/uploads/2018/04/Tese-NORMALIZADA-LENIR.pdf>.

United Nations Children's Fund 2001, 'The state of the world's children', <https://www.unicef.org/sowc/archive/ENGLISH/The%20State%20of%20the%20World%27s%20Children%202001.pdf>.

United Nations Children's Fund, 2017a, 'Orientações às famílias e aos cuidadores de crianças com alterações no desenvolvimento', <https://www.unicef.org/brazil/pt/orientacoes_criancas_com_alteracoes_no_desenvolvimento.pdf>.

United Nations Children's Fund 2017b, 'Metodologia para Multiplicadores. Estimulação de crianças com alterações no desenvolvimento no ambiente domiciliar e escolar. Curso para qualificação de profissionais de saúde, educação e assistência social,' <https://www.unicef.org/brazil/pt/metodologia_estimulo_domicilio_escola.pdf>.

United Nations Children's Fund 2017c, 'Projeto Redes de Inclusão. Garantindo direitos das famílias e das crianças com Síndrome Congênita do Zika vírus e outras deficiências', <https://www.unicef.org/brazil/pt/redes_inclusao2018.pdf>.

United Nations Committee on the Rights of the Child. 'General Comment No. 7: implementing child rights in early childhood', <http://www.refworld.org/docid/460bc5a62.html>.

van der Linden V, Pessoa A, Dobyns W, et al. 2016, 'Description of 13 infants born during October 2015–January 2016 with congenital Zika virus infection without microcephaly at birth — Brazil,' *MMWR Morb Mortal Wkly Rep*, vol. 65, pp. 1343–1348.

Weber, M. 2006, 'Bureaucracy', in Sharma, A., Gupta, A. (ed.), *Anthropology of the state: a reader*. Blackwell Publishing, Hoboken, NJ.

4 Zika in everyday life

Gender, motherhood and reproductive rights in Pernambuco State, northeast Brazil

Camila Pimentel, Ana Paula Lopes de Melo, Sandra Valongueiro Alves, Maria do Socorro Veloso de Albuquerque, Thália Velho Barreto de Araújo and Tereza Maciel Lyra

This chapter explores a set of critical questions in the intersection between Zika virus and wider issues of motherhood, gender, disability and reproductive rights in Brazil. We draw extensively from our participation at public hearings and meetings (as well as a workshop we organized on the social and economic impact of Zika) in the "epicenter" of the 2015–2016 Brazilian epidemic – the city of Recife in Pernambuco State, northeast Brazil.[1] The workshop itself, held in Recife in the beginning of 2017, brought together about a hundred people with very diverse backgrounds, interests and perspectives on how to manage the policy implications, emerging science and bodily impacts of the virus. This included, for example, different academic researchers (health, environmental studies, anthropology/sociology and epidemiology), representatives of international organizations (like UN Women and UNFPA) and public authorities (representatives of the Department of Health of Pernambuco State and Recife City); however, it also included representatives of emerging social movements that have been, in various ways and at different times, at the center of the global Zika response: the Brazilian feminist movement and a coalition of Congenital Zika Syndrome (CZS) affected mothers and their children.[2]

In order to explore the variety of perspectives and discussions we encountered during our workshop, we will discuss three issues: (1) how the social determinants of health (particularly sanitation and social inequalities) have played a role in the surge of Zika-related microcephaly cases since 2015 in Pernambuco State; (2) how the mothers with children affected by Zika have drawn upon sociocultural norms that reify motherhood in Brazil as they advocate for specialized health services and social policies to advance their interests and needs; and (3) how the feminist movement has responded to the Zika epidemic, specifically in terms of their own advocacy of reproductive rights and the social impact of arboviruses in the everyday life of women. In so doing, we draw on a number of interrelated social theories and social realities, as manifest in Pernambuco, to advance a theorization of *caring* in the age of Zika, from the standpoint of individuals, families, social groups and the state. Ultimately we believe our feminist critique of the Zika response in Brazil, in a context of state inefficiencies and rampant structural inequalities, has much to offer, specifically in how it calls attention to the need to reimagine theories of care and human rights engagement, and their moral consequences, in light of persistent gender and socio-economic marginalization that is endemic to Northeast Brazil and, arguably, remain the most important "risk factors" for Zika.

The emergence of a new disease: Congenital Zika Syndrome in Brazil

In 2015, Brazil became famous around the world – this time not because of soccer or carnival but because of the large number of unexpected cases of microcephaly of unknown origin in newborns. Pernambuco, a state in the Northeast region of the country, was considered the epicenter of the 2015–2016 epidemic.

Surprised by the sudden increase of babies with microcephaly that they began seeing in April 2015, the first cases were registered by local neurologists and medical doctors (Diniz, 2016b). These were reported to the State Health Department which, in turn, introduced a mandatory reporting protocol for new cases with immediate effect as an epidemiological surveillance tool. In little over a month, the number of microcephaly cases exceeded the number of cases in previous years,[3] accompanied by unusual patterns of brain calcification and arthrogryposis (Miranda-Filho, 2016). Task forces went into action on various fronts (epidemiological surveillance, health care delivery, public health outreach and scientific research) to find answers and investigate the risk factors associated with these new microcephaly clusters.[4] Reports of rash disorders in pregnancy among mothers of these newborns led health workers to suspect that it was associated with the Zika virus, a suspicion that subsequent studies confirmed (Araújo et al., 2016, 2017; Brito, 2015; Chan, 2016; Costa et al., 2017). The Brazilian Ministry of Health ordered compulsory reporting of cases throughout the country and declared a state of National Public Health Emergency in November 2015. By the end of the year, the Brazilian Bulletin of Epidemiology[5] reported a total of 399 suspected cases of microcephaly, across seven northeastern states, with most (268 cases, or 67.2%) from Pernambuco, as shown in Figure 4.1. Cases were reported throughout Brazil and by the end of 2017, 3,037 were confirmed, 65% of them in the Northeast region. As shown in Figure 4.2, these were spread throughout Pernambuco State.

The surge in microcephaly in Pernambuco sparked widespread concern in the scientific community and required government responses to what would subsequently be confirmed to be a new congenital syndrome characterized by a broad range of corporal and neurological alterations. Congenital Zika Syndrome (CZS) related to infection by the Zika virus in pregnancy, a condition that may also occur without microcephaly due to the wide range of clinical sequella. The words of one Pernambuco woman, who gave birth to a child with

Notification of Congenital Zika Syndrome cases in Brazil 2015 – 2017*

	2015		2016		2017	
	n	%	n	%	n	%
Under investigation	268	6.5	1,434	16.7	1,201	49.3
Confirmed	967	23.5	1,848	21.5	222	9.1
Presumable	46	1.1	143	1.7	121	5
Discarded	2,275	55.2	3,834	44.6	609	25
Inconclusive	83	2	99	1.2	13	0.5
Excluded	481	11.7	1,235	14.4	271	11.1
Total	4,120	100	8,593	100	2,437	100

Total number of confirmed cases (as of Dec. 2017)*

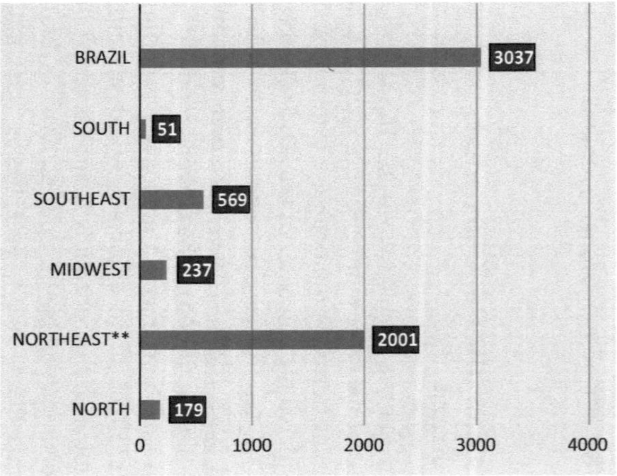

**Pernambuco - 438 cases

Figure 4.1 Cases of congenital Zika Syndrome in Brazil (2015–2017).

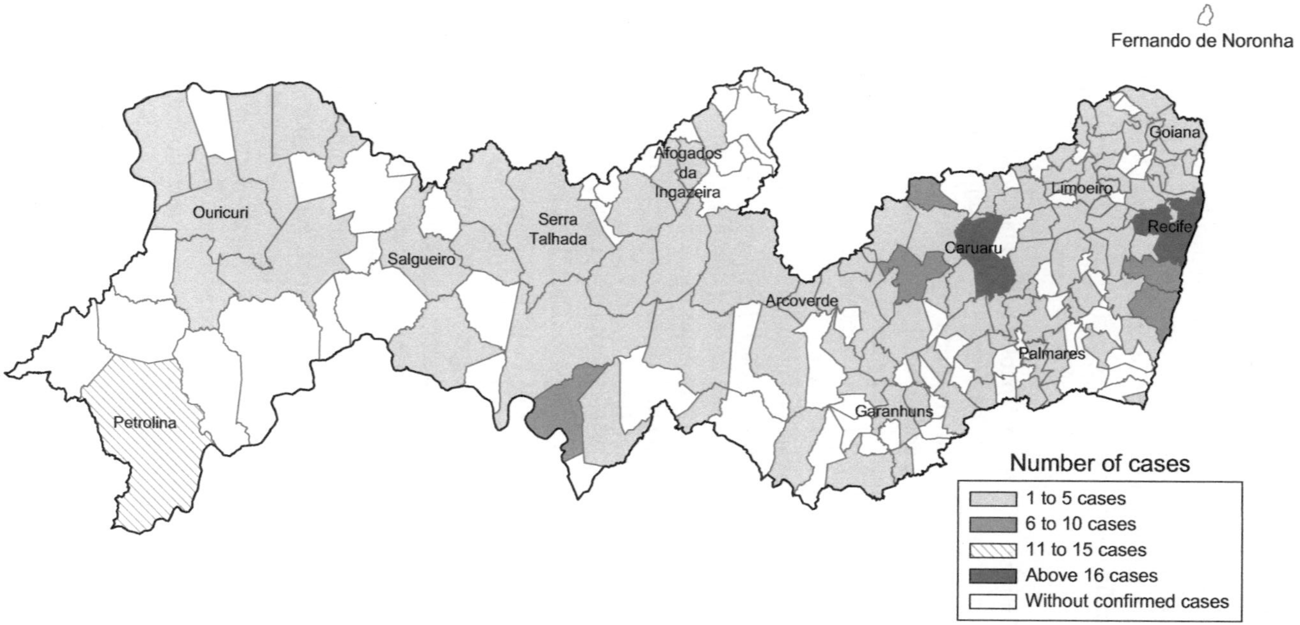

Figure 4.2 Spatial distribution of confirmed microcephaly cases in Pernambuco State (2015–2017).

microcephaly in the early stages of the epidemic, illustrates this complex clinical spectrum:

> My son is a Zika victim. He was born with microcephaly, ventriculomegaly, myopia and chronic encephalopathy. My pregnancy passed without incident, but in the third month, I woke up with an itch. I went to [the] emergency room and they told me that I had Zika, because itching is typical of Zika. They prescribed anti-allergy medication and did some ultrasound exams. Everything was normal and I continued my pregnancy. I took every test imaginable and nothing showed up. I only found out my son was sick when he was born and this was confirmed nine days later.
>
> (Fieldnotes, 2017)

By early 2016, images of "strange" babies with small heads were appearing regularly in the international and national news. Uncertainties about the scale of this new congenital infection, its cause(s) and the prognosis for this new class of newborns created national panic, adding to an already complex political situation in Brazil at the time, including the impeachment of President Dilma and austerity policies (including for health). Several hypotheses were put forward at the time as to the "real" cause of the spike in microcephaly: alleged side effects of vaccines given in pregnancy, use of larvicides used against mosquitoes, malnutrition and a number of conspiracy theories. These spread quickly on social networks without any substantial proof. To add another layer of complexity to the epidemic, Zika in 2017 was no longer an epidemic and cases of CZS had reduced to 15 confirmed cases.[6] This was despite the fact that cases were registered in almost all parts of the state between 2015 and 2016 (see Figure 4.2).

The need for an immediate response to an ongoing epidemic of a serious communicable disease about which little was (or still is) known led researchers, public authorities and funding bodies to focus their attention on the risk factors, the description of symptoms, characterization of the new syndrome, the creation of new laboratory tests, the accuracy of imaging exams to confirm cases, the testing of medication and vaccines and the need to prepare the health system to attend cases and to develop early childhood stimulation strategies for affected newborns. Such studies, based on the biomedical model, have shed much light on the pathogenesis of the new disease and possible clinical interventions and laboratory responses. As is so often the case with emerging infectious diseases, medical humanitarian response and biomedical research, relatively few studies have explored the sociocultural aspects of the disease and the context and discourses of those families – women, children and men in Brazil – who have been so significantly and severely affected.

Some researchers have raised the important question of the relationship between social inequalities and the epidemic of not only CZS but also other arboviruses such as Chikungunya and Dengue (Nunes & Pimenta, 2016; Castro, 2016). Dengue, for example, is endemic throughout Brazil, where it emerges in periodic epidemics that have been increasingly related to climate change (Ferreira, 2016); but, really, above all, Dengue in Brazil, and indeed throughout Latin America, is related more to the lack of social investment in basic sanitation and water supply, noxious and unequal living conditions and the disordered urban development of favelas and urban sprawl that are responsible for vector transmission (Associação Brasileira de Saúde Coletiva, 2015).

This is especially evident in Pernambuco, the epicenter of the CZS epidemic. As shown by the media images and journalistic tales of poverty, and clearly shown in regional statistics, families living in poverty were the group most affected by the disease (Souza et al, 2018; Lesser & Kitron, 2016). Pernambuco is a state in Brazil where 77% of the population lives below the poverty line and 54% of them are enrolled in government assistance programs for families whose income is half a minimum wage per person per month (about US $150/month). In the city of Recife, the state capital, 30% of people are subject to water rationing and do not receive water on a regular basis. In some neighborhoods, it is common for the service to be interrupted for a week at the time; in rural areas of Pernambuco, people can go for 30 days without running water. Approximately 97% of children diagnosed with the new "small head" syndrome (as it was sometimes called) were born in public hospitals. Although Brazil has a universal health system, the wealthy and middle class increasingly seek out private care; public services are mostly used by the poor (Paim, 2013).

It is also no surprise that women are most affected by arboviruses – data from the Ministry of Health show that about 56% of the reported cases of arboviruses occur in females. In Brazil, these are mostly poor Afro-Brazilian women of reproductive age, who are usually more exposed to mosquitoes by their (productive and reproductive) work and poor housing, often on the periphery of urban geographies (Scheper-Hughes, 1992). In the context of Zika, these women have also become the social group most affected by feelings of panic, fear and guilt as they struggle to cope with the possibility of transmitting the virus to their children. Lastly, any discussion about inequality and Zika needs to be situated within a broader appreciation of how the epidemic intersects with other challenges of motherhood in places like Pernambuco. Women are, historically, responsible for being caregivers on top of their professional and other livelihood work. Motherhood imposes responsibilities and identities that are socially imposed and constructed, and it is important to appreciate how these embedded realities influence everyday life for those personally affected by Zika.

By exploring these issues, therefore, this chapter seeks to raise a number of central questions regarding the social impact of Zika on the lives of women and divergent concepts of "motherhood" in Pernambuco, Northeastern Brazil. We do this by exploring two very different socially-embedded points of view: women with children affected by Zika and the Brazilian feminist movement.

Microcephaly, support groups and mother associations in Pernambuco

In order to understand how the Zika epidemic has affected women in Brazil, let us first start by exploring the perspectives of two associations of mothers of children with microcephaly that are active in Pernambuco and who participated in the workshop we organized in 2017. One of these associations – AMAR (an acronym that means "Alliance of Rare Mothers and Families" in Portuguese) – has been a point of reference for around four years for mothers of children with disabilities, especially those related to rare diseases. After the emergence of the CZS epidemic, this association was the first organization that the mothers of these children turned to for support and self-organization. In 2017, this association had around 420 members, about 150 of them mothers of children with CZS. The organization has extensive knowledge of Brazilian legislation and advocates for the rights of people with disabilities. Although it was already active prior to the emergence of Zika, it has since acquired greater visibility due to the increased media coverage.

The other association – UMA ("Union of Mothers of Angel," in Portuguese) – was founded in 2016 by two mothers of children with Zika-related microcephaly, who regularly met when visiting the doctor with their children and decided to set up a WhatsApp group, initially to exchange experiences, as a way of "*reducing the sense of loneliness and isolation*" (as they said) that they were experiencing. These women first allied themselves with the association mentioned earlier but then split from it, feeling the need for an organization specifically dedicated to the mothers (and families) of children with Zika-acquired microcephaly. This association currently (as of mid-2018) has around 400 mothers of children with CZS registered as members in various parts of Pernambuco State.

Both associations have their own headquarters, located in Recife: one (AMAR) was donated by the state government, while the other (UMA) was purchased with resources from an anonymous donor. The activities promoted by these organizations are diverse and include welcoming families, meetings with affiliates, participating in public hearings, conducting campaigns and marches, donating supplies (i.e. special milk, medicines, stimulus and rehabilitation equipment), as well as assisting with projects developed in partnership with universities, researchers, other non-governmental organizations (NGOs) and donor organizations. The experience of the Recife associations has become a point of reference for other parts of the country. Representatives of these associations have been invited to participate in events and share experiences, thereby helping women to organize in other states, such as Alagoas, Ceará and Bahia. These connections have helped to build up a national network and strengthen advocacy regarding the needs of these children and their families.

While advances in research since 2015 have shifted our understanding of Zika to account for a range of CZS manifestations, "microcephaly" and its medical and social impacts continues to dominate – in some senses symbolically – our perspective and understanding of this "strange" congenital malformation. As researchers, then, we see "microcephaly" as a *social fact*, in the sense proposed by Émile Durkheim (2007). In other words, it is something external – a social category, a label, a method of "otherness" – that is imposed on individuals in a coercive manner and performs a social function, conforming subjectivities, identities and, in some cases, stigma. In this sense, we also recognize as a social fact the way the epidemic was portrayed in the media, elaborating on specific symbolic meanings about affected children and their parents. The very term *microcephaly* occurs as an emic category, used by the mothers' movement (the association of mothers and affected families) as a discursive strategy, but also as a way of explaining the disease and building up appropriate meanings shared by group members. It is impossible to ignore how this infant disability has affected society in Pernambuco – not only because of its high occurrence but also because of the original "strangeness" of how "Zika's children"[7] came to be known. Families faced doubts about the disease and the meanings that came to be associated with it.

When looking at the political organization of these "activist mothers" (Pinheiro & Longhi, 2017) (most of them are mothers), we need to take into account the context of social turmoil associated with the epidemic and the way this sparked unexpected reactions, even among those working in the field of childhood disabilities. This can clearly be seen from the words of a representative of AMAR on this topic:

> In January 2016, we met various mothers seeking out our association as a 'cry for help.' They wanted to know what caused microcephaly. It was still not known that the cause was Zika. The look of desperation in these mothers was palpable. … We held a meeting with 158 women affected by Zika-related congenital syndrome. I had never seen so many babies with the same disease, even though I work with disabilities. This made a deep impression on me.
>
> (Fieldnotes, 2017)

It should be noted that these organizations were established by mothers who shared the same experiences and anxieties regarding the care of their children. Generally, in both, we find a reification of the social role of motherhood, a sacralization of children and the valorization of "overload" (multiple responsibilities) intrinsic to the position of the mother in Brazilian society (Pinheiro et al, 2009). These are expressed in a discourse that demands not only social belonging and acceptance but also government action through rights-based discourse. In this context, reification of motherhood seems to seek a re-recognition and validation of the role of the mother, a "super mother," who needs to redouble her efforts to address the care needs of a Zika-affected child. At the same time, in explaining their efforts, they also stress that they need care themselves. As stated by the vice coordinator of one of the associations during our workshop:

> We agreed to take these people on. It involves taking care of [those] who take care [of the affected children] and helping families feel they are part of a struggle for rights… caring for the caregiver is an important part of care. It is a cycle…We strive for *social belonging.* This is what a mother wants for her future life and principally for the quality of life of her child.
>
> (Fieldnotes, 2017)

At the heart of the ideology, in some senses, of CZS mother associations, motherhood is given a new meaning by, first and foremost, the experience of having a child with a disability that does not fit the image of a "normal" child generated, psychological and socially, during the months prior to birth. The public health emergency produced in these mothers an urgent need to redefine motherhood, seen now as having been transformed by the "gift" of a child with microcephaly. There was no time to mourn the imagined child; motherhood is viewed here as propitiation for this "gift of God." The children are sanctified as "angels" bringing special insights into life and all those who help are seen likewise:[8]

> When my son was born, my life changed, and not for the worse. It was a watershed in my life. Through him *I met wonderful people and I was able to help many others* and that is how the association began.
>
> (representative of UMA; Fieldnotes, 2017)

Marcel Mauss (2003), in his essay *The Gift*, argues that the exchange of gifts has a political dimension. We can see this in the sense of mission found in those who set up an association or political organization; with Zika, we also see this in the relationship established with other mothers and collaborators who participate in events and projects and provide donations and services. These partners are referred to as "guardian angels" and their "offerings" are also a way of symbolically forming a connection with the affected families.

The reification of motherhood evoked by the mothers associations involves a simultaneous rejection of negative feelings and burdensome life changes as well as a mechanism for social belonging; in so far that these associations support socially expected behaviors and discourse. The initial solitude of the victim of a "tragedy" is transformed by mutual recognition and the identity forged is that of mothers, real mothers, who now have a mission, a God-given opportunity to show what they are capable of "in spite of this":

> We decided to come out of isolation to fight for the lives of our children. We accepted God's challenge.
>
> (representative of UMA; Fieldnotes, 2017)

> Our children [are] the mission God has given us and we are in this to the end. If our children can't walk, we will walk for them. If they can't hear, we will be their ears. If they can't interact, we will fight for them. If they can't speak, we will be the only voice declaring that microcephaly is not the end of the world.
>
> (excerpt from a video presented by UMA during the workshop; Fieldnotes, 2017)

These associations play an important role as a network of social support, helping people deal with loneliness and social exclusion, poverty and despair. It is here that people fight together for their rights and those of their children, for better health services, social benefits, tolerance and so forth. Through these activities, they are also creating meanings of this very novel, very powerful experience:

> We found that, after the *Whatsapp* group, we became stronger. Because, when you meet someone else who is in the same situation, you feel strengthened

to confront the situation. The group has given me strength. It has made me become a special mother and that's where the true God-given mission came from. After that I told my family and friends about his illness, when he was three months old. I vowed that I would make the association my life. I seized the opportunity to seek out other mothers and relieve them of the isolation, sadness and anxiety that I once felt.

(representative of UMA. Fieldnotes, 2017)

A change of routine, making new friends, new ways of relating to health professionals and the continuous exchange of new information, contribute to integration among these activist mothers. During their visits and interactions with the health system as part of their caregiving, they have sparked a phenomenon that Diniz (2016a, b) has called "domestic science" – the informal comparison of symptoms, stages of development, medication, therapies and therapeutic progress that serve as sources of information and knowledge created by the women themselves. This strategy also feeds into the work of health professionals who are dealing with a syndrome still not well understood by the scientific literature, especially when they end up producing prognoses that contradict the true development of children as witnessed, day-in and day-out, by the mothers themselves.

We can see the role played by the mothers associations in providing a sense of shared identity, through confronting similar problems and sharing ideas regarding how to deal, socially, with their difficulties. Macro-sociologists, such as Goffman (1988; 2001) and Becker (2008), key thinkers from symbolic interactionism,[9] developed theories of deviance that are relevant here. From this perspective, the children with microcephaly are considered deviant according to biomedical norms. Because they are infants who cannot speak for themselves; however, it is the mothers who take on this role *for* them. They present them as "socially different" subjects undergoing a peculiar life experience that affects their subjective processes and interferes with the normal course of their lives. This leads the mothers to organize politically to provide visibility for their children, change social conceptions and campaign for access to health services and social policies that, so they hope, can meet their needs in the fragile and brittle context of health and living in Brazil.

For example, mothers present at our research workshop in Recife, early 2017, called attention to the impoverishment and lack of socio-economic security among women with children with microcephaly. This is a major concern in the lives of many women in Brazil. Most of these mothers have given up paid work to care for their children 24 hours a day. Some had their partners and the husbands abandoned them; one of the leaders of the associations has mentioned in public statements that about 70% of mothers of children with disabilities and rare diseases do not have husbands. However, it is important to note that being a "single mother" is a common situation in the daily lives of poor women in Brazil (PNAD/IBGE, 2016). A participant at the 2017 workshop underlined the need for policies that help these women get back to work. Women are fighting for places for their children in crèches with specialized facilities, and stressing the need to receive technical training in a profession that is compatible with their daily lives. As one stated:

> I hope my son lives a long life. But if, God forbid, 15 or 20 years from now, he passes away, who will give me a job after being unemployed for such a long time?
>
> (Mother of children affected with CZS; Fieldnotes, 2017)

From this view, disability, and the role the state can play in managing it, is not conceptualized narrowly as a "pathology" or "congenital defect" that merely needs to be fixed but extends to, as another mother told us, "the right to quality of life for our babies," which involves access to treatment but also social inclusion. This approach to disability contrasts with the traditional biomedical model, which views disability as an individual biological disadvantage requiring intervention to enable the "dis-abled" to fit into society. Members of these mother associations, however, suggested a more social approach to disability (Diniz, 2007; Gesser et al., 2012). This social experience of disability has often been discussed as a result of a system of "social oppression" that brands disabled people as generally "different" from others. But when these mothers concentrate their political campaign on public policy, inclusion and quality of life, they are breaking with the central focus of biomedicine (of intervening on/in the body) and enhancing the mental and physical capacities of individuals, by including other dimensions, such as removing barriers to social interaction and improving access to care (see Figure 4.3).

Now that the epidemic has passed its peak (in 2017) and the national and international public health emergency has subsided, the representatives of these associations have stated in interviews, public hearings and forums that they feel abandoned by the public authorities, who are providing less and less support as media interest in the plight of such families declines. As Diniz (2016b) vividly describes in neighboring Alagoas State, for these families Zika is an epidemic without an end: while the "emergency" and political panic may have subsided, the consequences of Zika have not. There is still a need for various therapies to enable children to interact, respond to stimuli and acquire enhanced neuro-psychomotor capacities. As the children grow, new requirements also emerge: such as the provision of adequately equipped schools and daycare centers to meet the specific needs of children, or social protection measures that minimize the vulnerability associated with poverty and poor living conditions, which are only exacerbated by the experience of living with a child with CZS.[10]

All of this shows that, in the case of these mothers and their children, the politics of care, which recognizes interdependence and autonomy, are central to social change and action. In the words of the director of the association that advocates for the rights of individuals with rare diseases (AMAR), whose disabled son is now 18 years old:

> It is as if you had a newborn child for the rest of your life. It reaches the point where you start taking more time to have a shower, simply to have some time

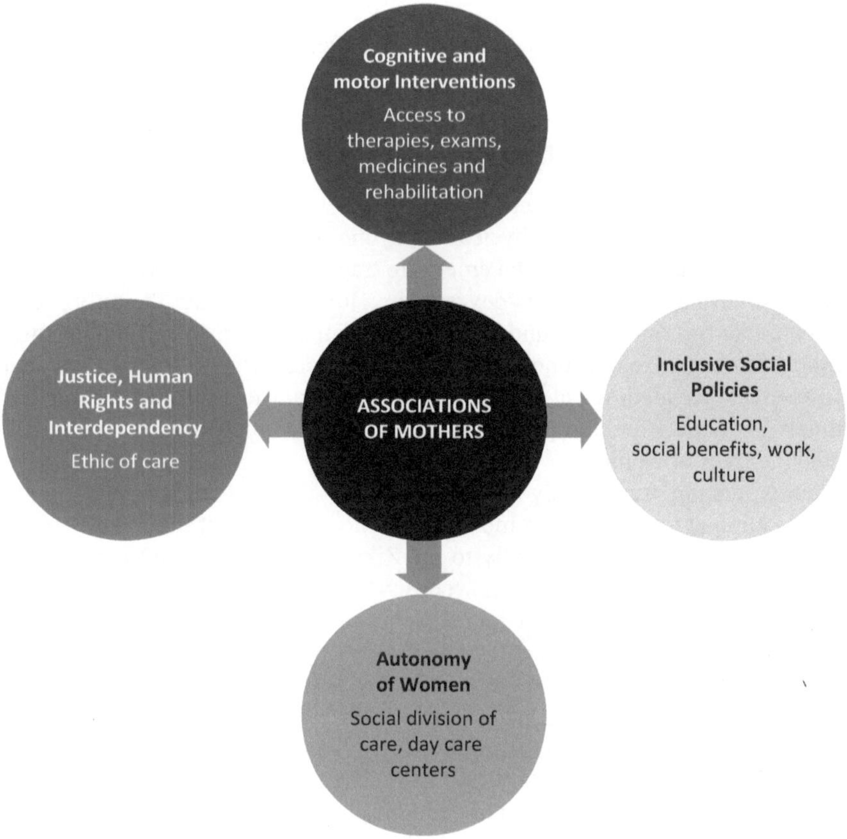

Figure 4.3 The demands of Zika-affected mothers, as discussed by mother associations, to address the burden of Zika in Pernambuco State, Brazil.

> alone. You want to go to the shops, just to get out of the house. Caregivers also need to be cared for.
>
> (Fieldnotes, 2017)

Interdependence, here, means being dependent on another person at some point in one's life. It is a condition that affects not only people with disabilities, but also their caregivers. This is an often-neglected aspect of the Zika epidemic: What about the psychosocial wellbeing of the caregivers? Who will care for the caregivers? Women (especially mothers) have, historically, assumed the role of caregivers and been required to meet the needs of others. This gendered conditioning has been accepted by public policy to the extent to which public authorities only deem themselves responsible when a female figure is absent (Guimarães, 2008). There is a need to show that interdependence is a condition intrinsic to human life, not only to that of women. Likewise, mothers of children with microcephaly need to be free to live their own lives. Recognition of this does not undermine the bond between mother and child. Quite the reverse! Figure 4.3 sums up the demands identified by the mothers associations in Pernambuco to address the burden of Zika.

The view of the Brazilian feminist movement

Grounded in the disability movement, the work of mother organizations to support children affected by CZS, physically, psychologically and legally, has been an important social response to the emerging tragedy of this new epidemic, and the social suffering brought by its devastation. However, it is not the only social movement that has formed around Zika. The feminist movement, which has historically been organized around a women and minority rights agenda, has also found a vehicle for ideological expression and practical socio-political action that continues to shape Brazilian perceptions of Zika, including how the virus has affected the lives of women.

In our workshop, we not only heard from mother associations; we also invited six NGOs aligned to the feminist movement, who were, at that time, working on different projects related specifically to the Zika epidemic and with arboviruses more generally. These organizations were invited because they have previously worked with some of the researchers in what became known as the "Zika Situation Room."[11] The Situation, Action and Articulation Room on Women's Rights was established in March 2016 by the UN system (UN Women and UNFPA) and civil society, in response to the Zika health crisis. It started with 25 entities, and (until the end of 2017) there were 40 institutions involved. Motivated by the epidemic, this collaboration allowed stakeholders to advocate for the improvement of basic sanitation with local authorities and to dialogue on sexual and reproductive rights. Programs emerged for these discussions, for the improvement of reproductive health services and greater access to information and contraceptives/reproductive planning and protection against the risk of sexual transmission of the Zika virus. This experience made it clear that the debate needed to be extended beyond academic circles to actors from organized civil society who were already in contact with vulnerable populations.

In the context of the Zika emergency, the representatives of the feminist movement pointed to the need to publicly reinforce debates on reproductive rights, specifically those related to the (non-)autonomy of women in family planning and the importance of issues of class, gender, race and age. According to them, those aspects are fundamental to elaborate a broader understanding about the consequences of the epidemic, as gender inequality is so much a part of the Brazilian reality. To highlight this perspective, we brought six Pernambuco feminist movement organizations to our workshop: SOS Corpo, Grupo Curumim, Gestos, Uiala Mukaj, Coletivo Mangueiras and Mirim Brasil. These organizations develop a variety of interventions at the community level and with public policies and advocacy. Some focus on Afro-Brazilian women, adolescents and/or young women. They work in reproductive health, sexuality, HIV/AIDS and/or gender inequality. Some focus on strengthening local women's social and economic support networks.

These organizations have been working for some time in the state (the oldest, for more than 30 years) and they had been meeting since March 2016 (face-to-face and online) to discuss the national response to the Zika virus epidemic. Since the formalization of the "Zika Situation Room," six meetings took place in different Brazilian states (until the end of 2017), including the last one, in Salvador, Bahia, in collaboration with Fiocruz.

The work of these organizations on the Zika epidemic continues a tradition of political action to defend rights and a general concern with health and sexual and reproductive rights in Brazil. A good example is the Program for Integrated Women's Health Care (PAISM in Portuguese) launched in 1983 as a result of dialogue with social movements, not only, linked to feminist perspectives. Assuming an integrated perspective on women's health, rather than isolated initiatives focused only on maternal-child issues, this program is still a challenge to the public authorities that failed to effectively (or holistically) implement it (Osis, 1998). In 2004, the program became national policy. In spite of this progressive move, many advances in the area of women's health – like control of fertility and increase in prenatal coverage – has remained difficult to address and programs have remained fragmented. In this sense, PAISM has had mixed results so far. Part of the reason for this has to do with the lack of educational efforts directed to health workers as well as the continued dominance of maternal-child health programming in the broader health and political agenda (Rattner, 2014).

Our workshop occurred shortly after the then director of the Brazilian Ministry of Health's Department of Communicable Disease Surveillance had publicly suggested that women should put off getting pregnant until the Zika epidemic was over, as a way of avoiding babies being born with microcephaly. This was also done in neighboring countries such as El Salvador and Jamaica during the peak of the epidemic in late 2015/early 2016. This pronouncement was widely criticized by the women's movement, which drew attention to a number of problems regarding the government's approach and created new and interesting dynamics for sexual and reproductive rights in Brazil.

A number of important, and yet controversial, points were raised by these organizations, which can be divided into three broad categories. First, they stressed that more focus should be placed on the empowerment of women in order to improve sexual and reproductive rights (SRRs). This includes women being able to negotiate conjugal sexual relations; address the lack or scarcity of contraceptive devices; strengthen access to family planning; and broaden the right to abortion. The second focus of these organizations involved an ideological commitment to social and environmental justice for the poor, often Afro-Brazilians, to access better sanitation, regular water supply, the right to dignified housing and access to the benefits and other welfare services allocated, at least in writing, by the state. Lastly, the feminist movement focused on improving health services. This included things like access to diagnosis (sometimes people access medical tests but do not have access to the results), compatibility of services with the needs of the population, health education and communication – including for mental health – in the age of Zika.

In our workshop, these feminist organizations continually noted the shortcomings of actions and campaigns developed by the public authorities, specifically to improve environmental sanitation. These interventions had become the main discourse of the state, framing the problem of Zika and its solution. In this narrative, what was needed was more of the same – to repeat interventions, attempted decades earlier, centered on eradicating the mosquito vector, principally through the efforts of private individuals (households) to exterminate stagnant water sources. Such elements, framed with symbolism that highlighted the need for greater individual responsibility and "behavior change," can be seen in much of the anti–*Aedes aegypti* campaign literature distributed in Brazil at the time.

As discussed by critical scholars, such as Marcos Cueto (2007) in his historical analysis of malaria eradication in Mexico, such campaigns, focused on eradication of the mosquito, tend to overlook the structural problems that persist in Brazilian society. The work of social movements, that draw on feminist perspectives, seek to underline the inequalities perpetuated by such strategies and how they can have a disproportionate impact on the lives of women. For example, some of the feminist NGOs present at the workshop believed that the feminization of responsibility for combating arboviruses was tied to campaigns focused on private domestic spaces as the principal locale for control of *Aedes*. However, unequal gender distribution of domestic work is a reality. For the political scientist and women's studies professor Joan Tronto (1997), it is especially important to bear this in mind when framing public policy and health promotion strategies because, as she put it, "caring is an activity governed by gender, both in the employment market and in private life. Women's occupations generally involve caring and women are responsible to a disproportionate degree for household care" (Tronto, 1997:189). This is even more striking in Brazil in the case of childcare, as the lack of public crèches means that caring for children often entails giving up productive work or resorting to care networks that involve, unsurprisingly, other women.

Care and the feminization of poverty

For a long time, and still today, care has been seen as an activity of lesser social importance and is typically considered to be the responsibility of women. This is why Joan Tronto (1997) argues that there is a need to view care from a feminist angle, as a way of revealing the social (and moral) inequalities between genders in this field of social life. This raises the question of the extent to which government action and health campaigns that focus on the mosquito and domestic hygiene are putting an extra burden on women, who are already overloaded with activities that are considered typically female.

Campaigns that focus on care of the home as the main strategy for vector control presuppose that there is someone available (and interested) to perform these activities. This was one of the main lines of argument of the feminist NGO participants:

> There is no public policy for confronting the epidemic. What we have is a transfer of responsibility from the state to the individual and this individual is a woman.
>
> (Fieldnotes, 2017)

Brazil's legacy of patriarchy and powerful culture of structural chauvinism (Saffioti, 2011; Aguiar, 2000) consistently reproduces, in the media, stereotypical gender roles that reinforce the feminization of household duties. Despite calls to address this through, for example, changing how women are presented in the media and advertising (Gill, 2008), women continue to be perceived as social actors who need to devote their time to care for the family and wider society, making it difficult for them to engage in paid work and, often, completely preventing them from working outside the home. This entails a problem in the development of democracy itself (Tronto, 2013), and leads us to reflect on the very notion of care: what it entails and the implications of the various ways of understanding it.

Care has traditionally been seen as a voluntary activity involving self-denial related to affection and love (Kleinman, 2015). There has tended to be an unfortunate dichotomization, however, between care work and the ethics of care, one that clouds the social and political dimensions involved in this kind of social action. According to Molinier and Paperman (2015), viewing care exclusively in emotional terms overlooks political issues present in the social world. This would appear to be the case in mosquito control campaigns. There is an appeal to the emotions: "*the mosquito isn't stronger than a whole nation*" and "*this mosquito kills.*" However, these are not emotions that spur or call for collective non-gendered action. On the contrary, when we realize that it is women who are responsible for care of the home, it is obvious at whom such campaigns are aimed. Feminists have historically called attention to this inequality, revealing what Tronto calls "*the indifference of the privileged.*" In other words, by failing to critique the notion of care, such media strategies and public campaigns serve only to reinforce the gender inequalities that structure Brazilian society. The act of caring (for other people or the environment) has an impact on the caregiver, in so far as it is presumed that she has the time to engage in this activity and is emotionally predisposed to do so. To continue to ignore the disproportion between the involvement of men and of women in such activities is, from a feminist point of view, to reinforce gender inequalities and reassert the classical, albeit problematic, division between the male public world and the female domestic sphere. This is why Tronto argues that there is a need for a feminist perspective on care:

> A feminist approach to care must start out by furthering understanding of what it means to care for others, both morally speaking, and in terms of the need to restructure broader social and political institutions, if caring for others is to constitute a more central part of the everyday lives of all members of society.
>
> (Tronto, 1997:200)

Aware that the categories of *caring about* and *caring for* should not presuppose the classical gender distinction nor even consider subjects only as individuals, this broader conception of care enables us to raise questions regarding the role of the state *as caregiver* in providing the basic conditions for a dignified life. Molinier and Paperman (2015) argue that we need to understand care as a *process*, extrapolating it interpersonally onto organizations and social institutions.

In government public health campaigns, the state does not appear as an entity responsible for caring for the environment, nor as a provider of essential services, such as basic sanitation (including collection and treatment of sewage and provision of a regular supply of water), dignified housing conditions and solid waste collection. This issue, addressed by the feminist movement in Brazil, and indeed globally, as a matter of environmental justice, was also raised during the workshop. One of the NGO participants called attention both to the inefficiency of urban sanitation and to inequalities in access to basic sanitation services by stating that:

> the epidemic was treated as if it were merely a problem related to cleaning your back yard. In fact, there is a serious lack of sanitation in this State and in the country as a whole. This chiefly affects more impoverished localities.
>
> (Fieldnotes, 2017)

The relationships between structural inequalities and Zika virus was also addressed by research groups studying environmental questions; these groups have, for a long time now, stressed the need to rethink vector control strategies.[12] Critical of government action, these groups reassert the need to concentrate efforts not only on environmental issues of an individual nature but more on structural challenges, such as reducing social inequality, providing dignified housing and democratizing access to basic sanitation – all of which are responsibilities of the public authorities.

These state inefficiencies are not, of course, distributed equally among socio-economic strata and from one geographical region to another (UNDP, 2017). The disparities in Human Development Index (HDI) between regions of Brazil are one indication of how inequality is produced and perpetuated; the South and Southeast regions have higher HDIs compared to the Northeast.[13] It is no coincidence, then, that the latter was the region most affected by the Zika epidemic and that the poorer parts of the Northeast States affected by the epidemic experienced the highest incidence. In the case of Pernambuco State, as elsewhere, Zika followed the fault lines created by social inequality. In what Castro (2016) has described as a state of structural inequality, the virus disproportionally affected economically underprivileged groups that live in areas where public services tend to be most lacking. A report by the Brazilian Department of Social Development, Children and Young People concluded in early 2016 that most families with children with CZS have a low household income and not all of these families have access to benefits, which is a right guaranteed by the Federal Constitution.[14] Even more worrying is the fact that, of the families affected by Zika enrolled in social programs, 77% still live below the poverty line.[15]

This structural inequality is related to another problematical facet of care as a predominantly female activity, which has become known as the "feminization of poverty" (Pearce, 1987). Pearce used this term to refer to the greater economic impact on women when they head households. In a world in which there is still a great disparity between men's and women's wages, even though this has declined slightly, the impact of Zika and CZS on the lives of women tends to impoverish them as workers, in so far as many of them give up work to care for their children.[16] Poor African Brazilian women with fewer years of schooling are the hardest hit. Within this ideological framework, the feminist movement has been critical of neoliberal policies that have contributed to this impoverishment of women, by ensuring that they remain underemployed, earn less than men and are, in many cases, forced to endure a triple work load: paid employment, housework, and care. What will it take to address this inequality? Perhaps a state apparatus that, oddly enough, *cares* enough about social inequality and the feminization of poverty? The severe economic recession in Brazil and ongoing political gridlock does not provide substantial hope that such concerted state interventions (as acts of *social caring*) will soon occur.

Health and sexual and reproductive rights during the Zika epidemic

A related point raised by the feminist movement workshop participants concerned the quality of health services to which women have access to and the lack of training of professionals to deal with the "new" reality of a triple epidemic. Early diagnosis (of both Zika virus infection and pregnancy) is still not available for most women who use the Brazilian public health system, known as the Universal Health System (SUS). Women who take the Zika test often do not receive the results. Despite the news headlines, the majority of health service staff are insufficiently informed regarding CZS and patients are unaware of the range of fetal malformations that may occur. According to feminist group representatives, these shortcomings may be so grave that they put women's lives at risk. In such cases, the right to a legal abortion should be considered, although a veil of silence still hangs over this issue in the Brazilian health services.

The non-viability of a fetus was also an issue raised by feminist organizations that question the paucity of interaction between health professionals and women who go through pregnancy with insufficient access to basic information that is vital for their physical and psychological well-being. With the emotional and psychological stress of Zika, this raises the question of the mental health of pregnant women who do not receive a diagnosis of microcephaly or those who are diagnosed as such but are unable to do anything to change the course of their pregnancy; prenatal care services still consider Zika infection a low-risk pregnancy, making it impossible for women (especially poor women) to exercise their autonomous reproductive rights. This concept is related to the right to decide freely on whether and when to have children, as well as to have access to the information and assistance for responsible decision making.[17] As with many countries in the LAC region, family planning programs in Brazil are weak, with various short-term contraceptive methods provided without any form of guidance and longer-term methods still not widely available.

For decades, women's movements across the Americas, with a strong presence in Brazil going back to the 1980s, have pointed out the lack of access to contraceptive methods, poor sex education, little information on women's rights and moral issues related to the patriarchal mentality that obstructs (and often denies) a woman's right to engage in sexual relations and plan her reproductive life as she sees fit. This can be seen in the results of demographic health surveys (DHS/PNDS), from 1996, and other studies made in subsequence decades, showing unmet demands for contraception (Coutinho et al, 2015; Lacerda et al, 2005; Hakkert, 2001). Women living in poverty are especially vulnerable to this; during the Zika epidemic in Recife and Belo Horizonte, for example, women of higher socioeconomic status reported having greater control over their reproductive wishes, including access to contraception (Marteleto et al, 2017). A national-level survey called "Born in Brazil" (*Nascer no Brasil*) has shown that around half of Brazilian mothers report that their pregnancy was unwanted; 25% would have preferred to wait longer and 30% said that they had not wanted to get pregnant at all (Leal et al, 2014; Brandão & Cabral, 2017).

While the Zika epidemic may have raised concerns about reproductive health issues, the government's response, centered on household-level mosquito control and the at times bizarre statements on the need to "delay pregnancy," show significant gaps in health policy (Bond, 2017). Even at the international level, in the official statements of the WHO and CDC, we find a marginalization and neglect of social facts. The first concerns the failure to see a closer link between gender and poverty in Brazil; the result of this is that policies and actions have failed to put the most vulnerable – women living in socioeconomically vulnerable circumstances – at the heart of the response in any meaningful way. A second crucial issue is the failure to address issues of gender violence. More specifically, delaying pregnancy is often not an option for women living in abusive relationships or contexts in which patriarchal values impede their freedom regarding contraception and free negotiation of sexual relations. Lastly, official agencies and the discourse of Zika control has tended to avoid the issue of contraception, both in terms of information and access.

The failure to raise the issue of gender in the initial stages of the epidemic and the disproportionate impact on the lives of women, principally when other factors, such as class and race were taken into consideration, is in some ways confusing. It was one of the motivations for us in bringing together representatives of the women's movement and academics to debate gender issues and Zika.[18] Sexual and reproductive rights have been on the agenda of the feminist movement for some time and have underlined the need for improved and more extensive all-round health care for women, involving primarily state intervention. Issues such as autonomy in decision making, reproductive self-determination, legalization of abortion and improved health services have guided the struggle for women's health care (Corrêa & Ávila, 2003). In the context of Zika, Brazilian feminists have highlighted how the virus recasts, and demands the rethinking of, social discourses on the issue of safe and autonomous motherhood, the unmet demand for contraception, especially long-term contraception, and the extension of the right to abortion.

Brazilian legislation is still highly restrictive in relation to legal options involving abortion: it is permitted in cases of rape, risk to the life of the mother and, recently (in 2012) cases of anencephaly.[19] In the aftermath of Zika, feminists sought ways of expanding the legality of abortion, and developing new arguments that address the new ways of experiencing pregnancy, marked by this new form of "Zika anxiety" and mental distress related to the fear of a positive diagnosis of CZS and concerns as to the viability of the fetus. These sentiments have coalesced around a movement for reproductive justice – one part of the broader involvement of the feminist movement in Pernambuco State, as summed up in Figure 4.4.

Discussion and conclusions

The workshop we organized, as engaged scholars and activists with decades of experience working in and around Pernambuco State, helped us build relationships. From this experience we are now working with the Zika and Social Science network, chaired by the president of Fiocruz, Nísia Trindade, and composed of national and international institutions, with several sources of financing. This network highlights the need to include social science perspectives for a broader understanding of the epidemic. In a democratic and participatory manner, we have built-up a strategic agenda of demands regarding not only the Zika virus epidemic and CZS but also the specific needs of women as a whole and children affected by CZS. The debates during our workshop in early 2017 drew attention to the advances made and challenges faced in drawing up strategies to improve information on scientific progress in the field, health services and rights in the age of Zika.

The national response has focused on clinical medicine and epidemiology and has made significant contributions to understanding the epidemic and the nature of the virus. However, strategies involving control of the mosquito touted in public campaigns presume that women are able, and willing, to use their time, already over-extended in socially determined care duties, to prevent pregnant female mosquitoes from making more mosquito babies. As we have shown here, those most affected by the new virus (CZS mother associations) and those with long-standing knowledge of the roots of gender inequality in Brazil that has driven the epidemic (feminist organizations) have criticized the lack of a *government that cares*.

The mothers of affected children, for example, complained of a lack of structural support to facilitate access to health services for their children's care and a paucity of reliable and intelligible information. The need to break the isolation of having a different experience of motherhood led some women to become advocates for their own and their children's rights, revealing the inadequacy of the public authorities in responding in a satisfactory manner to demands of this new reality, which are, in fact, issues that have long been debated in feminist circles, such as support and autonomy in motherhood.

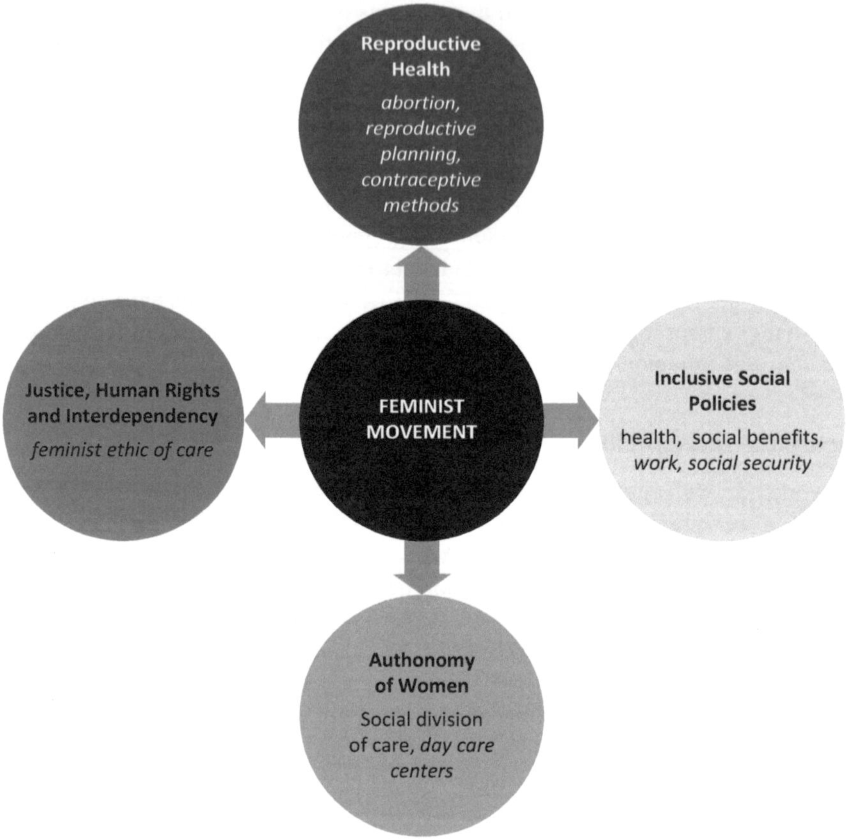

Figure 4.4 The demands and engagement of Brazilian feminist organizations in the Zika epidemic and its aftermath in Pernambuco State, Brazil.

As the Zika virus epidemic and the outbreak of microcephaly shadow inequality, care strategies that do not re-victimize or even blame the affected individuals are needed. In other words, we need to look again at theories of care, and their moral consequences, that lead care to be valued only because it is provided by women, thereby increasing the physical, mental and emotional burden placed upon women in their everyday lives. We have thus, throughout this chapter, espoused a feminist approach to care, as a way of drawing attention to the asymmetries and value judgments surrounding such activities, which should not be restricted to private life but instead involve revitalizing and challenging Brazilian social and political institutions to care for others, as part of their broader moral duty. It can thus be argued that the state should be responsible for caring for its citizens and, in the case of the Zika epidemic, the feminist and the mother of an affected children are speaking the same language.

As issues of race, class and gender make it even more difficult for individuals to act autonomously, there is a need to reflect on developing communication strategies regarding Zika that stress the need to defend human rights, without falling back into the classic emphasis on the private individual, which reinforce stigmas surrounding poverty, color and lack of schooling. Amidst the avalanche of scientific publications on Zika, therefore, we need to re-socialize the epidemic in order to produce more meaningful narratives that represent the actual experience of Brazilian women – narratives that are grounded in the long-standing, and often uncomfortable, historical and social facts of gender inequality in places like Pernambuco.

Notes

1 This workshop was organized as part of a multicenter mixed methods research project, funded by Welcome Trust, on the social and economic impacts of Zika in Brazil. The project was a partnership between researchers in Recife (Aggeu Magalhães Institute – Oswaldo Cruz Foundation and the Federal University of Pernambuco), Rio de Janeiro (Fernandes Figueira Institute – Oswaldo Cruz Institute) and London (London School of Hygiene and Tropical Medicine).

2 We are grateful to the CZS mother associations, the local and national feminist movements and the researchers from local and national universities and research centers who kindly attended this seminar.

3 The first bulletin alerting health professionals was circulated in October 2015 and 29 cases were registered in that month, compared to a mean incidence of 10 cases in previous years. Three days after reporting began, 90 new cases were registered in the state. See http://portalarquivos.saude.gov.br/images/pdf/2015/novembro/19/Microcefalia-bol-final.pdf

4 PERNAMBUCO. Secretaria Estadual de Saúde. Nota de Esclarecimento Microcefalia 01/12/2015. 2015b. See http://portal.saude.pe.gov.br/noticias/secretariaexecutiva-de-vigilancia-em-saude/microcefalia-sesinvestiga-casos-no-estado

5 See___http://portalarquivos.saude.gov.br/images/pdf/2015/novembro/19/Microcefalia-bol-final.pdf

6 According to Technical Inform from Pernambuco Health Surveillance Secretariat n. 3/2018, in the year of 2018 there were three cases of CZS. See https://docs.wixstatic.com/ugd/3293a8_4a678a55869042a5b6942409679841af.pdf

7 "Zika children" is an expression commonly used both by the mothers of children affected and by reports in the media.

8 Other studies, such as Barros et al. (2017) and Scott et al. (2017) have suggested the same.

9 A social theory characterized by an emphasis on interaction between subjects as an effort to understand the construction of the symbolic world of society and social arrangements.

10 The feeling of abandonment by the government was also highlighted by several human rights dossiers.

11 Two of us (CP & SV) were invited to join the situation room set up by the United Nations. From the outset, this initiative aimed to concentrate on social aspects, calling attention to issues of gender and race related to the epidemic. Sexual and reproductive rights issues thus guided actions that focused on the degree of information and political engagement regarding the epidemic, as a way of strengthening political impact on vulnerable communities.

12 One example of such a study is a special issue of one of the international WATERLAT-GOBACIT network's working papers devoted to microcephaly and structural inequalities. See http://waterlat.org/WPapers/WPSATGSA39.pdf

13 http://www.atlasbrasil.org.br/2013/pt/consulta/

14 Benefit of continuous rendering (BPC in Portuguese), created in 1993 by the Law 8,742/1993, guarantees a minimum wage, is guaranteed to the elderly over 65 years or for people with disabilities that make it impossible to fully participate in society. To obtain this benefit, it is necessary to prove that the income per person of the family group is less than one-quarter of the current minimum wage. Brazilian minimum wage, in 2018, is R$954 per month, approximately U$290 (at the time of writing). For more information: http://mds.gov.br/assuntos/assistencia-social/beneficios-assistenciais/bpc

15 Based on the World Bank's new poverty metric, which delimits US$5.5 per day per capita. An example of social assistance programs is "Bolsa Família," which is a program of income transfer aimed at the population living in poverty and extreme poverty to guarantee the right to food, health and education.

16 Early unplanned motherhood also contributes to the feminization of poverty, because of the lack of social structure and public policy to provide secure childcare and social support.

17 Since the Constitution of 1988, human rights constitute a guiding framework, obliging the state to comply with international treaties, including guaranteeing the means for free decision making in family planning. However, the restrained rules on abortion and its criminalization in Brazil are barriers to this decision-making autonomy. For more information, see Ávila (2003) and Vianna (2004).

18 Broader debate regarding gender is relatively recent. Two recent examples of this are the publications by Diniz (2016a) and Marteleto et al. (2017).

19 Anencephaly is a malformation of the neural tube of the embryo, causing absence or defective formation of the cerebral hemispheres, considered a condition incompatible with life. It is worth pointing out that Brazil is currently going through a wave of conservatism in relation to the human rights agenda, especially the rights of women. A parliamentary commission recently approved broad-scale criminalization of abortion on the grounds that life begins at conception. The decision still needs to be approved by a plenary session of deputies. However, we now have one of the most conservative congresses in the history of the republic, and it has shown little flexibility regarding broader debate of issues related to sexual and reproductive rights.

References

Aguiar, N. 2000, 'Patriarcado, sociedade e patrimonialismo', *Sociedade e Estado*, vol. 15, no. 2, pp. 303–330.

Araújo, T.V.B, Rodrigues, L.C., de Alencar Ximenes, R.A., de Barros Miranda-Filho, D, Montarroyos, U.R., de Melo, A.P., et al. 2016. 'Association between Zika virus infection and microcephaly in Brazil, January to May, 2016: preliminary report of a case-control study', *The Lancet Infectious Diseases*, vol. 16, no. 12, pp. 1356–1363.

Araújo, T.V.B., Ximenes, R.A.A., Miranda-Filho, D.B., Souza, W. V., Montarroyos, U.R., de Melo, A.P.L., et al. 2017, 'Association between microcephaly, Zika virus infection, and other risk factors in Brazil: final report of a case-control study,' *The Lancet Infectious Diseases*, vol. 18, no. 3, pp. 328–336.

Associação Brasileira de Saúde Coletiva. 2015, 'Nota Pública – Surto de Microcefalia: Emergência de Saúde Pública de Interesse Nacional', <https://www.abrasco.org.br/site/outras-noticias/institucional/nota-publica-surto-de-microcefalia-emergencia-de-saude-publica-de-interesse-nacional/14891/>

Barros, S.M.M., Monteiro, P.A., Neves, M.B., Maciel, G.T. 2017, 'Fortalecendo a Rede de Apoio de Mães no Contexto da Síndrome Congênita do Vírus Zika: relatos de uma intervenção psicossocial e sistêmica', *Nova Perspectiva Sistêmica*, vol. 26, no. 58, pp. 38–59.

Becker, H. S. 2008, *Outsiders: estudos de sociologia do desvio*, Jorge Zahar, Rio de Janeiro.

Bond, J. 2017, 'Zika, Feminism and the failures of health policy', *Washington & Lee Law Review Online*, vol. 73, no. 2, pp. 841–885.

Brandão, E.R., Cabral, C.V. 2017, 'Da gravidez imprevista à contracepção: aportes para um debate', *Cadernos de Saúde Pública*, vol. 33, no. 2, pp. 1–4.

Brito, Carlos. 2015, 'Zika virus: a new chapter in the history of medicine,' *Acta Medica Portuguesa*, vol. 28, no. 6, pp. 679–680.

Castro, J. E. 2016, 'Desigualdad estructural y determinación social', in Castro, J.E., Costa, A.M. (eds.), *Desigualdade estrutural e microcefalia: a determinação social de uma epidemia*. (articles in English, Spanish and Portuguese, Vol.3, n.9). Buenos Aires and Recife, Newcastle upon Tyne.

Chan, Jasper F. W. 2016, 'Zika fever and congenital Zika syndrome: an unexpected emerging arboviral disease?', *Journal of Infection*, vol. 7, no. 5, pp. 507–524.

Corrêa, S, Ávila, B. 2003, 'Direitos sexuais e reprodutivos: pauta global e percursos brasileiros', in Berquó, E. (ed.), *Sexo & Vida: panorama da saúde reprodutiva no Brasil*, Editora UNICAMP, Campinas.

Costa, F., Sarno, M., Khouri, R., Freitas, B. de P., Siqueira, I., Ribeiro, G. S., et al. 2017, 'Emergence of congenital Zika syndrome: view point from the lines', *Annals of Internal Medicine*, vol. 164, no. 10, pp. 689–691.

Coutinho, R.Z., Barros, J.V.S. e Carvalho, A.A. 2015, '30 anos de DHS: o que andamos pesquisando sobre fecundidade no Brasil', *Revista Brasileira de Estudos Populacionais*, vol. 32, no. 2, pp. 395–407.

Cueto Marcos 2017, *Cold war, deadly fevers: malaria eradication in Mexico, 1955–1975* Washington, D.C., Woodrow Wilson Center Press (Co-published Johns Hopkins University Press).

Diniz, Debora. 2007, *O que é deficiência*, Braziliense, São Paulo.

Diniz, Debora. 2016a, 'Vírus Zika e mulheres', *Cadernos de Saúde Pública*, vol. 32, no. 5, pp. 1–4.

Diniz, Debora. 2016b, *Zika: do Sertão nordestino à ameaça Global*, Civilização Brasileira, Rio de Janeiro.

Durkheim, Émile. 2007, *As regas do método sociológico*. trans. Paulo Neves; translation revised by Eduardo Brandão. – 3ª ed. Martins Fontes, São Paulo.

Ferreira, Henrique Santos 2016, *Clima Urbano e Dengue em Recife: influência climática sobre a formação das epidemias*, Dissertation, Universidade Federal de Pernambuco, Recife, PE, Brazil. <https://repositorio.ufpe.br/handle/123456789/18688>.

Gesser, M., Nuernberg, A. H., Toneli, M. J. F. 2012, 'A contribuição do Modelo Social da Deficiência à Psicologia Social', *Psicologia & Sociedade*, vol. 24, no. 3, pp. 557–566.

Gill, R. 2008, 'Empowerment/sexism: figuring female sexual agency in contemporary advertising', *Feminism and Psychology*, vol. 18, no. 1, pp. 35–60.

Goffman, Erving. 1988, *Estigma: notas sobre a manipulação da identidade deteriorada*, LTC, Rio de Janeiro.

Goffman, Erving. 2001, *Manicômios, prisões e conventos*, Editora Perspectiva, São Paulo.

Guimarães, R. 2008, 'Deficiência e cuidado: por quê abordar gênero nessa relação?' *Ser Social*, vol. 10, no. 22, pp. 213–238.

Hakkert, R. 2001, 'Levels and determinants of wanted and unwanted fertility in Latin America', in General Conference of the IUSSP. Salvador, Brazil.

Instituto Brasileiro de Geografia e Estatística. (IBGE). 2016, 'Mapa da população. IBGE [Online]', viewed 10 abr 2016, <http://www.ibge. gov.br>

Kleinman, A. 2015, 'Care: in search of a health agenda', *The Lancet*, vol. 386, no. 9990, pp. 240–241.

Lacerda, M.A. Miranda-Ribeiro, P., Caetano, A.J., Machado, C.J. 2005, 'Mensuração e perfis de demanda insatisfeita por contracepção nos municípios de Belo Horizonte e Recife, 2002', *Revista Brasileira de Estudos. Populacionais*, vol. 22, no. 1, pp. 113–129.

Leal, M.C. and Gama, S.G. 2014, Executive summary of the survey Born in Brazil (Nascer no Brasil). <http://www.ensp.fiocruz.br/portal-ensp/informe/site/arquivos/anexos/nascerweb.pdf>

Lesser, Jeffrey, Kitron, Uriel. 2016, 'A geografia social do zika no Brasil', *Estudos Avançados*, vol. 30, no. 88, pp. 167–175.

Marteleto, L.J., Weitzman, A., Coutinho, R.Z., Valongueiro Alves, S. 2017, 'Women's Reproductive Intentions and Behaviors during the Zika Epidemic in Brazil', *Population and Development Review*, vol. 43, no. 2, pp. 199–227.

Mauss, Marcel. 2003, *Sociologia e antropologia*, Cosac & Naify, São Paulo.

Miranda-Filho, Demócrito, Martelli, C.M., Ximenes, R.A., Araújo, T.V., Rocha, M.A., Ramos, R.C., et al. 2016, 'Initial description of the presumed congenital Zika syndrome', *American Journal of Public Health*, vol. 106, no. 4, pp. 598–600.

Molinier, P., Paperman, P. 2015. 'Descompartimentar a noção de cuidado?' *Revista Brasileira de Ciência Política*, vol. 18, pp. 43–57.

Nunes, João, Pimenta, Denise Nacif. 2016, 'A epidemia de zika e os limites da saúde global', *Lua Nova*, no. 98, pp. 21–46.

Osis, M.j.m.d. 1998, 'PAISM: um marco na abordagem da saúde reprodutiva no Brasil,' *Cadernos de Saúde Pública*, vol. 14, no. 1, pp. 25–32.

Paim, Jairnilson Silva. 2013, 'A Constituição Cidadã e os 25 anos do Sistema Único de Saúde (SUS)', *Cadernos de Saúde Pública*, vol. 29, no. 10, pp. 1927–1936.

Pearce, D. 1987, 'The feminization of poverty: women, work and welfare', *Urban and Social Change Review*, vol. 21, no. 1, pp. 329–337.

Pesquisa nacional por amostra de domicílios (PNAD/IBGE). 2016, *Síntese de indicadores 2015* / IBGE, Coordenação de Trabalho e Rendimento. - Rio de Janeiro: IBGE.

Pinheiro, D.A.J.P., Longhi, M.R. 2017, 'Maternidade como missão! A trajetória militante de uma mãe de bebê com microcefalia em PE', *Cadernos de Gênero e Diversidade*, vol. 3, no. 2, pp. 113–133.

Pinheiro, L., Galiza, M., Fontoura, N. 2009. 'Novos arranjos familiares, velhas convenções sociais de gênero: a licença-parental como política pública para lidar com essas tensões', *Revista Estudos Feministas*, vol. 17, no. 3, pp. 851–859.

Programa das Nações Unidas para o Desenvolvimento [UNDP]. 2017. 'Uma avaliação do impacto socioeconômico do vírus Zika na américa latina e caribe: Brasil, Colômbia e Suriname como estudos de caso', <http://portalarquivos.saude.gov.br/images/pdf/2017/agosto/16/UNDP-Zika-07–02–2017-Portuguese-WEB.PDF>

Rattner, D. 2014, 'Da Saúde Materno Infantil ao PAISM', *Revista Tempus, Actas de Saúde Coletiva*, vol. 8, no. 2, pp. 103–108.

Saffioti, H. 2011, *Gênero, patriarcado, violência*, Editora Fundação Perseu Abramo, São Paulo.

Scheper-Hughes, Nancy. 1992, *Death without weeping: the violence of everyday life in Brazil*, University of California Press, Berkley.

Scott, R.P. Quadros, M.T., Rodrigues, A.C., Lira, L.C., Matosm S.S., Meiram F., et al 2017, 'A Epidemia de Zika e as Articulações das Mães num Campo Tensionado entre Feminismo, Deficiência e Cuidados', *Cadernos de Gênero e Diversidade*, vol. 3, no. 2, pp. 73–92.

Souza, W.V., Albuquerque, M.F.P.M., Vazquez, E., Bezerra, L.C.A., Mendes, A.D.C.G., Lyra, T.M., et al. 2018, 'Microcephaly epidemic related to the Zika virus and living conditions in Recife, Northeast Brazil', *BMC Public Health*, vol. 18, no. 130, pp. 1–7.

Tronto, J. 1997, 'Mulheres e cuidado: o que as feministas podem aprender sobre a moralidade a partir disso?' in Jaggar, A.M. Brodo, S.R. (eds.), *Gênero, corpo e conhecimento*, Record/Rosa do Tempo, Rio de Janeiro.

Tronto, Joan C. 2013, *Caring democracy: markets, equality, and justice*, New York University Press, New York.

Vianna, A. 2004, *Direitos e políticas sexuais no Brasil: mapeamento e diagnóstico*, CEPESC, Rio de Janeiro.

5 Politics as disease in Venezuela

Vector control before and after the Bolivarian revolution

Roberto Briceño-León, Milady Guevara and Iris Terán

On Margarita Island, just north of South America, where luxurious five-star hotels coexist with the impoverished shantytowns that replaced fishermen's villages, malaria had disappeared. When occasional cases appeared, Venezuelan doctors on the island asked patients where they had traveled, and always got the same answer: the goldmines of Bolivar State in the Amazon. These patients were former workers that the economic crisis had pushed to the forest, returning to Margarita Island to visit their family with some money in their pockets, or prostitutes that had returned from working in the bars of the mines. But at the beginning of 2017, laboratory tests showed that patients had been infected with malaria without leaving the island. These were a different type of patient: they were local housewives and children.

In the Americas, arboviral diseases (like Zika and Dengue) coexist with endemic malaria, which has been steadily declining over the last few decades. In a recent report on malaria, the Pan American Health Organization (PAHO) reported that in 2015 there were 451,242 cases of malaria, a significant 62% decrease since the year 2000 (PAHO, 2017). However, the situation in all countries in the region is not the same. There are some, such as Venezuela, where the increase in malaria has been remarkable (see Figure 5.1). For example, the 240,631 malaria cases reported in Venezuela in 2016 accounted for nearly half (48%) of the total number of cases in the Americas (Oletta et al., 2018). Fifteen years earlier, however, Venezuela had contributed only 2.5%, a 12-fold increase. In 2017, cases nearly doubled (to 411,586) and estimates for 2018 are even worse (DGSA-MPPS, 2018).[1]

What has happened in Venezuela? There are eight countries in which malaria has increased since 2000: Venezuela, Colombia, Dominican Republic, Ecuador, Guatemala, Honduras, Nicaragua and Peru. But Venezuela leads the list, well above the others. With just 30 million people, Venezuela contributes more cases of malaria in the Americas than Brazil, a country with 207 million inhabitants (WHO, 2017).

What is striking about this change is that Venezuela had been one of the model countries for the control of malaria in Latin America. In the 1950s, the World Health Organization (WHO) declared Venezuela to be the first country where it had achieved localized eradication in a tropical country. An eight-year campaign with DDT had eradicated it from an area covering about half (49%)

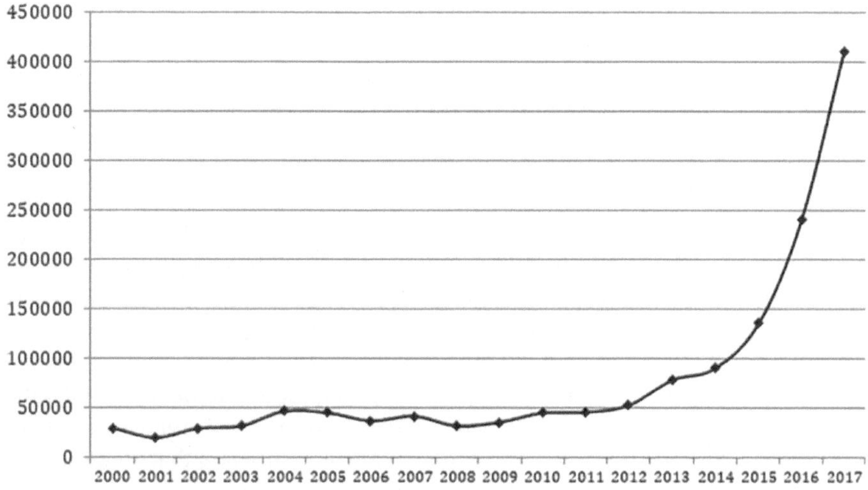

Figure 5.1 The rapid increase in malaria cases since 2010 in Venezuela. Note that the true number of cases may be much larger, due to issues of under-diagnosing and reporting. Source: WHO (2017).

of Venezuela's total population, between the Coastal Mountain Range and the Llanos region (Gabaldon & Berti, 1954).

Explanations for malaria resurgence, therefore, on Margarita Island and elsewhere in the Americas and the growing expansion of *Aedes aegypti* diseases, such as Dengue, Chikungunya and now Zika, are multiple (Benítez et al., 2004; Cáceres, 2011; Grillet et al. 2009; Torres et al. 2017; Hotez et al. 2017). We know that climate change, and El Niño and La Niña time cycles, as well as new vector dynamics and adapted parasite/viral strains have contributed to malaria resurgence and *Aedes*-borne epidemics, for example. But understanding vector-borne disease resurgence and emergence also demands some significant historical and socio-political explanations. In Venezuela, then, tracing the factors involved in the reappearance of malaria in areas where it was considered eradicated 50 years ago requires that we inspect the history of vector control programs in the country – their capacity, functioning, ideologies, effectiveness and motivations. Vector control is a public service, after all, and its inner workings are influenced by state ideologies and funding decisions. This is manifested in various ways. Political decision making can mean that funds are simply cut for vector control operations, and redistributed elsewhere, meaning there are less funds for insecticides, medicines and manpower. It can equally be the case that, while these essential commodities and human resources are in place, operating funds are not available – vehicles, gasoline and travel expenses to allow officials, doctors, entomologists and spray teams to travel from the office to the field. Funds can also be used wastefully, with ballooned staff numbers kept on the payroll for political profit. While all of these constraints have faced those involved in vector control throughout Latin America, the situation in Venezuela is striking, and insightful, because the slow decay of vector control efforts has, in some important ways, paralleled the country's rise (and now decline) in wealth, as a result of rapid oil price increases in the 1970–1980s and the early 21st century.

When we speak about "politics" we are really speaking about institutions, rules, roles and routines (March & Olsen, 2006; North, 1991; Peters, 2012) The ups and downs of vector control in Venezuela show the relevance of health policy institutions and their politics. In the 1940s, for example, health policy was orientated on building institutional capacities for malaria control, motivated by particular ideologies around health and state building that allowed technical experts to form strong relationships with political groups and generate financial resources. On the other hand, a health policy influenced by Bolivarian political ideology since the 1990s has generated an ethos of *institutional destruction,* so we argue in this chapter, that has led to the reappearance of communicable diseases that Venezuelans believed had disappeared. It is often said that politics is the most severe human disease. As this chapter will show, politics can contribute to health but it can also be an illness. As with all political approaches, understanding current events necessitates that we first look backwards, to some historical reflections.[2]

Malaria and World War II

In the Pacific battlefronts of World War II, it was known that malaria could end as many lives and disable as many fighters as enemy attacks. That is why warfare in the tropics had a major environmental sanitation component, having learnt from the building of the Panama Canal in the 1880s, when the French company *Nouvelle de Panama* abandoned their commercial effort due to engineering problems and excessively high mortality among workers and engineers. Ferocious attacks from the anopheles and *Aedes* mosquitoes played a central role. The new American company that took over from the French in 1904 invested in sanitation, roads, the screening of houses and drainage before starting more substantial engineering work. But in the 1940s, when such preparation was not possible and one had to act quickly in the context of war, the US Army instead turned to a very effective new chemical insecticidal spray to protect its troops. Due to its value in addressing malaria, the United States also kept it a military secret.

At the time, the American army requested the support of medical personnel with direct experience in the control of mosquitoes in the tropics, and in the treatment of malaria patients. Dr. Arnoldo Gabaldón, a Venezuelan doctor, was regularly invited to courses taught to Army doctors who would, after some preparation, serve in the Pacific against the Japanese empire. Gabaldón had spent several decades studying malaria and directed the malaria control program in Venezuela, where he had faced several epidemics. In one of these courses, a senior military officer, who had been Dr. Gabaldón's student at Johns Hopkins University, confided in him the secret of a wonderful new product called *Dichlorodiphenyltrichloroethane,* or DDT. The army wanted to use Gabaldon´s experience in the tropics to help design the best and most efficient insecticide application technique (Figure 5.2).

The product remained in the mind of the Venezuelan doctor. That is why, at the end of the war, he did not hesitate in asking the US Army to allow him to initiate an intense campaign to control and eradicate malaria in large endemic areas of his home country using DDT. Thus, the first-time application of DDT for purely civilian purposes could take place (López Ramirez, 1987). Venezuela had been an important, secure and politically friendly supplier of oil to the allies during World War II. The country also had sufficient income from oil sales that it could buy the new "wonder" insecticide, acquire the equipment and pay the salaries of the personnel needed for what became some of the first large-scale operations. Gabaldón formed a strong civilian army of doctors, entomologists, sanitary inspectors and insecticide sprayers who, in the following years, dedicated themselves to touring the country by car, horse and boat.

In October 1945, when everything was ready for the first application and the first shipment of the insecticide had arrived at the port, a coup d'état occurred. The president, who had lent his full support to the project, had been deposed, and a board of civilians and military officers replaced it. The worst was feared: that the anti-malaria campaign would be stopped because it lacked the necessary political support. However, the new acting president understood the relevance of stopping malaria for the country's health and economy and gave Dr. Gabaldón his full support. The president knew, moreover, that he could reap all the political fruits of such an action.

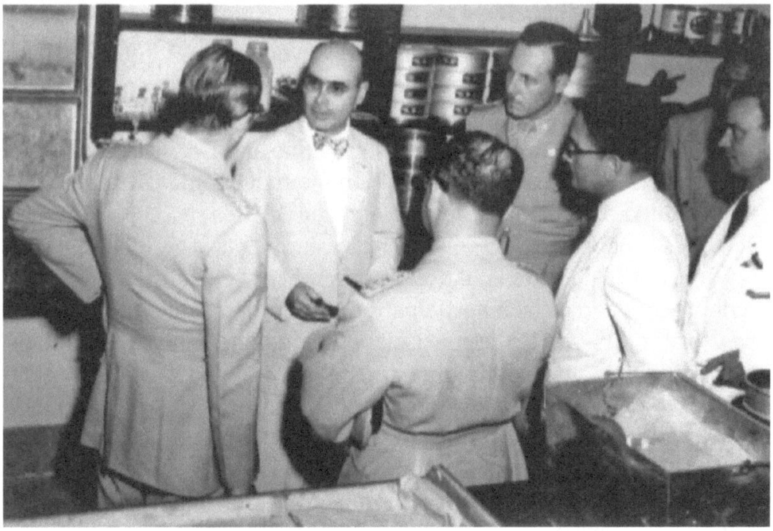

Figure 5.2 Arnoldo Gabaldón, at the center, explains the vector control plan to the Military Governing Board. Circa 1949.

A few months later, in December 1945, the vector control campaign began in Morón, Carabobo State, and covered large endemic areas along the coast, mountain ranges, the plains and on the border with Guayana, where the three most aggressive species of anopheles are found (*A. darlingi, A. albimanus* and *A. acquasalis)* and where the two main species of parasites that cause malaria circulated: *P. falciparum*, which can lead to death, and *P. vivax*, which causes significant suffering and morbidity. By 1949, the strategy to eradicate the disease in large areas of the country was already recognized as successful. The mortality rate by diagnosed malaria fell from 143 per 100,000 in 1942 to 8 per 100,000 in 1950 (Gabaldon, 1953); the technical key to this success was, in large part, the spraying of house walls with DDT (Gabaldon, 1949)

Vector control under military dictatorship

Systematic malaria vector control programs had already begun in Venezuela in the late 1930s after the fall of Dictator JV Gomez. Between 1931 and 1935, the death rate for diagnosed malaria cases was 164 per 100,000. With the beginning of the construction of the modern State of Venezuela, the Ministry of Health and Social Assistance and the Department of Malariology were founded (Yépez Colmenares, 1995). For some historians, this was the moment when the 20th century began in Venezuela. This process was the result of two factors: monetary resources derived from oil revenues that entered the central government and the existence of an elite who were dedicated to institutional construction and the creation of a bureaucracy of professionals and state workers (Briceño León, 2011).

The Department of Malariology began its activities with urban sanitation, with the construction of drainage for the reduction of the vectors and with the distribution of quinine to eliminate the parasite. The medicines were distributed through volunteers, who were not paid a salary, but were given national lottery tickets. This was a symbolic gesture, which cost little to the program, but could mean a lot of money if a volunteer was awarded the prize. As in many other countries (see Marco Cueto's [2007] history of malaria in Mexico and Eric Carter's [2012] work on Argentina), DDT had a major impact on the reduction of the anopheles population and resulted in a dramatic decline in malaria cases.

During the most intense phase of the antimalarial campaign with DDT, between 1945 and 1948, Venezuela underwent significant changes in the nature of the political process and citizen participation. Health and education services reached, often for the first time, the most dispossessed and traditionally abandoned population groups and communities. The government party had great popular support, which made it easier to continue the work of the Department of Malariology without major setbacks. In 1947, the first free elections were held, with numerous and many new political parties. They were the first direct and universal elections in Venezuela. In the election there were three candidates nominated by different political parties of different ideological currents: Rómulo Gallegos, by Acción Democrática, a social-democratic party; Rafael Caldera, for COPEI, which was a Christian-democratic party; and Gustavo

Machado for the Communist Party of Venezuela. In the election, the well-known novelist, R. Gallegos, who supported and praised the work of malariology, was elected with 74% of the popular vote and took office on February 15, 1948. His government was short-lived, however, as he was overthrown by a board of three members of the military in 1948. Despite this political crisis, the Department of Malariology continued, remarkably, in its work without major setbacks.

In November 1950, the new president of the Republic, C. Delgado Chalbaud, was kidnapped and murdered. Because the other two military members of the board, Marcos Pérez Jiménez and Luis Felipe Llovera Paez, feared that their ambitions would lead them being accused of the assassination, they decided to replace Delgado with a civilian puppet as head of the military government. Given the high visibility, popularity and significance of the malaria control program, they proposed that Dr. Gabaldón take charge of the presidency. Gabaldon had given the military two conditions to accept the appointment: the first was to be allowed to choose his government team and the second to investigate the strange murder of Delgado Chalbaud.[3] When neither of these was accepted, Gabaldón declined because he was reluctant to become a puppet and understood the trappings of political opportunism. Nor did he accept the position of Minister of Health that was offered later. As a result, he knew that his democratic positions and professional vision of work was unpopular with the government and feared that his political positions would affect the malaria control program

Gabaldón, therefore, resigned as head of the vector control department in order to preserve it. The military elite knew that those in charge of malariology were democrats, opposed to the regime, but they tolerated them, because they enjoyed the prestige and wanted to maintain their achievements. As a result, the vector control program continued during the dictatorship and those responsible carried out a detailed monitoring program that would allow them to comply with the protocols required to certify the eradication of the disease. In 1954, an article published in the *American Journal of Tropical Medicine and Hygiene* highlighted the achievements of malaria control in the country:

> After eight years of an extensive campaign, malaria has been eradicated in a large area where about half (49%) of Venezuela's population lives, being the largest area of a tropical zone where malaria has been eradicated. … This northern central zone, located between the Coastal Mountain Range and the Llanos region, the intensity of malaria was the highest in the tropical zone of America. … DDT was applied at the rate of 2 grams per square meter every six months … after exhaustive epidemiological investigations similar to those carried out in developed countries in the temperate zone, the following evidence was found. In an area of about 20,000 square kilometers no primary autochthonous cases have been found during the last three years. In another area of about 160,000 square kilometers, no cases of malaria have been observed during the last two years, with the exception of two cases near the edge of this area, which indicates that endemic malaria has completely

> ceased. ... With this experience it is expected that the eradication of malaria in almost all of Venezuela will be achieved in the near future.
>
> (Gabaldon & Berti, 1954: 795)

The continuity of the program remained despite political differences. From 1952, the Marcos Pérez Jiménez dictatorship acquired its most definite characteristics: on the one hand, the persecution and repression against the opposition, imprisonment and assassination of political and social leaders, and on the other, the alliance with other military dictatorships that governed countries in the region, such as Gustavo Rojas Pinilla in Colombia, Rafael Leonidas Trujillo in the Dominican Republic, Anastasio and Luis Somoza in Nicaragua and Juan Alfredo Strossner in Paraguay. The police monitored those responsible for malaria closely, but did not interrupt their duties. Thus, it was possible to continue the entomological surveillance and the control of anopheles vectors. Some studies, tests and control activities were started for *Aedes aegypti*, to address yellow fever, and of *Rhodnius prolixus*, for Chagas' disease.[4]

During the 1950s, the dictatorship was able to enjoy the economic fruits of the expansion of the world economy, which Hobsbawn has called the "golden age" of capitalism (Hobsbawn, 2001). This was a period in which oil income increased, because the United States stopped being an oil exporter to become a net oil importer. Venezuela became the world's leading oil exporter. That oil income allowed the construction of large public works and the expansion of health and education services. At the time, Venezuela, with its highways and tall buildings, was an emblematic country, a poster child for modernization. The per capita income was higher than in many European countries; it was a preferred destination for migrants from Europe and even America. However, corruption and political repression led to the collapse of the regime, while changing economic fortunes brought an end to the optimism of 1950s growth.

Controlling vectors in the time of an emerging democracy

After the fall of the military dictatorship in 1958, the three main parties (Unión Republicana Democratica (URD), Acción Democratica (AD) and the Christian-Social Party (COPEI) reached an agreement, calling for universal and free presidential and congressional elections. The candidate who was elected was R. Betancourt, who knew of and had supported the anti-malaria campaign that took place between 1945 and 1947. Due to his familiarity with the program, he appointed Dr. Gabaldón as his Minister of Health and, given the new democratic climate, Gabaldón readily accepted.

As can be imagined, the political situation was complex. The nascent democratic government faced two main enemies: the military and guerrillas. On the one hand were the military groups, who refused to let go of the power they had enjoyed for over a century, during which time almost all Venezuelan presidents had been from their ranks. On the other hand were the guerrillas that, inspired and supported by the Cuban revolution, had installed several guerrilla fronts in rural areas of the country. These two groups represented the ideologies that threatened democracy in the context of the Cold War. Both groups, with their weapons, had large influences on Latin America for several decades. The military represented a nationalist orientation and a defender of private enterprise following US-style capitalism. The Marxist guerrillas, by contrast, were connected to the Communist Party of Venezuela (PCV), a party linked to the Communist International and the Soviet Union, and by the *Movimiento de Izquierda Revolucionaria* (MIR), a youth fraction that split from the Acción Democrática party. In 1967, this group organized what became an unsuccessful invasion from Cuba, with Venezuelan and Cuban guerrillas landing on the Venezuelan coast of Machurucuto.

In this context, the vector control program became once again a political tool to increase support for the new government and reduce the social support of the guerrillas. No other social program had more visibility and political importance (Briceño León, 1996). Due to the presence of its staff and the size of its buildings throughout the country, it surpassed the Ministry of Health in a practical and symbolic sense. In those years, some people joked that what existed in Venezuela was not a malaria department that was part of a health ministry, but a Ministry of Health within a Department of Malariology.

There were three components to the government's anti-guerrilla policy, aimed at getting support from the peasants to defeat the guerrillas. The first was an Agrarian Reform Law, started in 1960 that facilitated the distribution of land parcels to the peasants, as well as an Agricultural Credit Program created in 1970 to increase their production. The second was a rural education plan, which involved both adult literacy and the installation of rural schools for children. And the third was a rural sanitation program involving the control of vectors, such as mosquitoes but also *Rhodnius prolixus*, with residual insecticides, the construction and improvement of rural housing and the installation of rural aqueducts.

It is important to emphasize that the rural housing program that began in Venezuela was implemented by the Department of Malariology of the Ministry of Health, not the government agency in charge of housing. That is, the housing program had a very clear sanitary purpose of improving health conditions and promoting the control of vector-borne diseases, especially Chagas' disease, which was endemic in much of the country. The traditional wattle and daub, palm-roofed houses were easily colonized by *R. prolixus*. In endemic areas, traditional peasant housing could contain up to five thousand blood-sucking insects that fed on the family living there (Rabinovich, 1985). The purpose of the plan was to replace wattle "ranchos" with a house with plastered walls and a sheet metal roof, where the vector of Chagas disease could not be so easily lodged and hidden (Briceño-León, 1990) (Figure 5.3).

These programs were successful at many levels. Despite the reduction in revenue from oil exports that forced the devaluation of the national currency and lowered the salaries of public employees by 10% in 1960, such health and social programs were still maintained. The vector control program reduced the population of *Anopheles sp.* and malaria cases, even in areas where the vector became resistant to the lethal action of the insecticide (Carquez, 2007). It also decreased the presence of *R. prolixus* in rural dwellings and new cases of Chagas' disease;

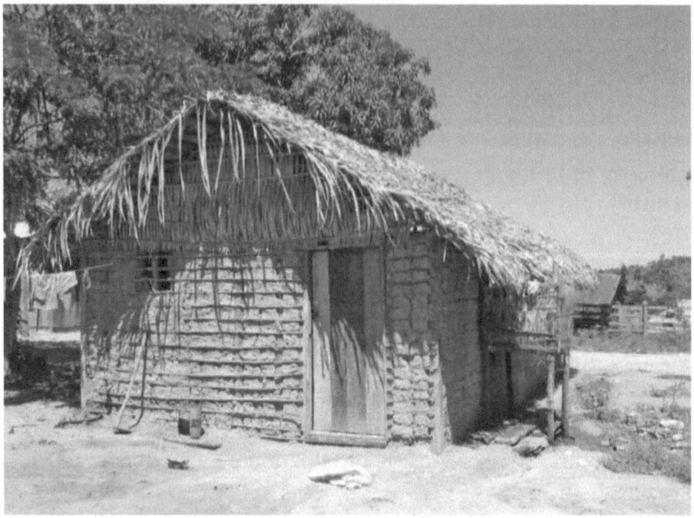

Figure 5.3 Housing structures and Chagas disease.

and with the reduction of *Aedes aegypti*–breeding sites came a reduced risk of new cases of yellow fever.

In the middle of the political crisis that faced the democratic government, the health policy sector was not neglected. On the contrary, health was prioritized and integrated into the plans of general social welfare. During this period, the government of Rómulo Betancourt (with Dr. Arnoldo Gabaldon in charge of the Ministry of Health) focused heavily on preventive medicine and environmental and basic sanitation, seeking to increase life expectancy at birth, which increased from 59.2 years in 1960 to 62 years in 1965. A balance was established between preventive and curative medicine for the allocation of budgetary resources, responding to epidemiological criteria. Mortality from infectious diseases decreased significantly for children, especially in regards to gastroenteritis. The general mortality rate reduced significantly as well during this period.[5]

As a result of these social policies, the guerrillas did not find support in many rural areas among the peasants, or in urban society. In the elections of 1963, although the guerrillas called for abstention, the civilian country voted in the midst of the armed conflict and elected Raúl Leoni, of Acción Democrática. The guerrillas were then defeated, and their leaders, to varying degree, joined the formal political and electoral process.

The emergence of rent-seeking behavior

The consolidation of democracy came slowly, as did the recovery of the economy. In the 1960s and 1970s, a program of industrialization based on import substitution, a strategy that Argentina, Brazil and Chile had already done decades before, was launched. However, the central mechanism of operation was completely different. For the Southern Cone countries, industrialization during World War II was a way of saving scarce foreign currencies, while for Venezuela it was something radically different: it was to find a way of spending the abundant foreign exchange that the oil revenue generated. This difference marked the type of industrialization that occurred in Venezuela, but also the rest of social life, including social policies and health policies, such as vector control.

Three circumstances marked the fate of vector control during the boom years: the loss of importance of vector-borne diseases due to the success of control operations; the existence of lots of money for programs; and the substitution of health goals for political goals. That is to say, it was not a question of using health targets to underpin political goals, as had been done before, but to misrepresent health goals to achieve political party goals.

It was believed that the great nightmare of malaria had passed. It was a battle that had been won by destroying the vector and the parasite. The slogan that had been developed, following the Latin expression, was to end the disease: *Malaria delenda est.* As that goal had been achieved, the Ministry of Health, with the legitimate pride and satisfaction of the work carried out, concluded: *et delete fuit malaria.* The same had happened with yellow fever and the breeding grounds of *Aedes aegypti.* In Venezuela, and the region, the idea spread that the goal of eradication had been achieved. But this triumphalist attitude, even if it had a reasonable basis, weakened the ideological support for the program. Politicians began to wonder: why maintain a program that serves to control a threat that no longer exists?

The second issue was the increase in oil revenue. The 1973 oil embargo by the Arab countries, begun as a response to American support for Israel in the Yom Kippur War, boosted oil prices in a hitherto unknown manner. The price of a barrel of oil doubled and then tripled in a few months, and with it the tax income that the government of Venezuela received was transformed. In 1974, the national budget tripled in relation to the previous year. That is, the new government of President Carlos Andrés Perez had three times more resources to spend than the previous one. And the money came without planning or notice. The new government party, Acción Democrática, managed to obtain a majority in the congress and this one granted extraordinary powers to the president to make the changes that were necessary, in the financial and economic policy of the country, to be able to spend the abundant wealth that arrived so quickly.

This could be interpreted as an unexpected blessing, and indeed it had been, but it was also a source of conflicts and perversions. A sudden infusion of oil cash changed the habits and attitudes of government authorities and institutions, and replaced politics as usual with a social behavior that has been called "competition for oil income" (Baptista, 1997; Briceño-León, 2015). Health policy and vector control ceased to be guided by epidemiological or entomological goals and became oriented towards the appropriation of the new oil wealth.

In the Department of Malariology, a mantra was repeated that malaria could end, but not malariologists. The affirmation referred to the continuing relevance of those personnel specialized in environmental health and in the control of other diseases transmitted by vectors in the tropics. And it was true. However the combination of these two factors, a triumphalist attitude and the big money in the public coffers, perpetuated a set of perverse practices that ended up distorting social attitudes and practices. Let's look at some examples.

The vector control program for Chagas' disease in Venezuela began in the 1960s with entomological inspection and intra-domiciliary spraying of a residual insecticide. The main vector causing the disease was *R. prolixus*, which is a wild triatomine that lives in palm trees and tropical forests, no higher than 1,500 meters above sea level. The insect hides during the day on the walls and palm roofs of peasant homes and goes out at night to feed on the family while people sleep. The program developed an ingenious system, which consisted in placing an envelope behind the front door of the house. In the envelope was placed a registration card, with the date and results of the visit. The inspectors left a small glass jar with a lid and instructed families to capture any of the insect Chagas vectors that they encountered. After some time, between three to six months, the entomological inspectors returned, checked the envelope, and if there were insects in the bottle, wrote it on the card and took the insects to the laboratory to confirm if they had the parasites. This strategy worked quite well, because it allowed health officials to identify the foci of reinfection and to apply the insecticide in the places where it was necessary. However, once the oil money came pouring in and the government's budget tripled, bosses had to find ways to distribute the expanded budget. Entomological inspections began in places where the disease had not been detected, including in areas where the presence of the vector was not possible due to weather and elevation. For example, in our own investigations in the Andean mountains, we found peasant houses that had envelopes with visiting cards and bottles located at more than double (3,000 meters) the elevation above sea level where the vector is known to survive (Briceno-Leon & Mendez, 2007).

The rural housing program of Venezuela, initiated in 1958 as part of the government's overall vector control approach, built more than half a million houses in its 40 years of existence. The program included the construction of housing, the installation of septic tanks and latrines and the provision of drinking water with rural aqueducts. The aspirations of the program went beyond the control of communicable diseases, as it represented an improvement of the conditions of rural life in general. But its purpose, at least originally, was clearly sanitary and rural. In times of financial abundance and the reduction of the threat of disease, however, housing began to be built in non-endemic areas and in non-rural areas. In some cases, the distortion was so great that housing was built for suburban middle-class families or in tourist areas, where they quickly changed ownership. The reason for this was political. Government officials needed to obtain political support, paying for loyalties, or making electoral propaganda without any relation to vector control or environmental health. For the population, this represented a way of obtaining a part of the distribution of the oil income, as housing was almost given away.

Employees of the public sector also had ways of competing for oil revenue. The union of the Ministry of Health employees had a contract stating that people should be paid travel expenses when they were ordered to work outside their normal place of work. It is a reasonable measure and applies almost everywhere; if someone is employed in a city and sent to work temporarily in another city, they must be paid those extra expenses through per diems. However, at one point the union decided to request a change in the rules and demand that travel expenses be paid when leaving the "office" instead of the "usual place of work." The consequence of this change was that entomological inspectors or insecticide sprayers, whose usual place of work was in endemic areas, could now be paid per diems when leaving the office. Therefore, if they had to cross the street in front of the office to check out *Aedes* breeding sites, they charged per diems. This change was approved, as it was a matter of guaranteeing political loyalties, and there was ample money to pay for it. Problems only began when there was not enough money for travel expenses.

Under these conditions, malaria outbreaks began to occur in different parts of the country, and in 1989 a Dengue epidemic hit. Authorities were baffled and ministers were trying to hide the situation. What had happened in Venezuela? The experts of international organizations were beginning to ask questions. Dr. Gabaldón, who by that time was working in his malaria laboratory at the Central University of Venezuela, had an ironic answer that we heard, personally, from him in his lectures: the increase of malaria was the fault of the air conditioners. And why air conditioners? The explanation was not entomological, nor related to mosquitoes, but to the work culture that had caused the oil wealth. The answer was simple: since the government had put air conditioners in the headquarters, the staff stayed in their offices and did not go out to study or fight mosquitoes in the heat and humidity of the tropics (Briceño León, 2011). Competition for rent had won the battle for vector control.

The Bolivarian revolution and the destruction of institutions

At the end of the 20th century, there was a strong demand for political change in the Venezuela. The economic boom that had begun in 1973 was reaching its end. While oil crises had generated abundant government revenue during this time, they proved to be short-lived and generated many expenses, waste and corruption.

For example, at the end of the seventies, a second oil crisis precipitated by political events in the Middle East again boosted prices and the rent economy. The "Islamic revolution" in Iran (1979) removed Mohammad Reza Pahlevi from power, the Shah of Iran, and turned the country into a theocracy under the direction of Ayatollah Khomeini. When the war began a year later, between Iran and Iraq, both exporting countries, the price per oil increased and the abundance of resources returned to Venezuela. However it was short-lived. The world economy had taken energy saving and production measures to protect itself from oil dependence. From this, a decline in oil prices began that led to a deterioration of Venezuela's economy and a sustained fall in real income. This has continued into the present.

The average Venezuelan could not easily understand the changes in the world economy that caused the reduction of oil prices and Venezuela's income. And just as politicians never explained to the population that the oil wealth, that in many ways facilitated populism, came from circumstances outside the country and not from their policy work, so too they could not explain that scarcity was the fault of others and not of themselves. Therefore, the national feeling was that if there was no money to distribute, it was because the politicians had stolen it. This was not entirely false, but neither was it the real cause of the drastic reductions in the national government's budget.

The system of two main political parties, Acción Democrática and COPEI, with which democracy in Venezuela had functioned, no longer represented the views of the population. Anti-political sentiment was widespread. For the 1998 presidential elections, the two parties that had ruled the country for 50 years lost popularity, and disenchanted voters declined to participate in elections. Voters wanted someone other than a traditional politician to govern. Sympathy grew for the mayor of Chacao, one of the municipalities in the Caracas capital city, Irene Saez, who had won the international beauty pageant Miss Universe. A well-known figure, albeit one discussed more in sports and celebrity circles, she appeared likely to become the future president. However, two facts changed that destiny. First was the loss of sympathy of the county's mayors because she accepted the support of one of the traditional political parties (COPEI), and the second was the appearance on the political scene of an ex-military man called Hugo Chávez, who had been imprisoned after a failed coup attempt in 1992. This altered the electoral landscape. Putting aside weapons to wield votes, Chavez became President of the Republic.

From 1999, then, the political situation changed radically. However, the oil and statist model remained in place, becoming also the model of the new regime. The new government raised the population's hopes for change and social improvement, and the charisma of Hugo Chávez, coupled with a good media campaign, placed the "Bolivarian Revolution" in the spotlight. For many, this change also brought hope in the new health policies that Chávez intended to implement. The most ambitious were proposals to establish a universal and free public health system, develop as far as possible the primary health care and prevention system, and reinvigorate the now noticeably declined environmental and community vector control programs.

As oil, the country's main export and income, was trading at around US$10 a barrel, the government started with limited resources and with a proposal for diversification of the non-oil economy. However, over the 2000s there was a steady increase in the price of oil, eventually topping over US$100 per barrel. This increase was the result of economic expansion in China and India, which increased their oil consumption, and a crisis in the prices of other commodities, which led financial capital to move towards oil, boosting the increase in prices to levels never seen before. Figure 5.4 shows the relationship between oil prices and political changes and the implications for mosquito-borne disease.

That increase meant that the national government had ten times more resources at its disposal. With the abundance of money in the coffers from the sale of oil abroad, domestic production and civil society became, again, insignificant.

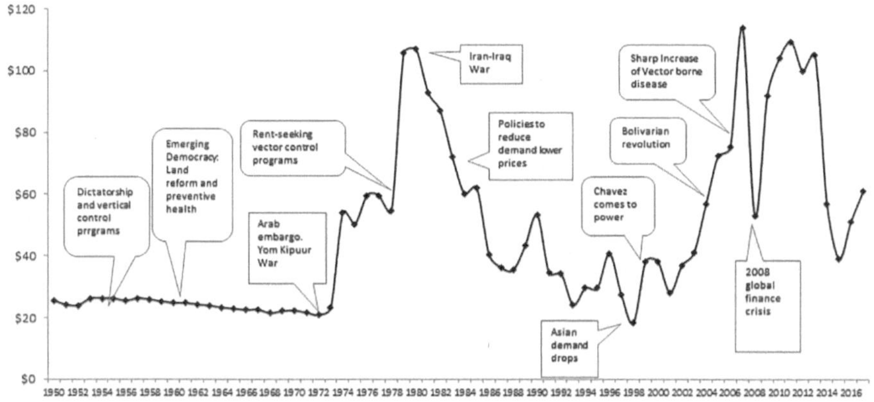

Figure 5.4 Key events in Venezuelan politics and vector control (1950–2017) related to fluctuating oil prices and government revenue.

Additionally, the presidency of Chavez gained increased powers due to the intermixing of high oil revenue and a compelling ideology that was systematically broadcasted to the rural population, where he held his powerbase. Eventually he succeeded in controlling all aspects of legislative, judicial, and military power. The president had all the power and all the money he needed. The state, that is, the government, assumed that it could dispose of everything and decide on everything in society. The old separation and autonomy of the judicial and legislative powers proper to democracy that, although with its limitations, had existed in the country, completely disappeared and presidential power became almost absolute.

But oil revenues entail a paradox. This wealth, created on the international market, needs to be spent, in large part, on the same international market. In a globalized world economy, there is no way of spending most, or at least a large quantity of it, in the country itself, since there are insufficient goods produced domestically to buy. An oil state does not produce cars, electronics, clothes, diamonds or other luxury or consumer goods. Therefore, oil money necessitates foreign transactions, cycling back outward to the global market. Understanding this political economy is essential to appreciating the contradictory health policies applied in those years.

In the 20th century, Venezuelan politics had little formally defined "conservative" or "right" political parties. Rather, most political ideologies were generally variations on traditional social democrat or Christian democrat positions. From its beginnings, however, the Chavez government, with its Marxist-Leninist ideology, assumed that everything that had been done in the past was bad and had to be destroyed. Repeating the slogan of the French Revolution that it was necessary first to destroy *l'ancien régime* before the new one could be built, the government set about dismantling the vector control program. Certainly this program had many shortcomings and problems – there was inefficient oversight, and a suspicion of management corruption, for example – but it also had experience, a professional staff and a valuable history that should not have been so easily discarded. The government's new health and vector control policy only managed to destroy structures that had existed for more than a decade, without building something different with which to replace it. After 18 years in power, the government failed to make a health policy or vector control system that was either new or better.

Throughout this process of institutional and anti-political destruction, there was military dominance in government. It was not a military government like the dictatorships of Argentina, Chile or Uruguay. But it was very different from what had been the discrete role, largely confined to the barracks, that the military had taken since the 1950s. Although President Chávez defined his government as a "civic-military" alliance, the weight of military officials in important government positions was remarkable. Many institutions, such as Ministry of Food, Citizen Security, Health, Education, Finance and Oil were in the hands of retired or active military personnel. This military presence played an important role in health programs, as senior staff were not only doctors who had assimilated into the military but also military personnel who had had no training or experience in health. Between 2007 and 2013, all health ministers were from the military.

Parallel to this, the Cuban presence in the country, given the ideological similarities between Chavez and Castro, increased in a very important way in the healthcare sector. Rather than model the Venezuelan system on the Cuban model, which has some of the highest health indicators of a low-income country and is lauded for this, the oil money created a situation of dependence, of exporting patients and importing expertise. According to official declarations, there were an estimated 31,700 Cuban aid workers in 2012: 11,000 doctors, 4,931 nurses, 2,713 dentists, 1,245 optometrists and 11,544 unspecified (Marcano, 2014). By 2015, the number had jumped to 46,000 (Telesur, 2015). At first, the government of Venezuela bought health, education and sports services from the government of Cuba. In 2004, an airplane was leaving Caracas every day, with more than 300 patients, who were taken to have eye surgery in Cuba. Although there are no reliable statistics, the official figures of the governments of Venezuela and Cuba mention hundreds of thousands of patients operated on for eye problems in Cuba with the so-called *Misión Milagro* (Telesur, 2015). A primary health care system, called the *Misión Barrio Adentro*, was installed, which operates in parallel to the Venezuelan health system but with Cuban personnel. Remarkably, this was run under the orders of a Cuban deputy minister who was not accountable to the Ministry of Health of Venezuela. In 2010, the policies of Dengue prevention and control presented by the officials of the vector control program in Caracas were discarded. By presidential order, the policies proposed by the Cuban advisers were assumed. This double policy also led to the existence of two parallel health statistic systems, which informed the ministry's epidemiological department. Official government statistics appeared alongside the alternative statistics offered by the *Misión Barrio Adentro*, that is, the government of Cuba. This situation led to conflicts, because diseases of international notification, such as syphilis, Dengue or malaria, were not reported to the ministry, but instead were sent directly to Cuba. These statistics arrived at the Ministry of Health only after being processed and delivered by the Cuban Ministry of Health to the president's office.

Although from the outset the government attacked private medicine, its practitioners and hospitals, and extolled the mandatory public nature of the health system, government ministries and the oil industry offered hospitalization insurance, surgery and maternity care with private insurance companies to state employees, as labour benefits. The consequences was that these individuals and their families (which numbered into the millions) went to private hospitals instead of public ones, strengthening the private health system and weakening the public system.

The reasons for these erratic health policies were political. The goals were not to improve the health of the population but to guarantee the political support of the voters before an election or a referendum. The sustainability of programs did not matter. In the end, not even the public health system was relevant, except that it caused public employees to have loyalty for the prevailing power and to vote for the government candidates in races for mayors, governorates or members of parliament.

This is why malaria reappeared in Venezuela with a force unique to the Americas. For these same reasons, after years of reducing *R. prolixus* vector transmission of Chagas' disease, cases of vector and oral Chagas transmission have also increased in urban areas. In Caracas, a secondary vector of Chagas' disease, *Panstrongylus geniculatus*, is now found throughout the city (Noya et al., 2009). And in the Chacao municipality of Caracas, which has the best economic and social conditions in the country, there was an outbreak of acute Chagas' disease in one school, in which a child died and several dozen children and some teachers contracted the disease. Investigators found that this was caused by the ingestion of guava juice, where an infected *T. cruzi* parasite had been liquefied (Noya et al., 2010).

Political conflicts and vectors

The national office of vector control has been located in the city of Maracay, capital of Aragua state, located in the north of the country and separated by a high mountain from the Caribbean Sea, for over 70 years. However, it is also one of the cities with the most cases of Dengue fever and, more recently, Chikungunya (Barrera et al. 2000; Camacho et al. 2016). In a recent study carried out in two of the three municipalities that make up the city, 21% of houses had breeding sites positive for *Aedes aegypti* and *Aedes albopictus* larvae/pupae (Guevara & Teran, 2017). The first reported cases of human deaths caused by Chikungunya in Venezuela were reported in this city (Torres et al., 2015), although these were immediately denied by the authorities. The president of the city's medical association, Dr. Angel Sarmiento, who had made the complaint, was charged with trying to create a "state of anxiety"; to escape persecution, he had to leave the country and flee to neighboring Colombia.

When local elections, for mayors, were held in late 2013, government party candidates managed to win 16 of the 18 municipalities in Aragua state. Maracay, the capital city, has 1.2 million inhabitants, and is made up of 5 municipalities. In one of these municipalities, an opposition candidate, Delson Guarate, was elected, representing an exception to political domination. The spread of Dengue in previous years had been closely linked to the trash and debris that accumulated in homes and streets as a result of irregular garbage collection. Failure to collect garbage had been part of the population's demands, and the new mayor promised to fix this problem. After he began his term, however, clashes between the new mayor and the state and national government transformed garbage collection into a political tool. In 2015, the governor seized the garbage trucks they had assigned to the mayor to prevent them from doing their work; then the mayor obtained other informal trucks to collect the garbage. In response, the government's political activists diverted trucks picking up garbage from other municipalities on their way to the landfill site and unloaded them in the streets of the opposition municipality. Garbage and Dengue had become a tool of political attack.

But as Mayor Guarate resisted, the national government sent police to arrest him in his office in September 2016, accusing him of "environmental crimes," because, the government argued, the mayor had not collected the garbage that had accumulated in the municipality causing an increase in *Aedes* mosquitoes transmitting Dengue, Chikungunya and Zika. He was detained in prison for the next 14 months without formal accusation; the initial hearing before the judge was deferred 10 times in 1 year. During this time, the national government wanted to legitimize elections for mayors to which opposition political parties had refused to participate because they did not comply with national laws. To increase the semblance of legitimacy, the government proposed to several imprisoned opposition mayors that they could be granted parole if they accepted to register as candidates in these elections. It was another legal violation, because it makes no sense to grant parole to anyone who is neither accused nor condemned. Two mayors accepted these political conditions, among them Mayor Guarate in Maracay. And so it was that in November 2017, he left the political prison to register as a candidate and campaigned for one month until the day of the elections, on December 13, 2017, when he fled the country to request political asylum in Colombia.

Gone were garbage, environmental crimes and Dengue and Chikungunya. That was never the problem, nor the real concern of the Bolivarian revolution. Only political control and the destruction of everything that could mean independence, autonomy or dissidence. That is why not only malaria or Chagas disease expanded, but also the diseases transmitted by *A. aegypti*. In 2014, for example, the country registered 3,750,698 cases of acute fever with no apparent explanation, and the great majority of these cases occurred between week 23 (June) and week 44 (November), at the peak of the Chikungunya epidemic. At some points, there were more than 200,000 cases each week, which has led to an estimated excess of 2,203,198 acute febrile cases, which can only be attributed to an explosive epidemic of Chikungunya. This is not surprising. In 2011 the House

Index (HI), which reports on the presence of *Aedes* vectors in homes, was never below 5%, the maximum allowable limit according to PAHO. In 2014, this index reached 17.4% nationwide (Oletta et al., 2014). Vector control faded in the midst of the country's political crisis.

Discussion and conclusions

The remarkable and early success of vector-borne disease control in Venezuela, as well as its recent decline, shows the relevance of political processes in vector control. Other factors, such as climate and available financial and human resources, and even geopolitics are equally important (Orsenna & de Saint Aubin, 2017). But the handling of any of these factors occurs in a social context that links health actions with the country's political orientation and decisions. From this experience, there are some factors we find important to understand, that are Venezuelan-specific but also have wider relevance to the region in the context of Zika, old resurgent diseases like malaria and future hitherto unknown ones.

In the Venezuelan context, the politics of vector control, and the political narratives underpinning them, have relied both on proclamations of success as well as threats of the recurrence of disease. Vector control policies have to be proven successful, for that is their purpose, and political leadership needs success in order to justify the resources allocated and reap the fruits. But, if success has been achieved, why should we continue to invest in vector control? This dilemma has arisen since the 1950s in the discussion between eradication and disease control in the World Health Organization (Litsios, 1998). The thesis of eradication expressed a valuable social ambition and a trust in technology, but it created an illusion of permanence that has proven to be epidemiologically incorrect and politically dangerous. Political management of the dilemma between success and permanent risk in vector-borne diseases has not been adequately communicated to the political leadership or to society.

The lack of resources to carry out vector control programs has been an important constraint for health ministries in many countries. However, the experience of Venezuela over several decades shows that an overabundance of resources can also lead to harmful consequences; namely, in the proliferation of unnecessary tasks, wastes of money and corruption and accompanying declines in motivation and purpose based on notions of social betterment. Overabundance, at least without civic oversight and good public management, promotes a culture of passivity.

The sustainability of health goals also requires the participation of communities at risk, and that is only possible if people believe that their actions are relevant and have the real possibility of contributing to health improvements. If people do not believe that their actions can prevent disease, why do something? There are two reasons why people may believe that their actions are not important in the prevention or control of vector-borne diseases. The first is frustration, having tried and never achieved anything. The second is passivity and apathy: if the goals are achieved solely through the effort and work of others, such as state officials or the politician of the day, why try? Where citizens assume that, given all the cash, vector control is the sole responsibility of the government, who must pay the officials to do the work of eliminating vectors, this may itself lead to passivity and apathy.

Politicians regularly face the dilemma of balancing recognition of health problems (by raising alarm bells and calls for action) with minimizing the problem, hiding it or even censoring information. Recognizing an epidemic or a re-infestation can be interpreted as recognizing a failure and can jeopardize political prestige and the government's position. However, hiding it can mean a late response, and can make the problem even greater. The difficulty for politicians and communities is to recognize that there is a problem and that the problem is "their own." There is a temptation, however, to interpret the problem as "somebody else's" and so it can be ignored or overlooked by authorities, civil society and families. The balance between recognizing successes and raising attention to threats must be guided by the political purpose of maintaining a sense of shared responsibility in society.

Since its origins, vector control programs have had two competing orientations: one military and vertical, and one civil and horizontal or participatory. In the former approach, for example, an entomological surveillance officer identifies the presence of disease vectors in homes by quickly inspecting houses and yards at a set time period. In the latter model, surveillance can also engage family members who live there 24 hours a day. The organization of malaria programs was the clearest expression of the military model. As part of this, sanitary programs and large-scale insecticide spraying programs were implemented by authoritarian governments, often among rural populations with high illiteracy. The entomological inspection team or the house sprayers arrived with a military authority that imposed the activities and applied the insecticide without asking the family for consent. However, society in Venezuela and elsewhere has changed dramatically; citizens have studied and learned their rights, governments became democratic, and restrictions have been placed on the exercise of arbitrary authority. The dilemma between authoritative military programs, which can be very efficient in their execution, and educational and participatory programs, which can guarantee the sustainability of the achievements, remains a relevant paradox.

Consistent with the controversy between a civilian or military approach to vector control, there is also the dilemma between centralized and decentralized management. Military and vertical vector control in Venezuela functioned in the past within a centralized system in the national government that had delegates in the different regions of the country. As in an army, the decisions were taken by central officials and met little comment or protest in the different regions. Changes in government systems and ideological forms in the Latin American political landscape has now led to a push for decentralization, which brings with it a transfer of responsibilities to provincial governments (states or departments) and municipalities (Yadon et al., 2006). The goal of decentralization is to bring the exercise of government closer to communities, so that there can be greater efficiency and a greater possibility of monitoring and demanding the fulfilment of programs by citizens. Decentralization has been carried out very irregularly in Latin America.

Responsibilities have been transferred, but not the resources for their execution. Some politicians in Venezuela have voiced, in public and private, that vector-borne diseases and health problems increased as a result of decentralization. To be successful, decentralization, at its core, requires a wider distribution of power in society. But military and authoritarian governments want to concentrate power, not distribute it. That is why in Venezuela President Chavez declared that centralization was returning, and that the country's health problems would be over when decentralization was reversed. Centralization and de-centralization are two political strategies with advantages and disadvantages; there is no single answer. Decentralization, with its proposal of carrying out vector control from the smallest and closest government bodies, such as the municipality, is attractive, but it requires local technical capacity and honesty and transparency so that it can work.

Lastly, the experience of Venezuela shows the conflicts and tensions between the perspectives of communities and vector-control departments. While communities think of health in a holistic way, as general welfare, vector-control programs often look only at particular diseases. This difference creates an issue between the goals of the Ministry of Health and the demands of the population. For politicians in charge of vector control, their responsibility is to reduce or eliminate the vector and thereby control the disease. For the population, malaria, Dengue fever or Zika is just one problem among many.

In communities where we have worked between 2015 and 2018, in the municipalities Francisco Linares Alcantara and Mario Briceño Iragorry, in Maracay, Aragua State, Dengue fever and Chikungunya can be a major annoyance, but more important for daily life is not having enough water to cook, clean or drink. In focus groups we conducted in 2017 with pregnant women at risk of Zika, the risk of congenital fetal malformations was considered of great concern, but it was of no less importance than the problems they face securing enough food to survive in the present. So, when people are forced to choose between keeping water in tanks and preventing Dengue fever, they do not hesitate to choose: water. For Amazon miners searching out gold in the precarious circumstances of the post-Chavez economy, malaria may be a resurgent problem that reaches into the international news, but these people are, really, more concerned about snake bites, robbery or abuse by the military.

In Venezuela, the Bolivarian revolution has converted one of the richest countries in Latin America into one of the poorest, and in so doing it has also transformed the country's effective national vector control system into dysfunction and led to rampant disease reemergence. This social and health calamity is the consequence of wrong policies in the economy, institutions and society at large. In the economy, policies have destroyed national production and a diversified business class through expropriations and subsidized imports, with the goal of reducing the social class of business leaders and owners. In society, policies have destroyed the social fabric of civil engagement by dividing the population into rich and poor, friends and enemies, into patriots and foreign agents and fomenting the struggle of classes and groups. And all of this has been accomplished in the name of a revolution that has destroyed the economy, the social fabric and rule of law.

Venezuela in 2018, then, is a nation defined by hunger, poverty and disease. In a national representative survey carried out by three universities, 72% of those interviewed stated that they had lost weight the previous year. Inflation is the highest in the world, estimated at more than 3,000% in 2017 and the average monthly salary does not reach US$20 per month (Encovi, 2018). The population does not receive medical attention; private or public insurances have a coverage that, due to hyperinflation, hardly serves to cover a laboratory test or an X-ray. Patients cannot find the most common medicines for hypertension or diabetes in hospitals or pharmacies, so they have to buy them on the black market or, if they are wealthy enough, import them directly from abroad. This has made out-of-pocket spending on health in Venezuela among the highest in the world (Encovi, 2018). The fact that Pfizer, in 2016, donated acetaminophen to assist with the Zika epidemic, something that was commented on in international news, shows how tragic the situations has become. As there is a lack of food for sale on supermarket shelves, a large part of the population depends on a box of imported food distributed by the government. And university professors, schoolteachers and policemen have abandoned their positions. More than 20,000 doctors have left the country. Workers and the unemployed from all social sectors are preparing to emigrate, in what is considered the largest migration exodus ever experienced in the Americas. For those of us who remain, including the authors of this chapter, there are more and more mosquitoes.

Notes

1 The annual incidence rate went from 122.9 per 100,000 inhabitants in the year 2000 to 775.5 per 100,000 inhabitants in 2016.

2 The research on which this text is based received financial support from the International Development Research Centre (IDRC), Canada. The opinions expressed do not necessarily reflect those of IDRC.

3 His murderer had requested asylum in the Nicaraguan embassy. However, he had been taken from the embassy by the police and was killed while on route to jail. The police alleged that he had tried to escape.

4 In an alliance with private business, experiments were begun on the construction of "healthy houses," and a "construction manual" of mud dwellings that preserved the health of its inhabitants. With the construction of houses, the control of the transmission of Chagas disease was mainly sought, but also to create a healthy habitat that would prevent intestinal parasitic diseases, schistosomiasis and yellow fever. The work was interrupted because the entrepreneur, Eugenio Mendoza, who promoted the initiative, had to leave the country due to political persecution in the final months of the dictatorship.

5 The general mortality rate reduced from 21.1 per 100,000 in 1941, to 13.7 per 100,000 in 1950, and then 6.6 per 100,000 in 1971 (Paez Celis, 1974).

References

Baptista, A. 1997, *Teoría Económica del Capitalismo Rentístico*. Ediciones IESA, Caracas.

Barrera, R., Delgado, N., Jiménez, M., Villalobos, I., & Romero, I. 2000, 'Estratificacion de una ciudad hiperendemica en dengue hemorragico', *Revista Panamericana de Salud Pública*, vol. 8, pp. 225–233.

Benítez, J. A., Rodríguez, A., Sojo, M., Lobo, H., Villegas, C., Oviedo, L., et al. 2004. 'Descripción de un Brote Epidémico de Malaria de Altura en un área originalmente sin Malaria del Estado Trujillo, Venezuela', *Boletín de Malariología y Salud Ambiental*, vol. XLIV, no. 2, pp. 93–100.

Briceño-León, R. 1990, *La Casa Enferma. Sociología de la Enfermedad de Chagas*. Acta Científica Venezolana,Caracas.

Briceño-León, R. 1996, 'El DDT y la modernización de Venezuela', *Boletin de la Dirección de Malariología y Saneamiento Ambiental*, vol. 36, no. 1/2, pp. 44–50.

Briceño-León, R. 2011, *Arnoldo Gabaldón* (Vol. 130). El Nacional, Caracas.

Briceño-León, R. 2015, *Los Efectos Perversos del Petróleo*. Libros EL Nacional,Caracas.

Briceño-Leon, R., & Mendez, G. J. 2007, 'The Social determinants of Chagas disease and the Transformations of Latin América', *Memorias do Instituto Osealdo Cruz*, vol. 102, no. suppl.1, pp. 109–112.

Cáceres, J. L. 2011, 'La Malaria en el estado Bolívar, Venezuela: 10 años sin control', *Boletín de Malariología y Salud Ambiental*, vol. 51 no. 2.

Camacho, D., Celis, A., Moros, Z., Osorio, J., & Araujo, R. 2016, 'Circulacion de virus Chikungunya en el estado Aragua (Venezuela) durante el año 2014', *Boletin de Malariología y Salud Ambiental*, vol. 56, no. 2, pp. 122–130.

Carquez, F. 2007, *Paludismo, Petróleo y Desarrollo Nacional*. Venezuela Siglo XX. Universidad de Carabobo, Valencia.

Carter, E. 2012, *Malaria, environment and development in Argentina*. The University of Alabama Press, Tuscaloosa.

Cueto, M. 2007, *Cold War, Dedly Fevers. Malaria Eradication in Mexico 1955–1975*. The John Hopkins University Press, Baltimore.

DGSA-MPPS. 2018, *Reporte Epidemiológico de Situación de Malaria*. Ministerio del Poder Popular par la Salud, Dirección Genral de Saneamiento Ambiental. MPPS, Maracay.

Encovi. 2018, *Encuesta Condiciones de Vida de la Población Venezolana*. UCAB-UCV-USB. UCAB, Caracas.

Gabaldon, A. 1949, 'The nation-wide campaign against malaria in Venezuela', *Transactions of the Royal Society of Tropical Medicine and Hygiene*, vol. 43, pp. 113–164.

Gabaldon, A. 1953, 'Importancia de la mortalidad sin diagnóstico medico en los datps boiestadisticos referentes a la malaria en Venezuela', *Boletin de la oficina sanitaria Panamericana*, vol. XXXV, no.1, pp.10.

Gabaldon, A., & Berti, A. Sept de 1954, 'The first large area in the Tropical Zone to report malaria eradication: North Central Venezuela. *The American Journal of Tropical Medicine and Hygiene*, vol. 3, no. 5, pp. 793–807.

Grillet, M.-E., Martínez, J. E., & Barrera, R. 2009, 'Focos calientes de transmisión de malaria: implicaciones para un control orientado y efectivo en Venezuela', *Boletín de Malariología y Salud Ambiental*, vol. 49, pp. 193–208. Obtenido de http://www.scielo.org.ve/scielo.php?pid=S1690–46482009000200003&script=sci_arttext&tlng=pt

Guevara, M., & Teran, I. 2017, *Estrategias de Liderazgo Municipal Intersectorial para el control de dengue y Chikungunya y Zika en los Municipios Francisco Linares Alcántara y Mario Briceño Iragorry. Estado Aragua, Venezuela*. Universidad de Carabobo, Maracay.

Hobsbawn, E. 2001, *Historia del Siglo XX*. Crítica, Barcelona.

Hotez, P. J., Basáñez, M.-G., Acosta-Serrano, A., & Grillet, M. E. 29 de Junio de 2017, *Venezuela and its rising vector-borne neglected diseases*. Obtenido de PLOS neglected tropical diseases. DOI:10.1371/journal.pntd.0005423.

Litsios, S. 1998, 'Arnoldo Gabaldon's independent path for malaria control and public health in the tropics: a los "paradigm" for WHO', *Parassitologia*, vol. 40, pp. 12, pp. 231–238.

López Ramirez, T. 1987, *Historia De La Escuela De Malariologia Y Saneamiento Ambiental De Venezuela*. Direccion General De Malariologia Y Saneamiento Ambiental, Ministerio De Sanidad Y Asistencia Social, Caracas.

Marcano, C. 2014, 'Las relaciones desmedidas', *El Pais*, 30 de marzo de.

March, J. G., & Olsen, J. P. 2006, 'Elaborating the "New Institutionalism"', En R. Rhodes, S. A. Binder, & B. A. Rockman (eds.), *The Oxford handbook of political institutions*. Oxford University Press, Oxford, pp. 3–22.

North, D. 1991, 'Institutions', *The Journal Economic Perspectives*, vol. 5, no. 1, pp. 97–12.

Noya, B. A., Díaz-Bello, Z., Colmenares, C., Ruiz-Guevara, R., Mauriello, L., Zavala-Jaspe, R., et al. 2010, 'Large urban outbreak of orally acquired acute Chagas disease at a school in Caracas, Venezuela', *The Journal of Infectious Diseases*, vol. 201, no. 9, pp. 1308–1315.

Noya, B. A., Díaz-Bello, Z., Colmenares, C., Zavala-Jaspe, R., Mauriello, L., Díaz, M. P., et al. 2009, 'Transmisión urbana de la enfermedad de Chagas en Caracas', *Revista Biomed*, vol. 20, pp. 158–164.

Oletta, J. F., Orihuela, Á. R., V, C. W., Godoy, O., Carvajal, A. C., Castro, J., Pena S, Barreto A. 2014,*Estudio de la densidad de vectores como factor determinante de la magnitud y diseminación de la epidemia de CHIKV*. Obtenido de Analítica: http://www.analitica.com/bienestar/salud/chikungunya-en-el-continente-americano-al-cumplirse-1-ano-de-su-introduccion-y-transmision/

Oletta, J. F., Walter, C., Orihuela, Á. R., Pulido, M., Carvajal, A. C., Castro, J. and Pena S. 18 de 03 de 2018, *Análisis preliminar del Informe Mundial de malaria, caso de Venezuela*. Obtenido de Revista SIC: http://revistasic.gumilla.org/2017/analisis-preliminar-del-informe-mundial-de-malaria-caso-de-venezuela/

Orsenna, E., & de Saint Aubin, I. 2017, *Géopolitique du moustique*. Fayard, Paris.

Paez Celis, J. 1974, *Ensayo sobre demografía económica de Venezuela*. Dirección General de Estadística y Censos Nacionales, Ministerio de Fomento, Caracas.

PAHO, P. A. 2017, *Epidemiological alert: increase in cases of malaria*. Pan American Health Organization. PAHO, Washington, DC.

Peters, B. 2012, *Institutional Theory in Political Science*. The New Institutionalism. Continuum, New York.

Rabinovich, J. 1985, 'Ecologia Poblacional de Triatominos', En R. U. Carcavallo, J. E. Rabinovich, & R. Tonn (eds.), *Factores Biológicos y Ecológicos en la Enfermedad de Chagas*. Centro Panamericano de Ecología y Salud, Buenos Aires, pp. 12–147.

Telesur. 30 de octubre de 2015, *Telesur*. Recuperado el 16 de marzo de 2018, de Telesur: https://www.telesurtv.net/news/Cuba-y-Venzuela-15-anos-de-fructifera-cooperacion-20141030–0008.html

Torres, J., Leopoldo, C.G., Castro, J.S., Rodríguez, L., Saravia, V., Arvelaez, J., et al. 2015, 'Chikungunya fever: atypical and lethal cases in the Western hemisphere: a Venezuelan experience', *IDCases*, Vol. 2, pp. 6–10.

Torres, J. R., Orduna, T. A., Piña-Pozas, M., Vázquez-Vega, D., & Sarti, E. 2017, *Epidemiological characteristics of dengue disease in Latin America and in the Caribbean: a systematic review of the literature*. Obtenido de DOI:10.1155/2017/8045435.

World Health Organization 2017, *WHO World Malaria Report 2017*. WHO, Geneva.

Yadon, Z., Gutler, R., Tobar, F., & Medici, A. 2006, *Descentralización y Gestión del Control de las Enfermedades Transmisibles En América Latina / Descentralización and Managament ff Comunicable Disease Control in Latin America.* Organización Panamericana de la Salud, Buenos Aires.

Yépez Colmenares, G. 1995, 'El impacto del paludismo en Venezuela y la organización de la Dirección Especial de Malariología en 1936 / Impact of malaria in Venezuela and the organization of the dirección especial of malariología en 1936', *Tribuna del investigador*, vol. 2, no. 1, pp. 16–26.

6 Tracking *Aedes aegypti* in a hotter, wetter, more urban world

Capacity building, disease surveillance and epidemiological labour in Ecuador

Anna M. Stewart-Ibarra, Rebecca Rose Henderson, Naveed Heydari, Mercy J. Borbor-Cordova, Yui Fujii and Kevin Bardosh

Introduction

At the height of the Zika epidemic in 2016, investigators from the Center for Global Health and Translational Sciences of the State University of New York (SUNY) Upstate Medical University received a US National Science Foundation (NSF) Zika Rapid Action grant to study transmission dynamics in a "high burden" region of Ecuador. The central site of the study was to be Machala, Ecuador's fourth largest city of 280,000 people, also known as the "banana capital of the world." This coastal city is located close to the border with Peru, making it a site of frequent cross-border transit where bananas, shrimp and gold mining make up the local economy. All four Dengue virus serotypes had been co-circulating in Machala for many years before Zika, disproportionately burdening those living on the outskirts of the city where garbage collection is limited and interruptions of the water supply are are common occurrence. The projected risk of Zika transmission was thought to be high.[1]

While funding mechanisms like the Zika Rapid Action grant are meant to provide agility in response to an emerging pathogen, being a successful grantee – winning the grant – requires considerable informal infrastructure, networks and skill. The ability to implement meaningful rapid research – a type of funding that is becoming more common in the world of epidemic response – is dependent on long-term relationships and groundwork that is simultaneously invaluable and yet often invisible, or at least marginal, to funding applications and formal publications.

Just as social forces shape the lives of *Aedes aegypti* (where they *breed* and who they *bite*) in an increasingly dynamic world impacted by eco-social forces, they also influence the efforts of scientists, policy-makers and vector control staff. In this sense, understanding the sociability of *Aedes aegypti* involves a great deal of labour to understand the eco-social forces influencing the mosquito while also navigating the (all-too-human) social world of global health funding, capacity building and the politics of policy.

Tracking mosquitoes in a changing world is particularly difficult and relies on an assortment of entomological data, statistical reasoning, mathematical models and GIS maps. A range of social, environmental and climatic phenomena, operating at different scales, needs to be brought together. But contextualized datasets and pathways for model calibration and validation are frequently lacking, calling into question the trustworthiness of scientific models and their representations (Braks et al. 2013). The lack of long-term epidemiological series data (> 30 years) means that researchers often have to work with shorter timescales (<10 years of data), a major impediment given the nature of the earth's climate which operates across seasonal, interannual, decadal and long term time scales. As discussed by Brisbois and Ali (2010), opposing interpretations can emerge of short-term meteorological data, and such ambiguities make causation and attribution very challenging. Ensuring that the science is useful outside academia, through acts of translation and engagement with the worlds of policy and day-to-day government vector control, is also fraught with troubles. Working in Cameroon on emerging zoonoses, Judson et al. (2018) explored the utility of disease models, constructed mostly by outside academic groups, for public health experts and found that most of the experts were unfamiliar with the academic models. The models typically lacked essential contextualized (local) knowledge that would have made them more detailed and accurate; for instance, of environmental boundaries and basic administrative regions. As Leach and Scoones (2013) argued, models of vector-borne diseases have social and political lives.

The few publications on disease models have examined the forces impacting model adoption at a national and international level, rather than the local forces that impact modeling groups. In this chapter, we take a slightly different route and examine the ways that disease-modeling projects are socially embedded in day-to-day practices, and how scientific research in global health – in this case, of *Aedes agypti* – is made real through what we call *epidemiological labour* in Machala, Ecuador.

Scholars of science and technology studies (STS) have long showed how the production of scientific knowledge takes place in a context and is the result of relationships (Janes and Corbett, 2009). Individuals and groups work together to gather data, and a diversity of viewpoints, backgrounds and interests shape the scope of science and how data are collected, analyzed and displayed. Social networks, and formal and informal relationships, also shape how knowledge is mobilized and made real through policy and social actions.

Despite clarion calls for capacity building and the creation of networks and "networks of networks" in global health, the description of science networks rarely describe the informal efforts of scientists out in the world, interacting with their local policy champions, friends and collaborators. Anthropologists have become interested in the idea of global health labour, for example, in the work of community health workers (Maes and Kalofonos, 2013) and field assistants (Biruk, 2012) and more broadly in the nature of transnational research partnerships (Crane et al., 2018). This work tells us that the mobilization of resources to collect scientific data, the creation of a locally skilled scientific workforce and collaborations with national scientific and government actors all have profound effects on the settings in which knowledge is produced and transformed.

An emerging disease crisis, like Zika, offers a unique opportunity to understand the social and political labour of global health. The humanitarian and medical emergency literatures are replete with the mantra of capacity building as a form of prevention for calamity (Lakoff, 2017). In reality, though, and in an era of new, unfolding geopolitical change and anti-globalism, most funding follows the epidemic curve. Projects are funded from epidemic-to-epidemic, or emergency-to-emergency, where atmospheres of fear and uncertainty co-exist with an urgency to act, to do something now. The challenge is this: acting in these contexts requires having informal social and biophysical infrastructures already on the ground, something that is often insufficiently acknowledged, unrepresented, underfunded and invisible.

In this chapter, we expand on these ideas and explore the decade-long history of collaboration, partnership and scientific labour of a US-Ecuadorian disease surveillance group working on *Aedes agypti* transmitted diseases in the city of Machala. Using reflections from team members gathered through auto-ethnographic writing as well as unstructured interviews, we describe the ways in which this group has participated in social worlds in order to build capacity at local and national levels and to maneuver in the world of science, policy and public health. This includes tracking the creation and texture of scientific partnerships, the mobilization of health resources and capacity building efforts, the work of entomology teams and the consequences of science for public policy. A socially-embedded science is particularly important to connect climate change to *Aedes*-borne illnesses; in order to track the complex, long-term changes that are impacting vectors and viruses in a hotter, wetter and more urban world, we need equally long-term partnerships to transform the landscapes of science, policy and public services.

Informality and earthquakes: Launching an *agile* research network in Ecuador

As mentioned earlier, the seamless implementation of "rapid" Zika surveillance in Ecuador was not as rapid as one would at first assume; rather, it was built on the effort of a formal and informal infrastructure that was already on the ground. Although the work of the Center for Global Health and Translational Sciences at SUNY had been ongoing in Machala since 2012, one of the project's lead investigators, Dr. Anna Stewart-Ibarra, a dual US-Ecuadorian citizen, was established in the region in 2007. As a graduate student in systems ecology, a professor of Anna's connected her with Dr. Mercy Borbor-Cordova, an Ecuadorian environmental scientist who was finishing a postdoctoral fellowship at the National Center for Atmospheric Research (NCAR) in the United States. At the time, relatively few groups were doing research on Dengue fever in the region, and even fewer were doing field studies to look at the interactions between climate, social vulnerability and Dengue. Mercy proposed that they start investigating this important area of emerging research.

Together, Mercy and Anna began meeting with researchers and practitioners in the climate and health sectors to identify health priorities and who was doing what in Ecuador: such as the National Directorate of Epidemiological Surveillance of the Ministry of Health (MoH), the National Vector Control Service (SNEM), and the National Institute of Hydrology and Meteorology (INAMHI in Spanish), among others. The idea of linking climate and health was novel and challenging given traditional departmental and disciplinary siloes. Dengue provided a malleable scientific subject, in that the incidence, severity and distribution of Dengue fever were increasing at the time in Ecuador, while malaria declined year after year in the 2000s. There was public and policy interest in Dengue. In the early 2000s, the first cases of Dengue hemorrhagic fever were reported, resulting in hospitalizations and deaths. A clear opportunity emerged for Anna and Mercy: to conduct scientific studies on the basic epidemiology, etiology, and ecology of Dengue that linked climate and health outcomes through social-ecological modeling that would help inform public health interventions.

This period involved much "door-knocking" and "elevator pitches." Mercy's prior experience in government in Ecuador as the Province Director in the Secretary of Risk, which eventually led to a senior position in the Ministry of Environment, and Anna's Ecuadorian family roots played important roles. Unlike other scientists, Anna and Mercy wanted to connect science with the public sector, an approach not often taken by traditional academic scientists. In 2007, a fortuitous family connection helped Anna to meet with the head of SNEM, the national agency responsible for Dengue control and vector surveillance. This opened the doors to conduct a small collaborative study with SNEM one year later, to study *Aedes aegypti* and social risk factors in peri-urban communities in the coastal tropical city of Guayaquil, the largest city in Ecuador, and a hotbed of Dengue transmission. This project was possible through pilot funding that Mercy received from NCAR. This productive partnership with SNEM in Guayaquil eventually led to the establishment of the Machala research program in 2010 in El Oro province, in partnership with local SNEM staff, as part of Anna's doctoral research.

El Oro province experienced the biggest Dengue epidemic in 2010. Over 2,000 cases were reported from the city of Machala, almost 1 out of 100 hundred people reported Dengue in this city with a population of 240,000 people – the true number of infections was likely much higher. Young people under 20 years of age accounted for 58% of all cases.[2] At the time, there were few scientific studies published on basic *Aedes* entomology or Dengue epidemiology in the country, let alone research looking at the links between urbanization, climate and Dengue transmission. Initial research in Machala, capital of El Oro Province, started with some nominal funding to Anna from a Fulbright Fellowship, and the local SNEM provided significant support, including two full-time staff and two half-time staff to assist with field and laboratory work, transportation, logistics and coordination with communities and the public health sector. These early studies with SNEM provided the first evidence for the effects of climate on Dengue and *Aedes aegypti* in Ecuador, and documented community perceptions of social-ecological risk factors.

The subsequent disbanding of SNEM in 2015, and decentralization of vector control activities, led some of Anna's collaborators to assume faculty positions at the local public university, the Technical University of Machala (UTMach). As the only university in El Oro province, UTMach plays an important role in supporting public health capacities, by training physicians, nurses and biopharmaceutical technicians, among others. As a result, UTMach emerged as a central partner in the Machala research program. INAMHI had greatly advanced the agenda in Ecuador on climate variability and change and also became a permanent collaborator at this time.

Research linking climate and health requires special attention to capacity building in places like Machala, Ecuador. The work is inherently trans-disciplinary, involving complex causal pathways and nonlinearity. Developing methods of assigning causal contribution to climatic influences, to link Dengue to weather patterns, for example, demands that we reason several steps removed from the health outcome of interest (McMichael, 2015:51). This level of causal disconnection requires teams of entomologists, epidemiologists, social scientists, physicians, climate scientists, statistical modelers and ecologists, to name a few. It requires access to health and vector data, climatic data and geospatial data on demographics. And it requires skills of interpretation, of re-interpretation, and political skills in translating these scientific interpretations – statistics, maps and models – into something that local collaborators understand, need and want.

The first five years of work in Ecuador (2007–2012) represented a time when *formal* institutional and project footprints did not exist in Machala. Without the established backing of institutions or large grants, the enthusiasm of graduate research, the support of local SNEM leaders and the emerging importance of Dengue played important motivational forces in establishing friendships, trust and a sense of camaraderie in this group of scientists and public health experts. The Dengue epidemic in 2010 coincided with a time of political tension and violence in Ecuador, including the national police going on strike and the president being held hostage, which also bonded the group together during late nights in the SNEM lab and community meetings on Dengue prevention, organized with out-of-pocket money and unpaid overtime.[3]

From this emerging collaboration came a set of long-term goals that the team frequently discussed together, and which ultimately, over time, provided leverage for the short-term aims of the Zika Rapid Response Fund in 2016–2017. These are summarized in Table 6.1, and included a focus on building partnerships, generating multidisciplinary knowledge, sustaining legitimacy and trust and maintaining a long-term presence on the ground. These goals, one could call them a code of conduct or even an ethical framework for engagement, created the agility to respond to Zika in Machala. But it also created the motivation and capacity for other forms of agility: to respond to humanitarian need and study the impact of Zika transmission dynamics after an earthquake, for example.

Just after the WHO declared Zika a public health emergency of international concern (PHEC) in February 2016, a magnitude 7.8 earthquake struck the north coast of Ecuador on April 16, several hundred kilometers north of Machala. In addition to the 660 reported deaths and 4,605 injured, the earthquake displaced over 30,000 people and left approximately 720,000 in need of humanitarian aid, without basic infrastructure and access to food, water, shelter and health care.[4] Many people experienced significant psychological trauma, which continued

Table 6.1 Informal infrastructure for capacity and surveillance strengthening

Approach	*Assets*	*Zika-oriented outcomes*
Committed long-term partnerships with local institutions	Early grassroots partnerships with Ecuadorian institutions and researchers Involvement of Ecuadorian public health professionals at every stage of the research process, including agenda-setting Creation of formal agreements with Ecuadorian institutions and universities through Memorandums of Understanding (MoU). This provided a solid foundation upon which to develop research and training collaborations. Everyone (local and international partners) brings unique assets to the collaboration. Flexibility and openness to partnering with a diversity of researchers and funding partners.	Ability to mobilize existing partnerships and relationships to respond to emerging Zika disease threat. Zika Rapid Response Grants and clinical trial capacity building
Social-ecological systems focus to assess biophysical, political, and other social drivers	Early studies prior to the emergence of Zika provided the evidence base for the effects of climate and social vulnerability on Dengue risk through a social-ecological systems approach – a transdisciplinary and participatory research framework. This departs from a traditional epidemiological biological model of disease transmission.	Participation in the creation of relevant national policy documents, such as the National Communication of Ecuador for the UN Convention on Climate Change, linking Zika and other *Aedes*-borne illnesses to climate change and socio-economic factors. Publications to forecast arboviral outbreaks using climate information (Lowe et al., 2017).
Timely research focused on public health priorities and solutions.	Close collaborators in Ecuador provide an engine of advocacy and legitimacy for the research, and continue to ensure that research is relevant for the country. Convening a group working to advocate for the implementation of the framework of climate services and health (WMO, 2014) Mobilization of the team in response to national crisis and emergency (earthquake in 2016).	Movement of team resources to document impact of natural disaster on Zika transmission dynamics in the midst of co-occurring epidemic and earthquake.

to be triggered during a prolonged period of strong aftershocks that lasted for months (Stewart-Ibarra et al., 2017).

In the immediate aftermath, the Machala team coordinated with the National Secretary of Risk and municipal government leaders in Machala, who were mobilizing humanitarian aid efforts for the communities affected in the north coast of Ecuador.[5] These relationships had been established as a result of a recent study that the team had conducted on flood risk in vulnerable peri-urban communities in Machala. The team (including the lab coordinator, project manager, Anna, her husband and driver) relocated from Machala to Bahía de Caráquez, a small city near the epicenter of the earthquake in Manabi Province. There were strong aftershocks and insecurity in the streets. At that point, two days after the earthquake, they assisted local public health professionals collect survey data on injury and damages. A school then invited them to establish a makeshift clinic in a classroom and they worked with Ministry of Health physicians and others to provide medical care to > 100 people per day, creating a functional pharmacy. They also coordinated the flood of donations of medications and supplies, including with donors and the US embassy. They distributed hundreds of gallons of drinking water, which had been sent from Quito by other scientist collaborators. As the efforts turned from short to long term, under the supervision of local ministry officials, the team collaborated with clinicians and government field teams to visit affected communities to provide primary health care and to collect more detailed health data that would aid in the relief effort (Figure 6.1).

After the earthquake, the Ministry of Health reported an increase of Zika cases, as well as Dengue and Chikungunya, as people faced increased exposure to *Aedes aegypti* due to inadequate shelter and increased water storage (Ortiz et al., 2017; Sorensen et al., 2017; Vasquez et al., 2017). The total number of ZIKV cases in

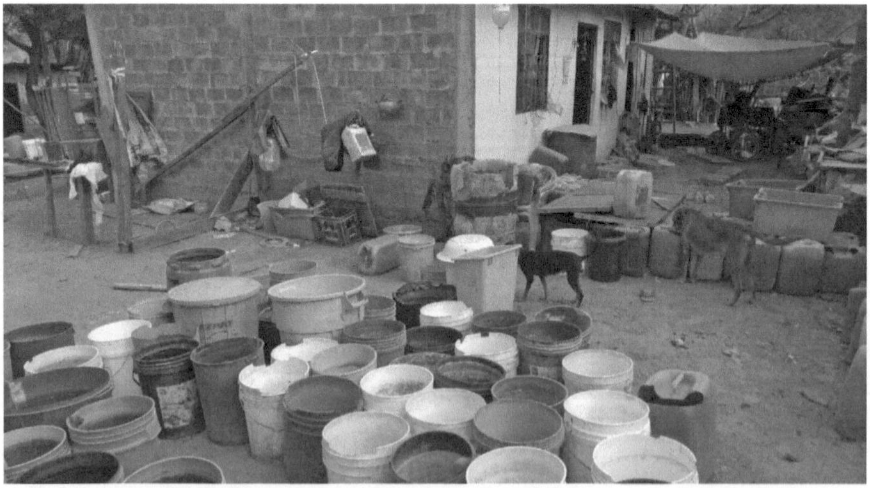

Figure 6.1 Water storage around homes in Bella Vista, Manabi Province, Ecuador in the months following the earthquake (Photo credit: A. Stewart).

Ecuador surged from 103 to 1,275 cases between epidemiological weeks 14 to 25 in 2016, in the aftermath of the earthquake. The majority (85%) of all cases in 2016 were reported from Manabí Province, near the epicenter. With Anna's team already working at the heart of the destruction, the ZIKV outbreak could be documented and explored in detail (Stewart-Ibarra et al., 2017). The team's ability to contribute to a coordinated earthquake response was the product of the interpersonal relationships and embedded commitments that emerged after a decade of local research and capacity strengthening. The temporary re-allocation of research resources towards recovery efforts reflected an overall agility that allowed for flexible shifts of focus and repositioning relative to specific on-the-ground needs and opportunities (Domachowske, et al. 2017). It also blurred the line between research, systems strengthening and humanitarian assistance.

The emergence of a global health partnership

The first major extramural grant project, begun in 2013 and funded by the Global Emerging Infections Surveillance and Response Program, was entitled "Capacity Strengthening in Ecuador: Partnering to Improve Surveillance of Febrile Vector-Borne Diseases" and was focused on the then-emerging threat of Dengue (Stewart-Ibarra et al., 2018). Scientifically, it established a passive and active surveillance system for Dengue infections in Machala, based on protocols developed in Thailand (Thomas et al. 2015). Working with a network of four sentinel clinics and the central hospital of the Ministry of Health, the team recruited study subjects who were clinically diagnosed with Dengue and visited their homes, as well as four neighbouring homes in each cardinal direction within a 200-meter radius. They visited these neighbours, and conducted clinical and household surveys and collected blood and adult mosquitoes in and around the home, that were later tested for viruses. The team was able to leverage other funding (in this case a study funded by the Ecuadorian government) and connect this epidemiological data to a network of automatic weather stations that had been installed by INAMHI across Machala.[6] Social-ecological information gathered at the household level allowed the team to analyze risk factors and link them to climatic data.

As global health embraces an equity focus, considerable efforts have been made to address the fact that local health researchers and academic institutions are often underrepresented or excluded entirely from health research projects (Adam et al., 2011). As Crane (2013) argued in her book *Scrambling for Africa: AIDS, Expertise and the Rise of American Science*, health research partnerships can come with major imbalances and power dynamics, for example, represented in the low indirect cost reimbursements from foreign US grants and high bureaucratic overheads, structures and expenses. As Musolino et al. (2015) summarized:

> Low-income and middle-income countries (LIMCs) lag behind in their ability to sufficiently reap the benefits from research and innovation partnerships for systems building, capacity strengthening, and economic growth ... global health research is not merely about global health but also about reinforcement

> of economic activity, research competitiveness, employment, and growth – a benefit package that today appears to stream more into high-income countries than into LMICs.

Equitable research partnerships involve, among other things, strengthening the capacity of local labs and universities (Larkan et al., 2016; Vasquez et al., 2013) and, as noted by Munung, Mayosi, and de Vries (2017), increasing access to training unavailable in country, support for research ethics systems, establishing research infrastructure and increasing access to funding and leadership positions. The Machala partnership has attempted to address many of these conventional critiques, although often in an organic, unscripted way: through trainings for researchers and public health practitioners (on research integrity and bioethics, geospatial analyses for public health and Dengue research), formal university collaborations, international training for local staff and research infrastructure development at the university and public hospital.

For example, the original 2013 project was presented directly to the Minister of Health for her approval, but the team spent an additional eight months going back and forth between Ecuadorian and US Institutional Review Board (IRB) committees before the protocol was approved. This process required patience and persistence to include the priorities and feedback of all parties. All of this was further complicated by the fact that the Ecuadorian government had recently established national norms for IRB committees and regulated human subject research. The Machala team did two things. First, in order to avoid lengthy revisions, they developed the habitat of designing protocols with local experts from UTMach but also members from the Ministry of Health in vector control, health promotion and epidemiology. This collaborative approach built shared values and purpose but also: (1) generated additional scientific knowledge in the form of access to local statistics and data of disease burden; (2) built capacity and networks by organizing meetings with local authorities; and (3) helped create legitimacy and visibility for implementation. By bringing a diverse number of Ecuadorian government and academic researchers into the scientific process, the team also included these key individuals as co-authors on multiple publications, creating soft incentives and motivations. Secondly, the team organized national-level workshops on bioethics, research integrity and regulatory considerations for human subject research, with participation by the senior leadership of the Ministry of Health, local universities and SUNY Upstate, including the directors of the Upstate IRB and research integrity committees. The trainings were conducted in Machala and the two largest cities of Ecuador (Guayaquil and Quito) over two years, with hundreds of participants from local universities and the public health sector.[7] Currently, an Ecuadorian member of the Machala research team is spearheading efforts to establish an IRB at UTMach.

This support and capacity building for research ethics was never an explicit part of any large and significant grant. Rather, it grew naturally from collegial discussions, meetings, casual conversations and a desire to be helpful and respond to emergent social expectations of a burgeoning partnership network. It was an act of solidarity. Within the 40-page protocol of the original study that outlined the study background, methods, potential risks, data assessment, there was a one-page section on *capacity strengthening*. It read:

> By strengthening the capacity of operative personnel of the MoH researchers, doctors, and students in the different steps of diagnostics, surveillance and control of vector borne diseases, the quality of surveillance information will improve, allowing for a more efficient response by the public health sector.

Although this objective represented a minor component of the formal IRB protocol, and of the total budget, it was a key part of the informal objectives of the team. To meet this objective the investigators also focused on university training, including an exchange program for health professionals, providing educational opportunities for local MoH field personnel, UTMach students and faculty, and regional researchers. These efforts represented capacity building as a necessary investment, and even by-product, to conducting high-quality longitudinal research that responded to local health priorities. Unlike the efforts of Sanchez et al. (2013) to strengthen infectious disease capacity through a formalized research-based graduate program at the National Autonomous University of Honduras, these efforts focused on mobilizing research resources to increase training opportunities.

SUNY Upstate's growing bond with UTMach and the MoH represented a mutual "win-win" relationship, especially as the university system in Ecuador was undergoing reform to increase research standards and greater emphasis on publications and international collaboration. In 2013, in preparation for the surveillance study, a basic clinical laboratory was set up in the MoH central hospital. Having a proper physical space in a shared setting made the team more visible and allowed for easier interactions and communication between the research team and MoH members. Starting in 2015, and continuing the following year, the project acquired space within UTMach including land to construct entomological huts to run semi-field trials, administrative offices, a laboratory to process mosquito samples and another space to grow adult mosquitos and conduct insecticide-resistant assays. In addition to the physical infrastructure growth, the team began to take on various student-interns to work for periods of two to eight weeks. Ecuadorian professors from the School of Medicine became increasingly active participants in mentoring both Ecuadorian and international medical students.

Like any healthy relationship, the costs and benefits flow two ways. The project accepted UTMach students to complete research practicum hours by conducting a combination of work in the field or labs, depending on requirements for their degrees; these volunteers were often hired by the team post-graduation. In fact, this process led to most project staff (there were five staff in 2018) being graduates from UTMach with most staff supported to pursue part-time Master's degrees. These graduates were attracted by the opportunity to work for an international research group, participate in a unique field of work with flexible and dynamic work expectations, and build their personal resumes. And it led to continuity in the team, allowing new projects to be informed by previous ones. Administrative offices and experimental huts for mosquito experiments were located in the School of Medicine at UTMach while entomology labs were located in the School of Chemical Sciences and Health, which increased access to faculty and students. In 2016, UTMach improved its national accreditation rating, in part due to increasing lab infrastructure, international collaborations and a strong publication record (all of which the *Aedes* research team was involved with), raising their profile and capacity to train students in research. The team also developed working relationships with universities in Quito and Guayaquil, expanding their capacity to conduct molecular analyzes of arboviruses in human and mosquito specimens in the country.

Urban Machala: Science landscapes and the social determinants of health

The science of the SUNY-Machala group, begun in 2007, has provided some of the most comprehensive social-ecological epidemiological investigations of *Aedes aegypti* transmitted diseases in the Americas. But this work depends on another set of infrastructures: fieldworkers and community members, operating in the physical landscape of Machala. Science is connected to the city (Figure 6.2).

As noted earlier, Machala is Ecuador's fourth largest city. It is off the beaten path, and one rarely sees any foreign tourists, or vacationing Ecuadoreans, there. Rather, it is a place known for its economic productivity due to agriculture and mining. The "banana capital of the world" sits on top of mangroves, and floods

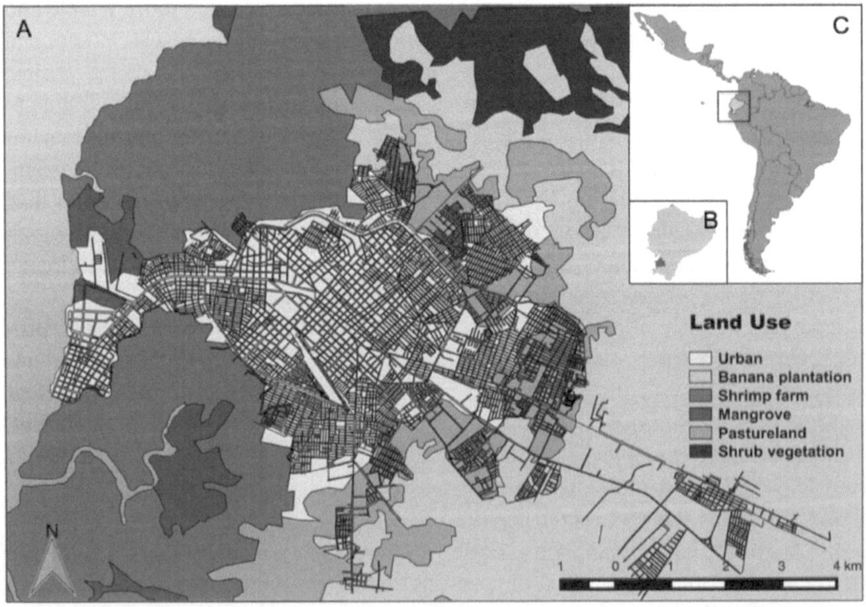

Figure 6.2 A map showing land use and land cover around the city of Machala (from Lowe et al. 2017 *The Lancet Planetary Health*).

annually with high tides and rains. Close to the border with Peru, it is a bustling city but with a small-town feeling about it, somewhat of a backwater. Why would you go to Machala, people ask?

The identity of Machala, however, has had important influence on the success of the research program. Historically, Machala is a place with limited scientific research, at least by academics. Unlike the larger cities in Ecuador, where scientists may look down their noses at vector control staff muddling through in the community, Machala's off-the-beaten-path culture contributes to a small town pride and, with the public health collaborators of the research group, a "can do attitude." It was this proclivity, to work hard with limited resources, that first cemented the chemistry between Machala public health leaders and Anna in 2010.

There are stark contrasts in social conditions in Machala, with wealthier families living in gated communities and low-income young families concentrated in the urban periphery, which lacks adequate sanitation. In the 2010 census, one-quarter of households lacked access to paved streets or sewerage, and one-third lack piped water inside the home (Stewart Ibarra et al. 2014b). Although Dengue, Chikungunya and Zika infect rich and poor alike, sickness has a greater impact on low-income families, due to lost wages and other costs associated with caring for the sick. Machala is a growing city, having officially added nearly 40,000 residents from 2010 to 2018, to 280,000 people. With the economic boom of the mid-2000s, the municipal government began ambitious urban renewal and gentrification in the city center, but national budgets were cut in 2015 following the decline in oil prices (which corresponded with a Chikungunya epidemic) reducing investments in infrastructure.

The early work of the research team investigated these social and ecological factors in relation to Dengue fever. Statistical modeling studies provided the first evidence that Dengue epidemics were associated with extreme climate events (El Niño) that resulted in warmer, rainier conditions (Stewart Ibarra and Lowe 2013). They found that rainfall did not affect *Aedes aegypti* abundance in all communities, due to differences in mosquito larval habitats (rain-filled abandoned containers vs. tap-water-filled domestic use containers) associated with differential access to piped water in the home (Stewart Ibarra et al. 2013). Studies showed that Dengue risk was unequally distributed across the community and the city. Entomological surveys revealed that 5–11% of homes contained 80% of mosquito pupae, posing a threat to neighboring homes (Stewart Ibarra et al. 2013). Using spatial analyses, they found that neighborhoods with high Dengue incidence were clustered, creating hotspots of transmission (Stewart Ibarra et al. 2014a). Using qualitative methods, the team found that local perceptions of Dengue involved a range of interrelated biophysical, political-institutional and community elements (Figure 6.3). People indicated that the lack of inter-institutional coordination and lack of social cohesion limited their ability to control Dengue.

The cooperation of community members can mean the success or failure of projects that seek to invade homes in search of mosquitoes, human blood, intimate health information or efforts to change human behavior and test the efficacy of new disease control strategies. These activities rely on trust and commitment on

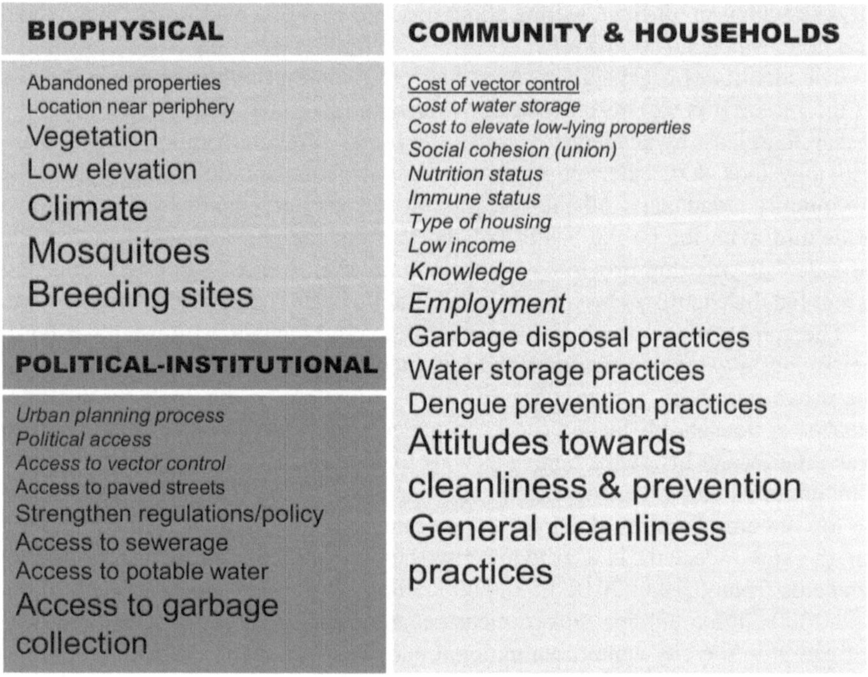

Figure 6.3 Key themes identified by periurban and central community members asked about Dengue risk factors in their neighbourhood. Text size indicates the importance of the theme (e.g., themes mentioned in more focus groups are larger). Themes in italics were identified only in the periurban community. Themes underlined were identified only in the central community (from Stewart Ibarra, et al. 2014 *BMC Public Health*).

behalf of community members who may otherwise feel that they have very little to gain from these efforts.

Community activities in the first large-scale internationally funded project, begun in 2013, were certainly influenced by the impact of the 2010 Dengue epidemic. Machala was hard hit by the largest Dengue epidemic on record in El Oro province. The Machala research team collaborated with local leaders and stakeholders (health promoters, neighborhood presidents, school principals and vector control fumigators) who advocated for the interests and needs of their communities.[8] The team organized educational meetings with community leaders, which allowed MoH staff to hear community concerns and voices. On the tail end of an epidemic, everyone was interested. Since then, the team has continued to emphasize building community buy-in and trust, which has included health outreach events and dialogues between communities, UTMach and the health sector.

People were interested in participating in these initial surveillance studies because they could be diagnosed and have same-day results, using rapid Dengue tests that were not available at MoH labs. The investigation included visiting neighbors, taking blood samples from them and alerting them to Dengue infections in their locality. Risk was seen, and discussed, as real and nearby. However, this level of community interest has not been the same with the cohort study, begun in 2016 and funded by the NSF Zika Rapid grant. This study takes blood from healthy volunteers and, due to challenges with diagnostics, has not been able to deliver rapid test results for Zika and Chikungunya. While the team conducted community meetings and talks in an engagement campaign, the lack of rapid test results has been a barrier to community interest and participation since molecular diagnostic (PCR) capabilities are not currently present in Machala.

Some elements of community inclusion took place on a more personal level. As part of any data collection, community members want to feel that their voices are heard and their humanity recognized, that they are treated not simply as sources of biological samples. However, this can be no easy task, especially when the field team is required to visit multiple homes in one morning. The cohort study required longitudinal visits to the same homes over a 3 year period. Interpersonal relationships between the field technicians and household members require energy, patience and time. This presented a conflict of priorities for field technicians attempting to build lasting relationships while managing multiple responsibilities and under pressure to meet data-gathering goals. These concerns came about during the weekly team meetings and the local team decided to decrease the number of households visited each day, and to allow more time at each home to converse. This gave participants the opportunity to better engage with the research processes, asking personal or project-related questions or enabling teaching opportunities about the spread of Dengue or habits of the *Aedes*

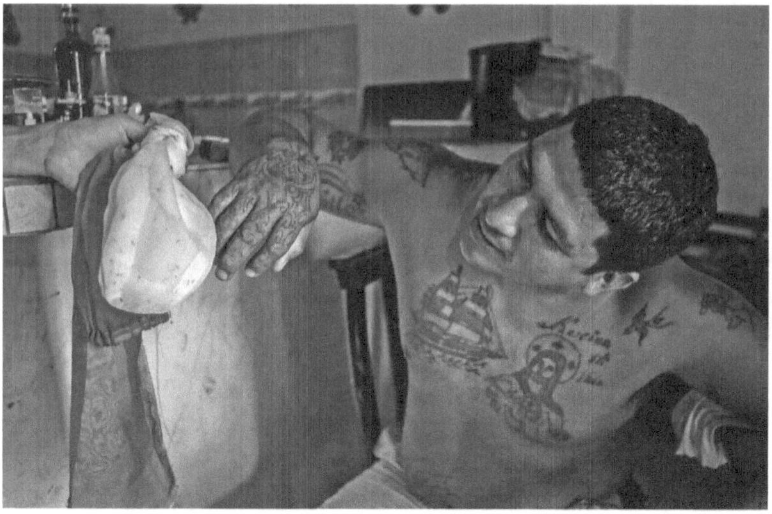

Figure 6.4 Local community member examining mosquitoes captured in their home, Ecuador (Photo credit: Dany Krom).

aegypti mosquito. For example, after aspirating mosquitoes, field technicians then had more time to show the captured mosquitoes and teach families to distinguish *Aedes aegypti* mosquitos (with their black-and-white striped legs and abdomen) from *Culex* and other species (see Figure 6.4). Friendly banter, including talking about changes in the city infrastructure and recent events, were important. Fieldworkers would frequently be invited for fresh tropical fruit or, if they were lucky, a shrimp ceviche. All of this likely increased the rate of retention of households participating in long term studies, and retention of field staff.

At the city level, the team has daily interactions with government employees as they share offices with ministry officials working on vector-borne illness. The local head of vector control in Machala likewise has been an active participant in several research projects and was included on multiple publications. However, there have been important limitations in the translation of the research into better vector control operations. The lack of vector control capacity in Machala is due to historical and policy decisions. As with other countries in the region, vertical and centralized vector control departments had been first established by the Rockefeller Foundation in the 1950s as part of malaria and yellow fever eradication efforts. These top-down programs operated somewhat independently from the MoH. While other countries, like Peru, had disbanded them in the 1990s, Ecuador did so only in 2015, integrating (in principle) vector control into primary health care systems and local municipal government. The rationale for the restructuring of vector control processes often centered on eliminating corruption and reducing the budget. What has happened in practice is that vector control faces serious capacity limitations (vehicles, field staff, materials and supplies), and medical entomological capacity has all but withered.

Soft money, hard problems

Maintaining the research activities in Machala is a constant balancing act. Difficulties, of course, come in many shapes and sizes but have included the central issue of juggling financial resources through a patchwork of projects from diverse funding sources, primarily from SUNY Upstate investigators.[9] The team has struggled to create a sustainable funding model in Machala. This has pushed the team to be nimble and able to respond to new funding opportunities, allowing the team to grow despite a tough environment for scientific funding. Efforts have been made to diversify funding, with periodic visits from SUNY investigators and international collaborators to the area, and a new ongoing pediatric respiratory study, which has helped to formalize the institutional collaboration between SUNY Upstate and UTMach. SUNY has also provided vital funding to fill gaps at critical points.

These grants have not, however, included covering the salaries of key collaborators at UTMach and the Ministry of Health – their efforts are considered in-kind contributions of the projects. Instead, extramural funds are effectively managed by a local community health NGO that supports the collaboration and research. These funds support UTMach and the MoH by covering the costs of training students and technicians, purchasing materials and research infrastructure that end up at the university and public hospital, such as the entomology laboratory and clinical research laboratory. In addition, the way the university system is set up prevents faculty from recovering their salary from grants and the local university is not currently set up to receive US federal grant dollars, although research visibility has now become a prerequisite for promotion. The MoH and UTMach have provided critical support such as laboratory space, student trainees, expert collaborators, access to data, and hosting annual research symposia. In this model, all institutions and collaborators bring valuable resources and expertise to the collaboration as equal parties.

The incentives, then, for UTMach staff center on knowledge exchanges, skills development, trainings, networks, publications and impact on their local communities. Many collaborators in Machala have a life-long commitment to community service, and the fact that the scientific work facilitates and strengthens academic-government-community relations is also seen as important.[10] In addition, the grants have provided faculty with the opportunity to present at and participate in relevant workshops, meetings and travel opportunities in the country, and collaborative conference and publication costs are paid for by the grants.

While funding grants have overlapped in many cases, current funding mechanisms designed to respond to specific diseases, epidemics and research questions do not facilitate the long-term maintenance of a vector-borne disease research and surveillance infrastructure, or of the capacity strengthening activities described earlier. Research and infrastructure has been entirely dependent on *soft money* and voluntary contributions by local partners (e.g., laboratory space at no cost).

While epidemics like Zika, and their surging public health fears, can be mobilized to support research and build capacity in places like Machala, this infrastructure is precarious and may crumble as fears and priorities recede. In 2016, in part as a result of the long-term presence of the SUNY team, Machala was chosen as one of the sites for an experimental Zika vaccine trial sponsored by the US National Institutes of Health (NIH).[11] This phase 2/2B multisite study was rolled out across Latin America and Caribbean to the evaluate the safety, efficacy and immunogenicity of the DNA vaccine in healthy adults. In order to enable this clinical trial to move forward, the team utilized their networks to approach national level MoH staff to facilitate formal support from the Ecuadorian government. The involvement of key ministry officials on past projects and publications facilitated buy-in on this clinical trial, and these leaders skillfully brought together key stakeholders at local universities and hospitals, such as Hospital Teofilo Davila, the provincial hospital in Machala. The SUNY team and UTMachala collaborators spent a year preparing for the clinical trial, a first to be conducted in the El Oro region and the first by the NIH in the Ecuador. In this context, the labour of science involved hiring and training six local staff and associate investigators (AIs) in clinical research coordination, recruitment, sample collection, data entry and data storage; renovating a new space adjacent to the hospital with new equipment for sample processing, storage and patient intake; and reexamining Ecuador's research approval structures to enable an international clinical trial to take place, given new regulatory frameworks. The site was reviewed in June 2018 by the National Agency for Health Regulation, Control and Surveillance (ARCSA), the

Ecuadorian equivalent of the FDA, and became the only site in Ecuador at that time with approval to do clinical trials.

However, all of this was on a strict time limit. Cases of Zika were rapidly diminishing, which meant that enrolling patients in the trial would be increasingly difficult. The study team knew there was a risk the NIH would pull funding once case numbers reduced to a certain threshold. But the team kept working for about one year in total. At the time, the hope was that this study would not only provide solid funding for a few years but that once the group had conducted its first NIH trial other studies and funding would follow. However, within one week of the projected start of study enrollment, the NIH canceled funding, which would have fully sustained the site for at least two years. This was a major setback for the team, highlight the fickle nature of soft funding for international research programs. However, SUNY stepped in and committed to support the team and site. UTMach and the MoH were unwavering in their commitments. This institutional stability was crucial to sustain the team. Today, the group has weathered this wave in funding, and have successfully received several grants that support ongoing research.

Policy and science: Impacting vector control in an era of climate change?

The need for researchers in the global south to produce locally relevant policy recommendations has been a key justification for health research capacity strengthening (Brownson, et al. 2009). The divide between science and policy also contributes to undervaluation of research at a national level, perpetuating gaps in funding by national governments. Within epidemiology and medical entomology, these problems are especially acute. Routine data collection and analysis emerging from government vector control department are often weak and fragmented, while scientific colleagues gear their labour and attention towards academic audiences. From the beginning, then, the goal of the Machala team was to generate good science, but good science that connected to capacity building and policy change. In this last section, we ask: what types of "impact" have emerged from this scientific labour?

In Ecuador, as in many countries, health policy is frequently created in a top-down, highly vertical manner, which makes researchers dependent on national ministries of health or environment, rather than local or regional offices. Despite the decentralization of vector control programs, there remains a rigid hierarchy that defines and structures budgets, personnel and activities. High-level changes require high-level connections. But in Ecuador, as elsewhere in Latin America, frequent changes in administrative staff at the national level limited efforts to form strong, sustained relationships with this policy world.

Nonetheless, the Machala team tried to build these relationships. An important shift occurred in national political culture that favored investment in science and technology with the election of the Ecuadorian president Rafael Correa in 2007, who was part of a wave of leftist governments in the region that included Hugo Chavez and Evo Morales. Correa's relatively long presidency (2007–2017) provided sufficient political stability to strengthen governmental organizations, after many years of short-lived presidents, political coups and economic crises (the flip side of this is that he rapidly grew the government; massive corruption scandals are now hot news topics in 2018). All of this brought increased prioritization of biomedical research and evidence-based policy, partially framed as a way to shift the base of the economy away from primary production and export (e.g., oil, bananas, shrimp, coffee). The Ecuadorian government began placing greater emphasis on research and higher education, establishing SENESCYT (National Secretary of Higher Education, Science, Technology and Innovation) in 2010, which is the equivalent of the US NIH and/or NSF. As a new agency, and for the first time, substantial funding for academic research and international scholarships were available between 2011 and 2015, until oil prices crashed and reduced government coffers.[12] This favorable political context, with respect to academic research, also helped the research program to become established and grow Machala.

In forming connections, the Machala and SUNY team recognized that there was frequent movement between the worlds of academic health research and health policy-making. By co-developing and co-implementing research studies with public health practitioners and local researchers the research team was able to create connections to future policy leaders, who were then presented with research created by colleagues they knew and trusted. These connections were also created through local forums, workshops and consultative meetings where the Machala team presented information in an easily understandable, digestible and usable format. The team crafted Spanish-language data narratives, drafting presentations and creating policy briefs. These focused on the effects of climate on Dengue risk, such as increased risk of epidemics during El Niño events. As another example, in 2016, the team organized a symposium in at UTMach where research posters that had been presented at international academic conferences were translated by SUNY student interns into Spanish for local researchers and public health practitioners in Machala.

One of the ultimate scientific goals of the Machala work was to generate the scientific data to develop an early warning system, or seasonal forecasts, for Dengue, thereby contributing to climate change adaptation measures to mitigate disease (Lowe et al., 2017). This was seen as a tangible way for the climate-health research to be applied and picked up in the policy world. To date, weather and climate information are rarely used to inform public health decisions in Ecuador, or more generally in Latin America and the Caribbean. As a first step, the research found clear connections between climate and Dengue, with El Niño events increasing the possibility of Dengue outbreaks. Surveillance studies showed that the burden of Dengue was higher than previously thought. For every Dengue case captured by a MoH clinic, there were an additional three cases in the community. These studies also found that Dengue virus in Machala was related to virus strains in neighboring countries, highlighting the role of human movement in the region in the spread of disease.[13]

Despite these advances, weather and climate information are rarely used to inform public health decisions in Ecuador, or more generally in Latin America and the Caribbean. The Machala team is applying the Global Framework for Climate Services (GFCS) for public health and has developed data collection with an eye to creating operational disease forecasts that consider climate and non-climate factors to predict disease outbreaks. These forecasts would form part of an epidemic early warning system (EWS). When a certain threshold is passed, an alert would be issued, triggering a sequence of predetermined actions to prevent the outbreak. If an EWS were developed, the public health sector would be able to make informed decisions about the allocation of scarce resources, such as personnel, and could begin alerting and mobilizing healthcare providers and local communities to take preventative actions and to identify the first cases of an outbreak. Actions include preventative vector control, education campaigns, retraining of medical personnel and purchasing of diagnostic supplies. In 2016, the team generated the first successful Dengue forecast, which correctly predicted an early Dengue following a specific heavy rainfall and flooding event (Lowe et al. 2017). The team is currently working to scale this up to the national level.

Although an early warning system has not yet arrived, the science in Machala has led to the group being invited to key national and international policy meetings and authoring the climate and health section of a policy report for the Ecuadorian government. It has raised the profile in national policy discussions, and opened the conversation about the siloed nature of policy decision making between sectors involved in health, including risks management, environmental control, housing development, water supply, sanitation, education, defense and others. By emphasizing the importance of local social factors in high-risk zones of disease transmission, the team attempted to make visible to policy-makers the ways that disease risk can be socially determined. Climate change consequences are not equally distributed across society. Members of the team were co-authors on the National Communications of Ecuador for the UN Convention on Climate Change, providing a Spanish-language synthesis of policy-oriented findings on climate and health.

Importantly, this scientific work has not changed day-to-day vector control operations or, really, controlled Dengue fever in Machala.[14] Rather, the impact of this scientific labour has been on strengthening a *culture of science* in Machala, of strengthening the scientific gaze in the collection, analysis and reporting of data. This has included data rescue, where historical MoH data has been cleaned and re-analyzed. It has included a general increase in the people's appreciation of the value of science in the public sector and significant influence on student experiences and career paths. And it has included raising the profile of MoH staff, who can now present their data locally and nationally. In short, public health staff have become more like scientists (and scientists more like public health staff). Let us end on an example: the political crisis in Venezuela led to a large influx of refugees in Machala in 2018 and worries about the importation of malaria, which has increased significantly in Venezuela in recent years. A number of imported and locally acquired malaria cases were confirmed in Ecuador-Peru border region, where a large number of people transit each day. The head of epidemiology in Machala, motivated by a writing workshop organized by the MoH, drafted a scientific paper on these cases in collaboration with the SUNY team, which has helped to raise the profile of the issue at a national level (Jaramillo-Ochoa et al. 2019). Slowly, so the hope is, scientific collaboration can promote evidence-based decision-making.

Discussion and conclusions

This chapter has meandered around various corners of global health that are all too often invisible to the end products of science but so essential to their success and inner workings. One of our goals was to move beyond the pretention that scholarship is divorced from the social contexts in which it operates, and that engaged global health science needs to think more about the labour of epidemiology in the real world, especially if we are to confront the challenges of climate change, urbanization and an increasingly globalized world. At the same time, we need to remain self-conscious and critical of the ways that these relationships can reproduce or undermine existing power structures. Scientists who hope to have an impact on society have the opportunity (and perhaps the responsibility) to expand the scope of impact of their research though capacity building at multiple levels. This is the informality of global health labour so important to making science relevant in cities like Machala.

Building a global health partnership around *Aedes agypti* and climate change demands navigating problems of money, priority and care in response to changing circumstances. Activities that depend on soft money engage with hard problems. Infrastructures, both physical and relational, bring with them the ability to respond to new diseases, to conduct innovative scientific research, after an earthquake or in the midst of an epidemic. The visible depends on the invisible labour of these groups, of global health scientists working – networking, writing and *lots* of traveling – in ways that are often unseen and unacknowledged.

This chapter has attempted to demonstrate the ways that long-term relationships, both formal and informal, may be productively established so that they are in place when a critical new crisis, like Zika, emerges. It likewise has attempted to highlight some of the ways that local capacity surrounding climate change and health research may be built in this context even without dedicated funding, again using informal relationships to transfer knowledge and skills and build institutional research strength. As the chapter has attempted to demonstrate, these informal actions are of vital importance in the creation of a robust research response to emerging pathogens in an era of climate change and urbanization. They are likewise vital in efforts to help local and national governments to grapple with the dynamic and expanding health threats wrought by climate change in a hotter, wetter and more urban world.

Notes

1 The first reported cases of Zika virus (ZIKV) infection in Ecuador were documented on 15 January 2016. By the end of 2017, a total of 912 cases of ZIKV in pregnant women had been confirmed, and there had been 15 cases of microcephaly associated with ZIKV and one case of *malformacion congenita* without microcephaly. As of the end of 2017, two neonatal deaths were associated with ZIKV, and there has also been

one case of encephalitis and two cases of Guillain Barre reported (Pan American Health Organization, 2017). The virus has since spread widely across the country, with distribution varying by region but remaining concentrated along coastal areas.

2 Epidemiological studies since then have continued to show that children bear the greatest burden of Dengue in the city.

3 There is very little funding available to SNEM to do community mobilization and education, despite PAHO and national policies promoting this approach.

4 See https://www.usaid.gov/sites/default/files/documents/1866/ecuador_eq_fs05_05-06-2016.pdf

5 These relationships were formed as part of a study (2014–2015) the team led on early warning systems for flooding and community responses in Machala, funded by the InterAmerican Institute for Global Change Research (IAI). This resulted in a strong partnership with the National Secretary of Risk and the municipal government of Machala. A major flood occurred in Machala in February 2016, which in some ways prepared the team to respond to the earthquake two months later.

6 The research group was awarded a national Ecuadorian grant for the project "Modeling of Climate and Dengue in Ecuador" (CLIDEN), funded by the Secretaria de Educación Superior, Ciencia, Tecnología e Innovación (SENECYT). As part of this project, the Instituto Nacional de Meteorología e Hidrología of Ecuador (INAMHI) assisted with the sophisticated sensor system to study the impact of climate on health. Machala was the first city in Ecuador with such a system.

7 Travel for SUNY participants in the workshops was paid for by the Research Office of SUNY Upstate, some expenses were covered by the GEIS grant and other expenses were covered by local partners who hosted the trainings. We also held multi-day trainings in geospatial tools for the public health sector in Machala and Guayaquil, with around 100 participants from research and health sectors. The trainings were free for participants. We contracted GIS experts to develop and run the workshops using local health data and open source GIS software (QGIS). We paid for this using GEIS grant funding. These trainings showed our strong commitment to our partners in Ecuador. By holding the workshops in three major cities, we also got a lot of visibility and press attention.

8 Prior to beginning data collection in a new community, the team would hold public meetings with local leaders, local Ministry of Health employees and community members to explain the research design and the protocol. Initially we had thought to pay the community members a nominal fee, but the study team felt that this was not culturally appropriate. Amendments to research protocols were made to include a non-monetary compensation to thank volunteers for their participation. Instead of gifting based on researcher's perceptions of what might be valued, the team held community meetings and asked participants, "What type of gift would be most useful?" The top answers were health kits and educational materials (most likely because the start of the school year was just around the corner) and so the group prepared and passed out over 250 health kits and 150 educational kits. The team also made a strong commitment to ensure that individuals received the results of all diagnostic tests done as part of the study. The field team also requested that all families receive mosquito nets at the end of the study, because they felt that this was the best way to shown gratitude for their participation and to lower the risk of disease (our recent study in Machala showed that homes that used mosquito nets had lower risk of Dengue infections).

9 This has included funding from GEIS, NSF, Deployed Warfighters Protection program, CDC, Clinical Research Management (a private CRO), IAI and others. US students have received competitive research fellowships to spend two months in Machala conducting guided global health research. Sources include Rotary club, Kean Fellowships of ASTMH, Fulbright and SUNY student scholarships, among others.

10 For example, in 2017, the SUNY team, with UTMachala, conducted Geographical Information Systems (GIS) training in Machala and Guayaquil, with close to 100 participants, including individuals from the local MoH epidemiology and vector control

units, and university students and faculty. Another training took place in early 2017 with US Centers for Disease Control & Prevention (CDC) staff, on insecticide resistance to *Aedes aegypti* mosquitoes. Such types of symposiums and trainings, done often over the years on different subjects, are excellent venues to take pride in mutual growth and share results with a wider audience. UTMachala provides space and computers in various auditoriums, classrooms, or labs, and capitalizes on inviting investigators from SUNY Upstate, University of Florida, University of Colorado and other international schools as guest speakers for conferences and events. Such events and scientific networking has also helped create Ecuadorian collaborations, for example, between UTMachala and the Escuela Superior Politecnica del Litoral (ESPOL) in Guayaquil, and the Catholic University (PUCE) in Quito. As part of the Machala project an important collaboration was also developed with the Escuela Superior Politecnica del Litoral (ESPOL), in particular with Biomedicine Laboratory, considered a leading public research university in the country.

11 In 2015, the first Dengue vaccine (Dengvaxia) was licensed by Sanofi Pasteur; however, the vaccine has proven to be quite controversial, and was never licensed in Ecuador, due to its limited efficacy.

12 Through the PROMETEO fellowship program, hundreds of PhD researchers came to Ecuador to conduct research with local partners. Anna was a funded Prometeo fellow for almost two years.

13 This is especially important today with the crisis in Venezuela and the mass movement of Venezuelan refugees into Ecuador.

14 That said, some steps have recently been taken. Vector control in Machala is based on chemical control but recent work, funded by CDC's Zika budget through the Machala group, has shown high levels of resistance to malathion. This will hopefully change the government's procurement decisions. The group in Machala has also piloted a school education program and tested a novel mosquito control device, both strategies that may, in time, assist with control efforts in the city.

References

Adam, T., Ahmad, S., Bigdeli, M., Ghaffar, A., & Røttingen, J. A. 2011, 'Trends in health policy and systems research over the past decade: still too little capacity in low-income countries', *PloS one*, vol. 6, no. 11, pp. e27263.

Biruk, C. 2012, 'Seeing like a research project: producing "high-quality data" in AIDS research in Malawi', *Medical Anthropology*, vol. 31, no. 4, pp. 347–366.

Braks, M., van Ginkel, R., Wint, W., Sedda, L., & Sprong, H. 2013, 'Climate change and public health policy: translating the science', *International Journal of Environmental Research and Public Health*, vol. 11, no. 1, pp. 13–29.

Brisbois, B. W., & Ali, S. H. 2010, 'Climate change, vector-borne disease and interdisciplinary research: social science perspectives on an environment and health controversy', *EcoHealth*, vol. 7, no. 4, pp. 425–438.

Brownson, R. C., Chriqui, J. F., & Stamatakis, K. A. 2009, 'Understanding evidence-based public health policy', *American Journal of Public Health*, vol. 99, no. 9, pp. 1576–1583.

Crane, J. T. 2013, *Scrambling for Africa: AIDS, expertise, and the rise of American global health science*, Cornell University Press.

Crane, J. T., Andia Biraro, I., Fouad, T. M., Boum, Y., & R. Bangsberg, D. 2018, 'The 'indirect costs' of underfunding foreign partners in global health research: a case study', *Global Public Health*, vol. 13, no. 10, pp. 1422–1429.

Domachowske, J. B., Stewart-Ibarra, A. M., Domachowske, E. T., & Reddy-Asiago, E. A. 2017, 'Chapter 9 global health clinical competencies', in Danielle Laraque-Arena,

M.D., FAAP and Bonita Stanton, M.D. (eds.), *Principles of global child health: education and research*, 1st ed, FAAP, In press.

Janes, C. R., & Corbett, K. K. 2009, 'Anthropology and global health', *Annual Review of Anthropology*, vol. 38, pp. 167–183.

Jaramillo-Ochoa, R., Sippy, R., Farrell, D.F., Cueva Aponte, C., Beltran-Ayala, E., Gonzaga, J.L., Ordoñez-León, T., Quintana, F.A., Ryan, S.J., & Stewart-Ibarra, A.M. 2019, 'Effects of political instability in Venezuela on malaria resurgence at Ecuador–Peru border, 2018', *Emerging Infectious Diseases*, vol. 25, no. 4, pp. 834–836.

Judson, S. D., LeBreton, M., Fuller, T., Hoffman, R. M., Njabo, K., Brewer, T.F., et al. 2018, 'Translating predictions of zoonotic viruses for policymakers', *EcoHealth*, vol. 15, no. 1, pp. 52–62.

Lakoff, A. 2017, *Unprepared global health in a time of emergency*, University of California Press, Oakland, CA.

Larkan, F., Uduma, O., Lawal, S. A., & van Bavel, B. 2016, 'Developing a framework for successful research partnerships in global health', *Globalization and Health*, vol. 12, no. 1, pp. 17.

Leach, M., & Scoones, I. 2013, 'The social and political lives of zoonotic disease models: narratives, science and policy', *Social Science & Medicine*, vol. 88, pp. 10–17.

Lowe, R., Stewart-Ibarra, A. M., Petrova, D., García-Díez, M., Borbor-Cordova, M. J., Mejía, R., et al. 2017, 'Climate services for health: predicting the evolution of the 2016 dengue season in Machala, Ecuador', *The Lancet Planetary Health*, vol. 1, no. 4, pp. e142–e151.

Maes, K., & Kalofonos, I. 2013, 'Becoming and remaining community health workers: perspectives from Ethiopia and Mozambique', *Social Science & Medicine*, vol. 87, pp. 52–59.

McMichael, A. 2015, 'Climate change and public health', in Levy, B., & Patz, J. (eds.), *A widening research agenda: challenges and needs*. Oxford University Press.

Munung, N. S., Mayosi, B. M., & de Vries, J. 2017, 'Equity in international health research collaborations in Africa: perceptions and expectations of African researchers', *PloS One*, vol. 12, no. 10, pp. e0186237.

Musolino, N., Lazdins, J., Toohey, J., & IJsselmuiden, C. 2015, COHRED Fairness Index for international collaborative partnerships. *The Lancet*, vol. 385, no. 9975, pp. 1293–1294.

Ortiz M. R., Le, N. K., Sharma, V., Hoare, I., Quizhpe, E, Teran, E., et al. 2017, 'Post-earthquake Zika virus surge: disaster and public health threat amid climatic conduciveness', *Scientific Reports*, vol. 7, no. 1, pp. 15408.

Sanchez, A. L., Canales, M., Enriquez, L., Bottazzi, M. E., Zelaya, A. A., Espinoza, V. E., et al. 2013, 'A research capacity strengthening project for infectious diseases in Honduras: experience and lessons learned', *Global Health Action*, vol. 6, no. 1, pp. 21643.

Sorensen, C. J., Borbor-Cordova, M. J., Calvello-Hynes, E., Diaz, A., Lemery, J., & Stewart-Ibarra, A. M. 2017, 'Climate variability, vulnerability, and natural disasters: a case study of Zika virus in Manabi, Ecuador following the 2016 earthquake', *GeoHealth*, vol. 1, no. 8, pp. 298–304.

Stewart-Ibarra, A. M., Hargrave, A., Diaz, A., Kenneson, A., Madden, D., Romero, M., et al. 2017, 'Psychological distress and Zika, Dengue and Chikungunya symptoms following the 2016 earthquake in Bahía de Caráquez, Ecuador', *International Journal of Environmental Research and Public Health*, vol. 14, no. 12, pp. 1516.

Stewart-Ibarra, A. M., & Lowe, R. 2013, 'Climate and non-climate drivers of dengue epidemics in southern coastal Ecuador', *The American Journal of Tropical Medicine and Hygiene*, vol. 88, no. 5, pp. 971–981.

Stewart-Ibarra, A. M., Luzadis, V. A., Borbor-Cordova, M. J., Silva, M., Ordoñez, T., Ayala, E. B., et al. 2014a, 'A social-ecological analysis of community perceptions of dengue fever and Aedes aegypti in Machala, Ecuador', *BMC Public Health*, vol. 14, no. 1, pp. 1135.

Stewart-Ibarra, A. M., Muñoz, Á. G., Ryan, S. J., Ayala, E. B., Borbor-Cordova, M. J., Finkelstein, J. L., et al. 2014b, 'Spatiotemporal clustering, climate periodicity, and social-ecological risk factors for dengue during an outbreak in Machala, Ecuador, in 2010', *BMC Infectious Diseases*, vol. 14, no. 1, pp. 610.

Stewart- Ibarra, A. M., Ryan, S. J., Beltrán, E., Mejía, R., Silva, M., Muñoz, Á. 2013, 'Dengue vector dynamics (Aedes aegypti) influenced by climate and social factors in ecuador: implications for targeted control,' *Plos One*, vol. 8, no. 11, pp. e78263.

Stewart-Ibarra, A. M., Ryan, S. J., Kenneson, A., King, C. A., Abbott, M., Barbachano-Guerrero, A., et al. 2018, 'The burden of dengue fever and chikungunya in southern coastal Ecuador: epidemiology, clinical presentation, and phylogenetics from the first two years of a prospective study', *The American Journal of Tropical Medicine and Hygiene*, vol. 98, no. 5, pp. 1444–1459.

Thomas, S. J., Aldstadt, J., Jarman, R. G., Buddhari, D., Yoon, I. K., Richardson, J. H., et al. 2015, 'Improving dengue virus capture rates in humans and vectors in Kamphaeng Phet Province, Thailand, using an enhanced spatiotemporal surveillance strategy', *The American Journal of Tropical Medicine and Hygiene*, vol. 93, no. 1, pp. 24–32.

Vasquez, D., Palacio, A., Nuñez, J., Briones, W., Beier, J. C., Pareja, D. C., et al. 2017, 'Impact of the 2016 Ecuador earthquake on Zika virus cases', *American Journal of Public Health*, vol. 107, no. 7, pp. 1137–1142.

Vasquez, E. E., Hirsch, J. S., Giang, L. M., & Parker, R. G. 2013, 'Rethinking health research capacity strengthening', *Global Public Health*, vol. 8, no. sup1, pp. S104–S124.

WMO. 2014, *Health Exemplar to the User Interface Platform of the Global Framework for Climate Services*. Global Framework for Climate Service, Geneva, Switzerland.

7 Arboviruses in Yucatan, Mexico

Anthropological challenges, multi-disciplinary views and practical approaches

Josué Villegas-Chim, Héctor Gómez-Dantés, Norma Pavía-Ruz, Ligia Vera-Gamboa, María José Rafful-Ceballos, Jimmy Emmanuel Ramos-Valencia and Pablo Manrique-Saide

Introduction

In Mexico, arbovirus epidemics (especially Dengue) have a long history, with public politics and social responses entangled with different discourses and practices. During the 20th century, basically two approaches for the control and prevention of mosquito-borne diseases have taken place, vertical interventions and horizontal ones. Although they followed different rationalities, they pursued almost the same objective: to eradicate mosquitoes. These battles were fought not just against "nature" but also between social groups, in "the culture."

Yucatan state, located in the south of Mexico, has had mosquito-borne diseases circulate since the pre-Columbian period (around 1480), where a Mayan Codex recorded a "blood vomit illness" called *xeek kik* (Góngora-Biachi, 2004). This could be the first reference to the presence of yellow fever in Mesoamerica. Mérida, the current capital city of Yucatan, has been an important center of trade, politics, science and art for a long time. It is one of the most important cities of the so-called peninsular region, where Mayan people have been the predominant cultural group for centuries. In the pre-Colombian period, it was one of the 16 Mayan provinces, known as *Ichkaansihó* (Five stones). With the arrival of the Spaniards in 1541, and upon finding most pre-Hispanic buildings abandoned, the modern city of Mérida was born. The history of this city is rich in important events, including a short independence period in 1841 when the Yucatan Peninsula separated from the rest of the Mexican Republic, although it was only for a short period (Cáceres et al, 1998). Later this area was divided into the states of Campeche, Quintana Roo and Yucatan during a process of armed and political conflict in the late 19th and early 20th centuries (Cáceres et al, 1998).

Another important historical event was the Caste War, in which the indigenous population revolted against the political oligarchy (criollos and mestizos) in 1847 (Reed, 2007, Cáceres et al, 1998). This ethnic resistance took place in the then main cities of Yucatan (especially in the south and east), but also had its repercussions in the city of Merida. One of these effects was of a symbolic nature and resides in the adjective "white city" with which Mérida is known today. This whiteness has nothing to do with the habit of painting house walls with lime but rather denotes the distinction of Merida as a city for the "whites." Outside the urban enclave was where the native population lived. Currently, Merida is still known as the "white city" but without any reference to the racial segregation of the colonial period.

Since then, the city has expanded significantly in population, with about 900,000 people in 2015. As it is a capital city, Merida attracts people from the rest of the state, searching for work and educational opportunities; likewise, people from outside the state have emigrated for similar reasons, resulting in the enrichment of multi-culturalism in Yucatán (Figure 7.1).

Merida also has ideal socio-urban conditions for the proliferation of *Aedes* mosquitoes and their related viruses. The city and its surrounding towns have been especially known as a place infested with mosquito-borne diseases since the 1980s. As part of an international *Aedes* eradication campaign from 1964 to 1970, *Aedes*-endemic places such as Yucatan (southern Mexico) was apparently free of this vector; but in the following years, rapid re-infestation took place, as well as the introduction and circulation of new Dengue virus (DENV) serotypes (Gómez-Dantés, 1991; Gómez-Dantés and Willoquet, 2009). Indeed, in comparison to other regions, the prevalence of Dengue in Yucatan from 1980s onwards has been increasing with major epidemics in 2011 and 2012. In 2014, Chikungunya virus (CHIKV) emerged in Latin America, with severe consequences for the Yucatecan population in the next year. In 2015, Zika virus (ZIKV) appeared as an emergent and controversial disease. In Table 7.1, we can see the reported cases for the capital city in Yucatan.

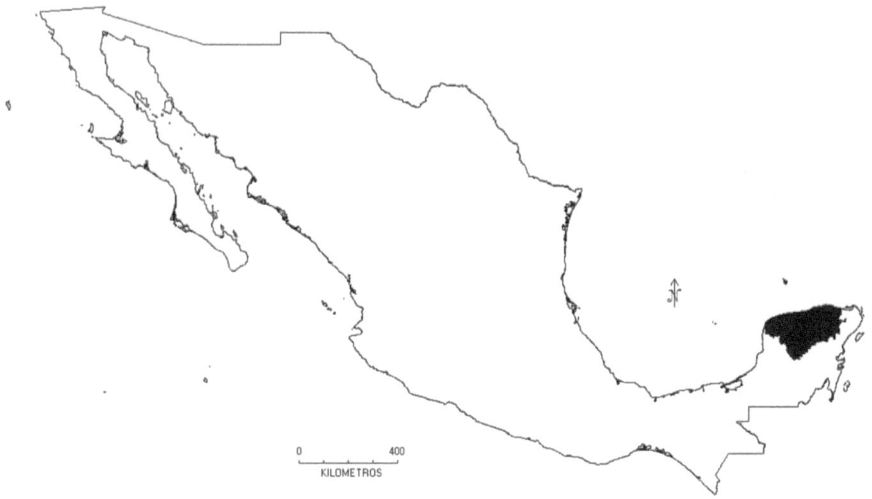

Figure 7.1 Map of Mexico (in white) and the State of Yucatan (in black).

Table 7.1 Cases reported in Merida, Yucatan, Mexico 2015–2017

	2015	*2016*	*2017*	*Total*
Dengue	5,391	2,387	173	7,951
Chikungunya	478	695	21	1,194
Zika	–	8,932	2,291	11,223
Total	5,869	12,014	2,485	20,368

Source: SINAVE.

Our anthropological team has been doing research, on different aspects and in different capacities, on *Aedes*-borne diseases (ABDs) for almost seven years now. In this chapter, we reflect on what we have found, both in terms of our research data and also through our personal experiences in public health interventions and research.[1] We draw upon this portfolio of studies, some past and some ongoing, to discuss the nature of multi-disciplinary approaches, the challenges of social research and the ways in which ethnography can have practical applications in the world of overlapping arbovirus epidemics.

Many of the results discussed here are under analysis for further publications. Therefore, the aim of this chapter is to contribute to the anthropological analysis, considering multi-disciplinary views, on the challenges of mosquito-borne diseases in Yucatan, Mexico. To achieve this objective, we will discuss several issues from different scenarios. First, we discuss the current portfolio of socio-anthropological research on ABDs in Yucatan and how these studies have shifted within a changing epidemiological situation. Second, we will analyze how recent outbreaks are changing the social perception of society about ABDs as well as prevention and control behaviors. Third, we make a call for an anthropological reflection on local vector control programs not just in Yucatan but also in the whole of Mexico; in this regard, we propose to view the existing surveillance system as a "system of meaning" with roles, social actors and normative practices that shape ABDs in Mexico. Finally, is also important to study how Zika virus is already changing practices, perceptions and prevention and control programs into a more complex reality given the role of sexual transmission and maternal risk.

The Yucatan portfolio: Anthropological research on *Aedes*-borne diseases

Yucatan has been the site of many anthropological studies for many decades, due to its links to Mesoamerican ruins and Mayan culture. One of the most pioneering anthropological studies in modern times was conducted by Robert Redfield, which focused on the socio-cultural transformation of Yucatecan society, specifically the transition from rural villages to a more urbanized existence (Redfield 1944). In the 1990s, applied anthropological research emerged on Dengue for the first time in Merida City with Rockefeller Foundation support and focused on cultural beliefs and practices and the development of a vector-control intervention grounded in community participation and health promotion strategies (Winch et al, 1991; Lloyd et al, 1992). A key finding from this early work was that local perceptions of Dengue (illness and symptoms) were very different from the scientific and biomedical discourse (see Table 7.2).

The impact of this work in public policies or governmental programs was not very clear since, when funding stopped, there was little follow-up. This is a persistent problem in social studies on arboviruses; research is often short term, with little time and room to engage in long-term perspectives and network building at the local level, which are needed to engage public policies and interventions. Nonetheless, these local classifications of Dengue fever, identified almost 20 years ago, gave us some clues for further anthropological studies on mosquito-borne diseases in Yucatan. In 2010, former members of that previous project and a new social science team started a new research as part of a World Health Organization (WHO) project aimed at addressing the social determinants of neglected diseases, including Dengue (Barrera-Pérez et al, 2010).[2] We, as part of these new projects, observed many similarities on the local classifications of fever mentioned in Table 7.2 in both rural and urban settlements. But we also found a greater emphasis, from the population, on the ways in which the social environment could shape the prevalence of Dengue. These new findings were likely the result of geographical and demographic changes, but were also likely influenced by theoretical shifts in the social sciences too that moved beyond sociocultural beliefs to pay more attention to the lack of public services, public insecurity, illegal drug activities and racism, for example.

Since this time, we have been involved in several projects, many of which have had a social science component. Normally for this kind of research, anthropological work is focused on three main aspects: to conduct a social analysis of the communities where the (biomedical or entomological) projects are planned; to assist with community activities to promote the interventions in collaboration

Table 7.2 Local classifications of fever and body temperature, Merida, Mexico

	Irritación	*Calentura*	*Fiebre*
Degree of elevation	Barely elevated	38–39°	Above 40°
Associated symptoms	Tiredness, sweating	Tiredness, weakness, cough	Delirium, convulsion
Causes	Hard work, vigorous exercise, begins in sun often followed by exposure to something cold	Same as *irritación*, failure to take care of *irritación*, winds	Failure to take care of *calentura*, infections
Recourse to cure	Home treatment	Home treatment, then doctor if not better in 3 days	Go to doctor first

Source: Winch et al (1991:4).

with entomologists, epidemiologists and medical doctors; and, lastly, to examine the social acceptance and perceived efficacy of the control tools. In all aspects, ethnographic observations are a key dimension for our work.

The project "*Aedes aegypti*–proof houses" formerly ran in Acapulco, Mexico (Che-Mendoza et al, 2015), was scaled-up in Merida in 2013 and the objective was to install insecticide-treated house screens on door-windows (Manrique-Saide et al, 2017).[3] As in many interventions with new methods for mosquito-vector control, this small-scale trial had to be evaluated from the communities' perspective. We applied a survey to a subsample of households; an important finding was that participants accepted the project because the screens were free and were perceived to be beneficial for their families in many ways: to avoid mosquito-human contact and reduce the risk of Dengue, which was perceived to be high at the time and in this particular community. This research was part of a huge effort of the Autonomous University of Yucatan and the federal Mexican government to reduce mosquitoes by using a new type of household intervention strategy. Currently, the project is being implemented in more neighborhoods in Merida.

In 2014, a cohort prospective study on Dengue infection began, funded by Sanofi-Pasteur. The main goal was to generate a statistically-robust baseline of Dengue epidemiology for planned vaccine field trials of Dengvaxia (Hladish et al, 2016; Pavía-Ruz et al, 2018; Rojas et al, 2018). A total of 450 families were enrolled for this project and social research was also done on local perceptions and behaviors around Dengue. Interestingly, and in contrast to the high perceived threat of Dengue found in the *Aedes*-proof house study, many aspects of the research findings found almost 20 years ago continued to be found during our research: a low risk perception of Dengue and few corresponding preventive practices being undertaken.[4] Nevertheless, this situation was about to change. The emergence of Chikungunya in 2015 and Zika virus in 2016 impacted health systems, social practices and social perceptions of Yucatecans about mosquito-borne diseases. Risk perception due to this new scenario changed the way people conceptualized domestic preventive measures such as the use of body repellent and cleaning of their properties and backyards.

Our multi-disciplinary team has been involved in two projects related to Zika virus, coordinated by the Autonomous University of Yucatan, in Merida since 2015. The first was funded by CDC in a rural village (Ticul) and in an urban city (Merida); the second one was part of an EU-Horizon 2020 funded initiative, called ZikAlliance (which involved the anthropology-team.). The first project, known as "Pregnancy without Zika," was aimed at timely detection of Zika cases, with emphasis on changes in the normal course of pregnancy and birth of children with microcephaly or other abnormalities. As part of these activities, we conducted three social science studies related to pregnant women: (a) socio-cultural factors associated with Zika virus; (b) in-deep interviews with pregnant women about how they lived and experienced the Zika outbreak; and (c) a social assessment of the perceived efficacy of the medical project, which included observing the clinical practices of health professionals, who were in charge of managing the intervention. This fieldwork provided some additional insights on the cultural meanings of Zika in Yucatan.

Lastly, we have also been involved a Wolbachia-based strategy for *Aedes*-vector control in Yucatan. The main difference here, in contrast to the other mentioned projects, is that the Mexican government is actively promoting this project. Key aspects of our activities for this project are networking with national and international entities (academic, governmental and private sectors) and a strong community engagement approach for local stakeholders and inhabitants from the mosquito releasing sites.

Clearly, Yucatan has become a focus for *Aedes* research, an assemblage of knowledge generation and one that is targeted towards translating research, including anthropological research, into public health intervention plans and policy. A part of this collaborative work, the Yucatan group has collaborated with many foreign universities (Emory University, Washington University, University of Florida, James Cook University, Sun-Yat-Sen University, and Michigan University State) and governmental institutions (Ministry of Health and, from Mexico; Center for Disease Control and Prevention, from the United States; and the Chinese government). An essential part of this collaborative work has been the stronger ties with the municipal and state governments. Another important collaboration has been in the creation of the State Committee for the Prevention and Control on *Aedes aegypti*, which aims to work closely across government, academia, private enterprises and society. Epidemiological and entomological issues have been the major concerns to address, rather than research and novel tools.

Global outbreaks, local concerns: Social perceptions and cultural responses in Yucatan

In Yucatan, as in many other *Aedes*-endemic places in Mexico, the presence of mosquitoes and of "fever" are often seen as both a symptom of disease and a disease itself. Historically, there has been a lot of focus on the therapeutic practices of the Yucatec Maya, including the classification of fevers and the traditional medical practices and hybridized categories (with biomedicine) that revolve around them.[5] In 2014, we conducted an anthropological study focused on social understanding of fever in Merida and found that despite individuals going to a clinical facility, they also look for self-medication. Dialogues with doctors are often limited because symbolic elements typical of local Mayan-speaking healers are not shared.[6] This can limit communication between patients and health workers. During our research, as well as in the earlier social studies in the 1990s, "fever" was not always associated with DENV, and small outbreaks were normally expected in the rainy season. In fact, despite the ubiquitous presence of mosquitoes, and the high circulation of arboviruses, social perception of Dengue risk was actually very low.

Our studies found that Dengue was not a very big deal at all for many families in Yucatan; they considered other illnesses such as pneumonia more relevant.[7] People are very accustomed to keeping buckets in their backyards for cleaning and drinking purposes and although they recognize that these are potential mosquito-breeding sites, they only wash them when they become visibly dirty. There is also a clear gender dimension, as mentioned in other studies in Latin America countries (Cepeda et al, 2017; Arenas-Monreal et al, 2015; Danis-Lozano et al, 2002; Davies et al, 2016; Guerra-Reyes et al, 2019). Some families collect "garbage" (small or medium-sized containers) for sale, storing these in their backyards, where they become mosquito-breeding sites. However, something changed in 2015 with the CHIK outbreak.

Before the CHIK outbreak in Yucatan, the state government, through the public health department, promised via media press that Yucatan was "bullet-proof" against the new virus. The explosive outbreak that ensued (see Table 7.1) demonstrated a different scenario. The disjunction between these official proclamations, which stressed confidence and safety, and the high CHIK infection rate as well as new debilitating symptoms and chronicities (like arthritis) led to a number of consequences. Distrust in authorities arose because of this false sense of security and took health services by surprise. Popular perceptions began to shift. Despite the widespread concern and attention to CHIK, a similar type of helplessness emerged as the appearance of this new disease was quickly "normalized," as had occurred with DENV previously (Chávez Arias et al, 2017). Chikungunya was seen as an additional sickness that festered in poor environmental conditions, part of "daily life" of Yucatecan society, especially for low-income families. One key informant reported, "There is nothing we can do. If you go to hospital you probably get infected because there are a lot of mosquitoes there; even the nurses and doctors have that sickness. So, tell me, why should I go there?" The problem was not with the low capacity to deliver health services in an outbreak situation; without a vaccine or treatment and given the rapid illness course, that typically lasted a week or less, there was little for the health services to do. The response of the government was to increase vector control activities, such as fogging in the streets and spraying inside houses when a positive case was confirmed. These epidemics have proved to be very challenging to the government.

In Yucatan, the social-ecology of *Aedes* breeding is intimately related to increased urban space. Since the fieldwork of Robert Redfield and others in the 1960s, the geography and economy of Yucatan has shifted dramatically, as it has in other areas of Mexico. The region has seen increased migration to cities and town; almost 50% of the entire population of Yucatan now lives in Merida (Fraga, 1991; Pérez-Campuzano et al, 2014; Fortuny-Loret de Mola, 2006; Pérez et al, 2014). In the south of Merida, for example, 40 years ago the land was occupied by forest without any human settlements and certainly no water supply services. But as people migrated from rural towns to seek employment, they have also built up mosquito-breeding sites. These include public spaces, especially open sewers. During our research, we have observed a tendency for people to lay blame for mosquito reproduction on others, either using the narrative of public habitats (without any owners but the municipal government) and private spaces that are neglected and uncared-for. These are seen as sources of disease spread. They are commonly associated, as Dengue itself is, as a "disease of poor people." So, if a household is recognized as a potential mosquito-breeding sites, it means that they are "a poor family." In both cases, locals say that mosquitos proliferate because the government is not doing their job.

Just as CHIK faded from social consciousness in 2016, another disease emerged: ZIKV, suddenly embedded in an even more political set of discourses. Once again, the particularities of the virus shifted social perceptions and responses, but in different ways (Manrique-Saide et al, 2018). In our research, we found that the recent ZIKV outbreak did not invoke the same level of social fear as CHIK for most people in Yucatan, something that is supported elsewhere by other studies (Bardosh et al, 2017). This may be confusing, if one follows the health communication scheme of the Mexican authorities or of international agencies like PAHO and WHO. Both viruses are thought to have infected large-numbers of the population, although the rates of asymptomatic infections are considered to be less for CHIK (~50%) than ZIKV (~80%). Another issue is the more severe, and more widespread joint and muscle pain of CHIK, some of which can last one to two months or longer. A final reason is that the number of natural abortions, and cases of microcephaly and other congenital consequences, have not risen to alarming levels in Mexico.

Another important sociocultural reason to take into account for the "low status" of Zika in Yucatan is the "feminization" of the virus. Our initial fieldwork shows that Zika is perceived as a disease that affects "only women", and more specifically, pregnant women and their children. This situation will bias the search for cases to young women, and neglect those infections in younger children and old males who are also bitten by mosquitoes and help transmit the virus. These findings challenge the very idea of an effective prevention program in Yucatan. The social understanding of this new virus changed the face of arboviruses because of its associations with additional cultural practices and beliefs related to intimacy and sexual taboos on top of transmission through mosquito bites.

The culture of vector-control evaluation: Some anthropological reflections

In a national meeting of vector control experts held in Yucatan in 2016, precipitated by the ZIKV epidemic, the following statement was made in one of the opening sessions: "the enemy is the mosquito." That is to say, the problem is the mosquito, whose very existence is a modifiable factor, through better and more organized vector control. This perspective is, in many ways, practical. It involves targeting the "guilty entity" in a way that mobilizes humans against the enemy – it is a form of public health militancy, grounded in historical experience. But it is neither an interdisciplinary perspective nor a holistic overview of the arbovirus problem.

In the Yucatecan context, the "social issues" of vector-borne diseases are often described as being related to "communities," "the population" and "local inhabitants" but almost never to the official institutions that lead prevention and control programs. In other words, these institutions also have "cultures" because they produce and reproduce social norms, values, hierarchies, status, social relations of power and, most importantly (and apparently not obvious to many of these stakeholders), they are part of local cultures with global connections due to collaboration with different governmental agencies, private companies and research centers. Here we have one of the biggest challenges from an applied anthropological point of view: to effectively communicate to, and facilitate changes with, the culture of public health programs. Governmental institutions, in an anthropological sense, are systems with cultural meanings. However, asking and obtaining permission from government agencies to study their cultural practices and inner-workings as an institution is very challenging, and requires asking some uncomfortable questions. As vector-borne disease researchers, the politics of access is, in many ways, congruent with the difficulties we face in asking permission from families to access inside their homes and community – for entomological inspections, for example, or to administer a questionnaire or conduct a focus group. In a sense, we can say that this lack of access is itself a "structural barrier" to the efficacy of prevention and control programs, albeit one that is rarely part of Venn diagrams or other typical frameworks.

In our daily ethnographic observations, we have noticed that very few of our colleagues (including biologists, medical doctors, epidemiologists, ecologists, nurses and technical and operative personnel) use any personal protection products to prevent mosquito bites, despite the fact that many of our projects and the official public health risk communication materials recommend these sprays to much less educated and wealthy "target communities." When we ask them the reasons for this discordance, our colleagues typically answer with various arguments justifying why they do not have repellents inside their bags at this very moment. They seem annoyed at having been "busted" or "exposed" by this inconsistency. This tells us something about how a "culture of evaluation" is seen as very important for "vulnerable population," but apparently does not apply to the scientific teams that promote those same preventive measures. Our anthropological team can only imagine what we would find if we asked these kinds of questions in a more systematic fashion and with a view to understanding the relationships between governmental institutions and *Aedes*-borne diseases in Mexico. Again, some informal observations have given us clues to the formal and informal management of the surveillance system.

In Yucatan, as in the rest of Latin America, there are many opportunities to improve the culture of public evaluation. There are key systematic reviews on the efficacy of different vector-control strategies (chemical control, environmental management, community participation, biological control) against the mosquitoes that evidenced different results regarding manifold variables such as functionality of vector control programs, building capacity, training operative personnel, community engagement-participation, public campaigns to promote actions, budget of the programs, following the guidelines, and so on; every method or mechanisms have their own efficacy and limitations and an integrated approach make more sense, due to several challenges, rather than apply just one strategy (Dusfour et al, 2019; Mendes Luz et al, 2011; Bowman et al, 2016; Erlanger et al, 2008; Horstick et al, 2010). Although authors like Bauman et al (2016) argue that there is still need for a more robust research focused on the evaluation of different vector control methods (i.e. insecticide susceptibility and resistance), the question here is: what will be the contributions from an anthropological perspective? First at all, the evaluation process on the efficacy of vector-control programs are indeed social practices embedded into wider cultural context, politics of diseases control, financial resources, interests of private companies on validation for the promotion of products, societal acceptance, and the way the prevention actions are deployed. Suárez (2004) calls the attention to the way the prevention-control mechanism is understood from public politics vs community-target, is key for the sustainable life of the interventions itself. However, it is important to remember Manderson (1998) that pointed out that there is a juxtaposition of science over 'local knowledge' in a wider public health field. Thus, the question here is: do the society really understand how every vector control method works, or, the so-called Integrated Intervention Management? Whiteford (1997), gave us an example of how things goes in the wrong or unexpected way in her study about the ethnoecology of Dengue fever as a way to link culture, history, and politics into the way people understand the failure or success of the prevention of Dengue infections in Dominican Republic; here, she identified that the concept of Mala union, uncovered that government failure is part of the context of a vector-control failure. There is a lot to be done towards a holistic approach for the evaluation of vector-control programs aimed to enhance the strategies for better results.

Dengue vaccine in an inter-epidemic context

Chasing urban mosquitoes with fumigators and finding their breeding sites in vases, tires and bottle caps has proved to be very challenging in Yucatan and elsewhere. One of the most important events in the history of Dengue control, therefore, has been the recent production and licensing (now in 19 countries) of an effective vaccine. There were many laboratories that pursued this apparently unachievable goal, which took almost 40 years to accomplish, but finally we have a vaccine against four Dengue serotypes based on the related yellow fever vaccine. Sanofi-Pasteur invested hundreds of millions of euros in its Dengvaxia® program since it began in mid-1990s (Guy et al, 2015).

While WHO sets the guidelines for the introduction and evaluation of new vaccines in endemic areas, international initiatives (Dengue Vaccine Initiative, DVI) and Latin American agencies support research and provide information required to evaluate the best scenarios for the introduction of vaccines (WHO, 2012, 2016). In the case of the only registered Dengue vaccine, Dengvaxia®, the results from randomized clinical trials in Yucatan (and other Latin American and Asian countries) have illustrated the merits of the vaccine (Capeding et al, 2014; Villar et al, 2015) and have promoted the recommendations from WHO's Strategic Advisory Group of Experts (SAGE). Nonetheless, international attention to Dengvaxia®, a live recombinant tetravalent Dengue vaccine, has highlighted the complex socio-political relationships between vaccine trials, national health policy, scientific knowledge and socio-cultural aspects of new vaccines, and the importance of pharmacovigilance after licensing.

In the case of Mexico, the advent of the vaccine promoted the creation of a Mexican Dengue expert group (MDEG). The exercise carried out by the MDEG was directed to the early adoption of a Dengue vaccine in Mexico, and included the proposal that Low and Middle Income Countries (LMICs) actively participate in the generation of evidence, the analysis of data from clinical trials, the estimation of the burden of disease and the use of national-level evidence by decision makers to create a sustainable immunization program with all the resources required for the adoption of the new vaccine (Betancourt-Cravioto et al, 2014). This exercise was designed to prepare the regulatory processes, epidemiological background information, economic evaluation and the logistical organization for the early registration, introduction and evaluation of the Dengue vaccine in Mexico. This process found uneven ground with academic groups questioning the safety of this vaccine since preliminary results demonstrated low protection to DEN2 serotype and potential risks of increasing hospitalizations (Hernández et al, 2016).

The emergency caused by the 2015 Chikungunya epidemic followed by Zika virus in 2015–2016 produced an unexpected amount of attention that displaced Dengue from the concerns of the community in Yucatan as well as from public health programs. The discourse around vector control (*Aedes aegypti*) transitioned from the hopes of a new vaccine to a more integrated approach focused on several arboviral diseases, instead of targeting only one: Dengue.

The vaccine itself has also played a role in this reconfiguring. Further studies have shown that the vaccine is not as effective as first thought, specifically in naïve populations (those who have never had Dengue) and children under nine years old. This has to do with pathogenic mechanisms and the immune enhancement produced by the combination of certain sequences of Dengue virus infections in some populations. This has generated a set of critical and precautionary warnings amid calls for its immediate introduction. WHO has subsequently issued interim guidance recommending the vaccine be used only in individuals with a documented past Dengue infection (WHO, 2016). The findings have led to cessation of a large public vaccination program in the Philippines, in which > 700,000 children aged ≥ 9 years were vaccinated in 2017, amidst widespread media coverage focused on the possible role that severe Dengue played in the deaths of several children who had received the vaccine.

This has not been the only element that has shifted the conversation. The anthropological challenge for us, with funding from Sanofi-Pasteur to explore issues of acceptability and implementation, was how to advocate for a "magic bullet" that targets one disease, instead of introducing a weapon (or refining existing vector control approaches) that deals with three infections that happen to be transmitted by the same vector: *Aedes aegypti*. It is one thing to do years of research and clinical trials but another very different problem to introduce a new vaccine to the global market and convince local governments to pay for it and citizens to take it.

The main goal of the project, *Familias sin Dengue* in Yucatan, funded by the Sanofi-Pasteur laboratory, was to evaluate the vaccine Dengvaxia®, approved by the national agency that evaluates and establishes pharmaceutical regulations (COFEPRIS). When *Familias sin Dengue* began in 2014, the remains of the 2012 Dengue outbreak lingered in Yucatan. This was fresh in the memory of local citizens. Although Dengue fever remains, from a community viewpoint, not really an "important disease" (as discussed earlier), governmental prevention and control programs of *Aedes aegypti* have had very different points of view on this problem. Previous work, in other countries, on the acceptability of a (hypothetical) DENV vaccine has shown widely differing results – for example, with very high acceptance (94%) of a potential paediatric DENV vaccination programme in an Indonesian survey (Hadisoemarto and Castro, 2013) but poor attitudes to vaccination in another Indonesian study, particularly among those of lower socioeconomic status and with poor knowledge of DENV (Harapan et al, 2016). Major barriers to participation in a DENV vaccine trial (lack of trust and information, fear of side effects and of exploitation) were also identified in Puerto Rico (Guerra et al, 2012). When we asked the participants of *Familias sin Dengue* about the acceptance of Dengvaxia®, 90% of the answers were, "Yes, I'll accept this vaccine." For the local community, remember DENV was not a big deal, but they were okay about the implementation of this new vaccine. Ethnographically, we have found that many families normally ask, in their medical consultation, for a vaccine rather than pills for all sorts of ailments and diseases, because they are viewed as more effective and less of a burden.

However, the situation changed with the CHIK and ZIKV outbreaks, as suddenly we have two new diseases in Yucatan and no available vaccine against these viruses. While some efforts were made at developing a ZIKV vaccine, with some advocates thinking that this could be developed relatively quickly, these statements were overly-optimistic. This made people in Yucatan wonder, "Why should I accept this dengue vaccine," many informants of our research reported. The same situation occurred when ZIKV emerged in 2016. However, our recommendation is to conduct more in-depth research on the socio-cultural complexity of this subject, as the initial studies were relatively limited in scope.

Towards a socio-political surveillance of *Aedes*-borne disease prevention

Decades of Dengue outbreaks, a widespread and very debilitating CHIK epidemic (from the perspective of local people) and the emergence of a new congenital syndrome (ZIKV), all followed in rapid secession, point us to some important questions that should be asked about the efficacy of the current vector control program and about local sociocultural logics. It is one thing to study topics such as social perceptions of risk and another very different activity to conduct a rigorous and critical sociopolitical analysis of *Aedes*-borne disease prevention programs, as Suárez (2004) and Nading (2014) pointed out as a key dimension for mosquito-vector control strategies. The complexity of reducing or eliminate mosquitoes is not just about what communities do or do not do, accept or reject, but also encompasses an institutional process, the bureaucratic rules in action and the informal ways that individuals manage vector control programs. In a sense, we need a new type of anthropological engagement, at least in Mexico and in Yucatan; in the words of public health, we need an "anthropological surveillance" of vector control programs, of their social and political forms, mechanisms, outcomes and impacts.

We can already anticipate some barriers to such an activity. There is a common complaint among anthropologists working in health, that no matter how illuminating our findings might be, they are not taken seriously by other colleagues (such as epidemiologists, medical doctors, biologists, etc.), government stakeholders or private entrepreneurs. The main reason is that "slow research" (as discussed by Adams et al, 2014) is in conflict with the hegemonic perspective of the perspectives that dominate epidemiology and entomology, at least in Mexico. Of course, when things get rapidly worse, as in an outbreak of Zika, Chikungunya, Ebola, cholera or whatever, there is a demand for rapid responses that quickly assess the situation; there is no time for years of research, for example, although there is certainly an opportunity to link the response with anthropologists who already have a high-level of cultural knowledge and experience.

So how can we transform the perception of public health practitioners about the value of anthropology and transform anthropological findings themselves to be more operationally relevant and concrete? As Kleinman (2010) stated, many anthropologists have spent a lot of time attacking biomedicine, of critiquing the power and control involved in bureaucratic and scientific knowledge forms, but it is important that such attacks are also constructive and, ultimately, transformative. To do such work, however, there needs to be some resources available for meaningful employment.

We can draw upon some examples from our portfolio of current research projects. We had the opportunity to study the Chikungunya outbreak in 2015 by observing 200 households in a semi-urban city, Ticul, in Yucatan. Although our data could not be of use during the outbreak itself, we systematically documented the social behavior and cultural responses that gave us important clues for future epidemic events. These included some important findings, such as changes in preventive practices, health-seeking behavior, social perceptions on how CHIK could spread within households and the different ways that these disease symptoms are normalized. When the Zika outbreak occurred in 2016 in Yucatan, we were able to repeat aspects of this research, this time interviewing 200 pregnant women in Merida, which allowed us to validate and deepen our previous findings and uncover additional cultural aspects that people associated to this new virus.

From these ethnographic observations, an important question about interventions is: who is responsible for the efficacy of these preventive programs? From the communities' perspective, the government is responsible and the failure of their actions is proof of this disappointing management. Nevertheless, we have found that the communities themselves have also ignored their responsibilities. This is to say, for many local inhabitants, carrying out preventive domestic practices is, simply speaking, not a priority. New interventions (for example, insecticide-treated screens in doors and windows or even new vaccines like Dengvaxia) can reinforce these attitudes because they are vertical interventions managed in collaboration with the local government of any kind outside of passive compliance and acceptability (these types of interventions are typically provided for free). As an informant highlighted during our fieldwork, "[i]f I have this intervention, why do I have to worry about doing other things by myself?" This is a central paradox of public health. Nevertheless, this could create a false sense of security because the interventions do not always work as they should due to many variables, not only social but also entomological and epidemiological ones as well.

Zika virus: New disease, new paradigm?

With the emergence of Zika, the very nature and notion of what a vector-borne disease is, how it is transmitted and how it affects people, has been challenged (Cepeda et al, 2017; Davis et al, 2016; Guerra-Reyes et al, 2019). This has pushed social scientists engaged with Dengue, like our team in Yucatan, to consider other kinds of topics in vector-borne disease research other than the classic focus on environmental health. This has included issues on maternal and child health care, contraception, abortion and women rights and sexual intercourse as a new mechanism for virus transmission of an *Aedes*-borne illness. Talking about Zika, therefore, expanded our idea of anthropological surveillance into other, sometimes uncomfortable areas, like abortion and disability. These are imbued with new cultural and moral values related to maternity, taboos on sexual intimacy, guilt or blame related to abortion and contraception practices and gender relationships of power. In addition, pregnant women and their families may have already started the process of resignification of mosquito-borne illnesses as well as the social appropriation of scientific-biomedical discourses about this emergent disease.

We identified that ZIKV is something "in-between" Dengue and Chikungunya and "something else", although easily confused with the "normal symptoms" of pregnancy. Pregnant women have access to information about ZIKV, but they are skeptical about some issues, like the relationship between ZIKV infection and "small-heads in newborns." At the time, there was much uncertainty and a feeling that access to information was limited and not always very clear.

Zika also bumps up against another cultural dimension long seen in the "old challenges" to HIV programs: sexual education. Here we have an unexpected dichotomy between vector control and now this very new world of sexual transmission. Thus, as we could say, to fight mosquitoes is not what it used to be. Combining the use of body repellents and condoms to prevent a mosquito-borne disease makes the work of prevention campaigns much more difficult. For example, cultural biases on sexual education in Yucatan have not been well addressed in this new scenario. A recent study demonstrated that two concepts are key to understand the wider context of HIV in Yucatan: social vulnerability and risk-groups (Quintal-López et al, 2014). These researchers focused heavily on indigenous immigrants as a high-risk HIV group, which offers an important frame for thinking about the social vulnerability of pregnant women to ZIKV. Religious beliefs can also have important impacts on vector-borne diseases. We found some insights into local discourses when people told us that it is God's will that their families have had, for example, Dengue fever. One interesting question to be answered will be: do pregnant women think in the same way about Zika virus in

Yucatan? As ZIKV vaccine trials began in a number of countries, it is also unclear how pregnant women will respond to separate Dengue and ZIKV vaccines, not to mention the complex immunological effects this may create.

Conclusions

There are important avenues for sociocultural engagement in arboviruses, both during endemic and epidemics periods, that are still emerging for anthropologists. As attention increases, and as more potential threats come into existence, how can we develop methodologies – or "gold standard guidelines" – for anthropological knowledge, focused on the improvement of *Aedes*-borne disease prevention and control in places like Yucatan? While an interdisciplinary approach, drawing together different disciplines, sounds like an ideal option, the real challenge is not about "bridging disciplines." In Yucatan, we have interdisciplinary teams where our anthropological inputs are valued and considered, but most of the attention we get from these recommendations are focused on "the community." This "community focus" is itself reinforced by common perceptions about anthropology; that is, it is a field focused exclusively on "the other" – often remote tribes, exotic peoples or Neolithic remains. In Yucatan, this includes a heavy focus on Mesoamericans.

But the social realities of *Aedes*-borne diseases are a complex reality that extends beyond the community; thus, we also need to see prevention and control mechanisms as social practices with rules, social norms, cultural values and power relations (Suárez, 2004). Public health policies on arboviral diseases are part of social discourses assembled in a larger discursive matrix. Anthropologists should not just be instrumentalist in how they approach collaborations with biomedical researchers and public health staff; they should also provide a critical praxis to efforts to reduce mosquitoes, educate the public about sex and protect pregnant women from congenital syndromes. This should include more of a focus on community participation, which up until now has remained a very poorly integrated element in mosquito-borne disease prevention and control in Yucatan. Here, the inclusion of anthropologists and the deep consideration and respect for what we bring to the table is not as developed as it is in more developed nations. Therefore, in the future, we seek to expand our focus, and to better develop some of the ideas we have outlined above, specifically for an anthropological platform for socio-political surveillance of public health activities to assist with pre-, inter- and post-epidemic events.

Notes

1 We would like to thank Dr. Kevin Bardosh for constructive editorial inputs and the Welcome Trust for funding the open access fee associated with this book chapter. The opinions expressed here of the authors do not reflect the view of their institutions or the financial agencies that provide funding for the studies mentioned in this chapter.

2 As part of the project, we organized several workshops with many types of participants. The interviewers and leaders of the peripheral communities or urban neighborhoods

(located in the South of Merida) were invited as well as different government authorities (health departments, education, natural resources and environment, and politicians), researchers and the public press.

3 Historically, there was no enough or solid evidence on the efficacy of the mosquito-screens installed on doors and windows in Mexico. Therefore, one of the main objectives of the project was to prove the efficacy of the method with some improvements. Since the trial intervention was implemented successfully, our lab (UCBE-UADY) has been working with the federal and local government to scale-up this intervention to more houses in Merida, especially in hot-spot areas where the number of mosquitoes is very higher (this data is provided by the government through the entomological surveillance system).

4 We found that risk perceptions were different in the *Aedes*-proof house intervention study (2013) in comparison to the Dengue cohort prospective study, which was conducted the next year (2014). The first study was performed in a small neighborhood (called Manzana 115) where risk perceptions were high largely due to the fact that Manzana 115 had been hard-hit by the Dengue outbreak in 2012. In contrast, the second study was done across all of Merida, in high-, medium- and low-risk transmission areas. Here, we found much lower risk perceptions.

5 All medical practices in Mesoamerica today respond to both diachronic and synchronic processes that together make up traditional healing methods and biomedicine, rooted in pre-Hispanic Mesoamerica models. One of the practices we documented in fieldwork consisted of the use of painkillers that were not ingested but prepared as a mixture with commercial unguent. The people put this mixture on the whole body to eliminate high fever. When we asked about the efficacy of this measure, some informants said that it works. Perhaps the "symbolic efficacy" is playing an important cultural association here but also the same interviewees reported that they went to see a doctor.

6 As an example of cultural limitations in health care we can refer to the management and care of fevers: "In Yucatec Maya, as well as in many other Mesoamerican languages, a subset of temperature terms is used to talk about sensory temperatures as well as categorical temperatures. Although the distinction between sensory temperature (non-marked) and categorical temperature (combined with kùuch 'load') seems a straightforward one, the term kùuch is not always mentioned in everyday conversations and speakers talk simply about 'hot' and 'cold' things (chokoh/síis ba'al) without explicitly mentioning 'its load/effect', which is implied. This is one reason why the distinction between sensory and categorical meaning is not always so obvious" (Le Guen 2015: 157–158).

7 Although they did consider fever, as a symptom, to be something to be taken very seriously.

References

Adams, V., Burke, N. J., & Whitmarsh, I. 2014, 'Slow research: thoughts for a movement in global health', *Medical Anthropology*, vol. 33, no. 3, pp. 179–197.

Arenas-Monreal, L., Piña-Pozas, M., & Gómez-Dantés, H. 2015, 'Aportes y desafíos del enfoque de género en el estudio de las enfermedades transmitidas por vector', *Salud Pública de México*, vol. 57, no. 1, pp. 66–75.

Bardosh, K. L., Jean, L., Beau De Rochars, V. M., Lemoine, J. F., Okech, B., Ryan, S. J., et al. 2017, 'Polisye kont moustik: a culturally competent approach to larval source reduction in the context of lymphatic filariasis and malaria elimination in Haiti', *Tropical Medicine and Infectious Disease*, vol. 2, no. 3, pp. 39.

Barrera-Pérez, M., Manrique-Saidé, P., Barrera-Buenfil, D., Wejebe-Shanahan, M., Rodríguez-Pavón, J., Magaña Canul, R., et al. 2010, *Study of the social determinants of neglected and other poverty-related diseases in Latin America and the Caribbean.* University Autonomous of Yucatán (México); Institute of Tropical Medicine (Antwerp, Belgium); World Health Organization (WHO). Research Report.

Betancourt-Cravioto, M., Kuri-Morales, P., González-Roldán, J. F., Tapia-Conyer, R., & Mexican Dengue Expert Group. 2014, 'Introducing a dengue vaccine to Mexico: development of a system for evidence-based public policy recommendations', *PLoS Neglected Tropical Diseases*, vol. 8, no. 7, pp. e3009.

Bowman, L. R., Donegan, S., & McCall, P. J. 2016, 'Is dengue vector control deficient in effectiveness or evidence?: Systematic review and meta-analysis', *PLoS. Negl. Trop. Dis.*, vol. 10, no. 3, e0004551.

Capeding, M. R., Tran, N. H., Hadinegoro, S. R. S., Ismail, H. I. H. M., Chotpitayasunondh, T., Chua, M. N., et al. 2014, 'Clinical efficacy and safety of a novel tetravalent dengue vaccine in healthy children in Asia: a phase 3, randomised, observer-masked, placebo-controlled trial', *The Lancet*, vol. 384, no. 9951, pp. 1358–1365.

Casares, G. 1998, *Yucatán en el tiempo. Mérida, Yucatán.* ISBN 970 9071 04 1.

Cepeda, Z., Arenas, C., Vilardo, V., Hilton, E., Dico-Young, T., & Green, C. 2017. *Dominican Republic gender analysis: A study of the impact of the Zika virus on women, girls, boys and men.* Oxfam GB, London.

Chávez Arias, N. P., Villegas Chim, J. E., Wejebe Shanahan, M., Barrera Buenfil, D., Rafful Ceballos, M. J., Ramos Valencia, J. E., Rodríguez Pavón, J., Barrera Pérez, M. A. (†), Pavía Ruz, N., & Gómez Dantés, H. 2017, 'Studying sociocultural factors associated with dengue fever in elementary school children in Yucatan, Mexico: An anthropological approach', *SAGE Research Methods Case Health*, http://dx.doi.org/10.4135/9781473998551

Che-Mendoza, A., Guillermo-May, G., Herrera-Bojórquez, J., Barrera-Pérez, M., Dzul-Manzanilla, F., Gutierrez-Castro, C., et al. 2015, 'Long-lasting insecticide-treated house screens and targeted treatment of productive breeding-sites for dengue vector control in Acapulco, Mexico', *Transactions of the Royal Society of Tropical Medicine and Hygiene*, vol. 109, no. 2, pp. 106–115.

Danis-Lozano, R., Rodríguez, M. H., & Hernández-Avila, M. 2002, 'Gender-related family head schooling and Aedes aegypti larval breeding risk in southern Mexico', *Salud. Publica. Mex*, vol. 44, no. 3, pp. 237–242.

Davies, S. E., & Bennett, B. 2016, 'A gendered human rights analysis of Ebola and Zika: locating gender in global health emergencies', *International Affairs*, vol. 92, no. 5, pp. 1041–1060.

Dusfour, I., Vontas, J., David, J. -P., Weetman, D., Fonseca, D. M., Corbel, V., et al. 2019, 'Management of insecticide resistance in the major Aedes vectors of arboviruses: Advances and challenges', *PLoS. Negl. Trop. Dis.*, vol. 13, no. 10, e0007615.

Erlanger, T. E., Keiser, J., & Ultzinger, J. 2008, 'Effect of dengue vector control interventions on entomological parameters in developing countries: a systematic review and meta-analysis', *Medical and Veterinary Entomology*, vol. 22, pp. 203–221.

Fortuny-Loret de Mola, P. 2006, 'Migrantes retornados: asechando su vida', In Cornejo Portugal, Inés (coord.), *Juventud rural y migración maya hablante*. UAM, Mexico.

Fraga, J. E. 1991, *La migración rural en la Península de Yucatán: 4 ensayos*. Mérida, Yucatán: CINVESTAV/IPN, Unidad Mérida, Mexico.

Gómez, H. 1991. 'El dengue en las Américas. Un problema de salud regional', *Salud publica de Mexico*, vol. 33, no. 4: 347–355.

Gómez-Dantés, H., & Willoquet, J. R. 2009, 'Dengue in the Americas: challenges for prevention and control', *Cadernos de saúde pública*, vol. 25, pp. S19–S31.

Góngora-Biachi, R. A. 2004, 'La erradicación de la fiebre amarilla en Mérida, Yucatán: una historia de tenacidad y éxito', *Revista Biomédic*, vol. 15, no. 4: 251–258.

Guerra, C. L. P., Rodríguez-Acosta, R., Soto-Gómez, E., Zielinski-Gutierrez, E., Peña-Orellana, M., Santiago, L., et al. 2012, 'Assessing the interest to participate in a dengue vaccine efficacy trial among residents of Puerto Rico', *Human Vaccines & Immunotherapeutics*, vol. 8, no. 7, pp. 905–915.

Guerra-Reyes, L., & Iguiñiz-Romero, R. A. 2019, 'Performing purity: reproductive decision making and implications for a community under threat of Zika in Iquitos, Peru', *Cult Health Sex*, vol. 21, no. 3, pp. 309–322.

Guy, B., Briand, O., Lang, J., Saville, M., & Jackson, N. 2015, 'Development of the Sanofi Pasteur tetravalent dengue vaccine: one more step forward', *Vaccine*, vol. 33, no. 50, pp. 7100–7111.

Hadisoemarto, P. F., & Castro, M. C. 2013, 'Public acceptance and willingness-to-pay for a future dengue vaccine: a community-based survey in Bandung, Indonesia', *PLoS Neglected Tropical Diseases*, vol. 7, no. 9, pp. e2427.

Harapan, H., Anwar, S., Bustaman, A., Radiansyah, A., Angraini, P., Fasli, R., et al. 2016, 'Community willingness to participate in a dengue study in Aceh province, Indonesia', *PloS one*, vol. 11, no. 7, pp. e0159139.

Hernández-Ávila M, Santos-Preciado JI, Grupo multidisciplinario de investigadores del Instituto Nacional de Salud Pública. 2016, 'Análisis de la evidencia sobre eficacia y seguridad de la vacuna de dengue CYD-TDV y su potencial registro e implementación en el Programa de Vacunación Universal de México', *Salud Pública de México*, vol. 58, no. 1, pp. 71–85.

Hladish, T. J., Pearson, C. A., Chao, D. L., Rojas, D. P., Recchia, G. L., Gómez-Dantés, H., et al. 2016, 'Projected impact of dengue vaccination in Yucatán, Mexico', *PLoS Neglected Tropical Diseases*, vol. 10, no. 5, pp. e0004661.

Horstick, O., Runge-Ranzinger, S., Nathan, M. B., & Kroeger, A. 2010, 'Dengue vector-control services: how do they work? A systematic literature review and country case studies', *Transactions of the Royal Society of Tropical Medicine and Hygiene*, vol. 104, pp. 379–386.

Kleinman, A. 2010, 'Four social theories for global health', *The Lancet*, vol. 375, no. 9725, pp. 1518–1519.

Le Guen, O. 2015, 'Geografía de lo sagrado entre los mayas yucatecos de Quintana Roo. Configuración del espacio y su aprendizaje entre los niños,' *Ketzalcalli*, vol. 2005, no. 1, pp. 154–168.

Lloyd, L. S., Winch, P., Ortega-Canto, J., & Kendall, C. 1992, 'Results of a community-based Aedes aegypti control program in Merida, Yucatan, Mexico', *The American Journal of Tropical Medicine and Hygiene*, vol. 46, no. 6, pp. 635–642.

Luz, P. M., Vanni, T., Medlock, J., Paltiel, A. D., & Galvani, A. P. 2011, 'Dengue vector control strategies in an urban setting: an economic modelling assessment', *The Lancet*, vol. 377, no. 9778, pp. 1673–1680.

Manderson, L. 1998, 'Applying medical anthropology in the control of infectious disease', *Tropical Medicine and International Health*, vol. 3, no. 12, pp. 1020–1027.

Manrique-Saide, P., Che-Mendoza, A., Herrera-Bojórquez, J., Chim, J. V., Guillermo-May, G., Medina-Barreiro, A., et al. 2017, 'Insecticide-treated house screens to reduce infestations of dengue vectors', in Márcia Aparecida Speranssa, (ed.), *Dengue-immunopathology and control strategies*. Dengue. In Tech. ISBN 978-953-51-3436-7, Print ISBN 978-953-51-3435-0.

Manrique-Saide, P., Che-Mendoza, A., Herrera-Bojórquez, J., Villegas Chim, J., Guillermo-May, G., Medina-Barreiro, A., Dzul-Manzanilla, F., Martín-Park, A.,

González-Olvera, G., Delfín-Gonzalez, H., Arredondo-Jiménez, J. I., Flores-Suarez, A. E., Pavía-Ruz, N., Jones, C. H., Lenhart, A., & Vazquez-Prokopec, G. 2018, 'An integrated intervention model for the prevention of Zika and other Aedes-bornediseases in women and their families in Mexico', In: Alfonso Rodríguez (ed.), *Current Topics in Zika*. Intech, London.

Nading, A. 2014. *Mosquito trails. Ecology, health and the politics of entanglement.* University of California Press, Berkley, CA.

Pavía-Ruz, N., Barrera-Fuentes, G. A., Villanueva-Jorge, S., Che-Mendoza, A., Campuzano-Rincón, J. C., Manrique-Saide, P., et al. 2018, 'Dengue seroprevalence in a cohort of schoolchildren and their siblings in Yucatan, Mexico (20152016)', *PLoS Neglected Tropical Diseases*, vol. 12, no. 11, pp. e0006748.

Pérez-Campuzano, E., & Gamallo Chaine, P. 2014, 'Tendencias recientes de la migración desde y hacia Mérida', In Ricardo López-Santillán (ed.), *Crecimiento urbano y cambio social: escenarios de transformación de la zona metropolitana de Mérida*. CEPHCIS-UNAM, Mexico.

Pérez S., & Fargher, L. 2014, 'Expansión urbana de Mérida: ¿integrada o marginada?', In Ricardo López-Santillán (ed.), *Crecimiento urbano y cambio social: escenarios de transformación de la zona metropolitana de Mérida*. CEPHCIS-UNAM, Mexico.

Quintal-López, Rocío, & Vera-Gamboa, Ligia. 2014, 'Análisis de la vulnerabilidad social y de género en la díada migración y vih/sida entre mujeres mayas de yucatán'. *Estudios de Cultura Maya*, vol. XLVI, diciembre, 2015, pp. 197–226. Centro de Estudios Mayas Distrito Federal, México.

Redfield, Robert. 1944, *Yucatán. Una cultura de transición*. FCE, México.

Reed Nelson. 2007, *La guerra de castas*. ERA, Mexico.

Rojas, D. P., Barrera-Fuentes, G. A., Pavia-Ruz, N., Salgado-Rodriguez, M., Che-Mendoza, A., Manrique-Saide, P., et al. 2018, 'Epidemiology of dengue and other arboviruses in a cohort of school children and their families in Yucatan, Mexico: baseline and first year follow-up', *PLoS Neglected Tropical Diseases*, vol. 12, no. 11, pp. e0006847.

Suárez, R. 2004, 'Dengue, políticas públicas y realidad sociocultural: una aproximación al caso colombiano', *Revista Colombiana de Antropología*, vol. 40, pp. 185–212.

Villar, L., Dayan, G. H., Arredondo-García, J. L., Rivera, D. M., Cunha, R., Deseda, C., et al. 2015, 'Efficacy of a tetravalent dengue vaccine in children in Latin America', *New England Journal of Medicine*, vol. 372, no. 2, pp. 113–123.

Whiteford, L. 1997, 'The ethnoecology of dengue fever', *Medical Anthropology Quaterly*, vol. 11, no. 2, pp. 202–223.

Winch, P., Lloyd, L., Godas, M. D., & Kendall, C. 1991, 'Beliefs about the prevention of dengue and other febrile illnesses in Mérida, Mexico', *The Journal of Tropical Medicine and Hygiene*, vol 94, no. 6, pp. 377–387.

World Health Organization. 2012, *Global strategy for dengue prevention and control. 2012–2020*. World Health Organization, Geneva. viewed 20 April 2016, <http://apps.who.int/iris/ bitstream/10665/75303/1/9789241504034_eng.pdf?ua=1>.

World Health Organization. 2016, *Summary of the April 2016 meeting of the Strategic Advisory Group of Experts on immunization (SAGE)*. World Health Organization, Geneva. viewed 20 April 2016, <http://www.who.int/immunization/sage/meetings/2016/april/SAGE_April_2016_Meeting_Web_summary. pdf?ua=1>.

8 Does belonging really matter?

Municipal governance, vector control and urban environments in a Colombian city

Tatiana García-Betancourt, Mauricio Fuentes-Vallejo, Catalina González-Uribe and Juliana Quintero

> I think that *Aedes aegypti*-transmitted diseases, like Zika, are an opportunity for Girardot's people. It is a chance to move forward … maybe we can see now, how paralyzed and resigned we are. It is a call to action.
>
> (Teacher, Girardot, 2017)

Belonging is an amorphous concept, but one with relevance to the control of mosquito-borne diseases. Public health authorities, in their quest to sever the ties of mosquito reproduction, aim to dislodge insect populations from "belonging" in their ecological niche. For *Aedes aegypti*, this means household water containers, and other habitats, in urbanized and urbanizing cities and towns of (mostly) tropical regions. On the other hand, implementing effective vector control interventions also means creating and maintaining human connections – of systems, staff and stuff, so to speak – that can "belong" and hold program goals together. This includes the motivation, meanings and shared cooperation that sustain, or disrupt, intersectoral action. Belonging, in all of its psychological complexity, is an important but often overlooked component to the process of community participation in vector control. In this chapter, we expand on the idea of belonging, as a concept, by exploring the physical and social landscape of a Colombian city – a stage for the drama of arbovirus infection.

The quote at the beginning of this chapter, from a leader of a local public university exemplified a citywide dilemma that, as public health researchers, we became aware of during our work, from 2005 to 2017, in the city of Girardot, Colombia. The dilemma related to the municipality's development plans and the relationships between government entities and local residents, resulting in a lack of "community" participation. Girardot was/is in a continuous, ongoing and uncertain process of developing an identity, something that heavily depends on current resources and politics, and past histories. Our foray into the city's identity politics began in 2005 when we lead a team of entomologists, anthropologists, epidemiologists and geographers to assess Dengue transmission, including vector density, community practices and people's knowledge and attitudes. Since then, we have conducted research in Girardot, under different research projects, which has allowed us to view the city through more than a decade of sustained change. Over time, and with our local interlocutors, we have gained insights into what *belonging* means to people in Girardot and how important these issues are for attempts to control mosquitoes.

Although it is common for social scientists to use the word "belonging," terminological ambiguities remain (Antonsich, 2010). Usually, the word is used as a synonym of identity and/or of citizenship. But belonging has individual (emotional) and collective (political) dimensions (Bauböck, 2005; Jones and Krzyzanowski, 2007; Krzyzanowski and Wodak, 2007). It simultaneously refers to the intimate emotion of feeling at home in a certain place (place-belongingness), and an official discursive resource used to construct or justify forms of social inclusion/exclusion (politics of belonging).

In the city, belonging also has physical, social and historical textures. Our interest in this chapter is to explore this, with a focus on individual and collective ideas of urban history, development and sociality in the small Colombian town of Girardot.[1] In other words, we seek to explore how "belonging" offers an opportunity to reinterpret the social and ecological interactions involved in mosquito-borne disease spread and vector control programs.

But why focus on cities? For the first time in history, more than half of the world population lives in urban areas (54% in 2016). From an urban health point of view, this imposes a triple health threat, especially for tropical countries: infectious diseases (such as HIV, tuberculosis, influenza and vector-borne diseases), non-communicable diseases (diabetes, cancers and heart diseases), and injuries related to traffic accidents and violence (WHO, 2010). Urban spaces are profoundly heterogeneous and the negative impacts of unplanned urban growth create and reinforce existing health inequities (UN-HABITAT & WHO, 2010). Colombia does not escape this trend. In 1937, only 29% the population lived in urban areas; but by 2005, it had risen to 75%, largely concentrated in the Andean and Caribbean regions (Universidad Externado de Colombia, 2007).

Girardot Aedes-Free: Approaches and activities of a participatory project

Girardot Aedes-Free was a project funded by the Special Programme for Research and Training in Tropical Diseases (TDR-WHO) in collaboration with the International Development Research Centre (IDRC). It sought to follow an eco-bio-social approach (as part of a broader EcoHealth approach), which had been previously developed by TDR and IDRC in six Asian countries, focused on improving community-based vector control through multi-disciplinary research groups and partnerships between academic institutions, communities, municipal services and NGOs (TDR, 2011). This served as our research framework, in which macro- and micro- factors are identified as both part of the problem and part of the solution for preventing arbovirus transmission. Rainfall, humidity, temperature, vector behavior, ecology, demographic change, urbanization, health systems, vector control and health services, political contexts, sanitation, sewage, garbage collection and water supply are all among the factors to be explored under this holistic research framework. Understanding how these factors overlap and reinforce one another in both the natural and human environment helps to determine the effectiveness of public health interventions.[2]

The project went through three distinct phases. In the first phase (2010–2011), we explored ecological, biological and social factors through different field studies. Large rectangular cement tanks (known as *albercas*) and large round plastic containers (tanks/barrels) were identified as the most productive *Ae aegypti* habitats, most of which were kept indoors. Seventy percent of all pupae were found in *albercas* and 24% in tanks/barrels, compare to only 6% in tires (Quintero et al., 2014). These findings suggested that any effort to reduce larvae/pupae should focus on the household level, with an important component on water storage practices. Despite the fact that water service interruptions have now become rare, a long history of water shortages and high water prices were one of the principal factors driving water storage (García-Betancourt et al. 2015).

In the second phase, a community-based intervention was designed, implemented and evaluated. This intervention consisted of the design of long-lasting insecticide-treated net (LLITN) covers for the most productive containers. Two types of covers were design: (1) aluminum frame covers for the *albercas*; and (2) elastic waterproof fabric covers for the large round plastic containers. A total of 354 covers were constructed and used in four clusters, approximately one per household. We then focused our attention on evaluation; the results showed a decline of 71% in the pupae-per-person index in the intervention group compared with a 25% reduction in the control group. We found that 60% of households reported a willingness-to-pay for the covers, 83% would recommend them to friends and neighbors and 90% would be happy to receive them again for free (Quintero et al., 2015). Furthermore, 26% reported less use of personal insecticide sprays.

The last phase of the project aimed to scale-up the intervention to 5,000 of the 25,471 total households in Girardot (DANE, 2008). This phase ended in September 2017 with 5,672 covers implemented in 3,900 households. As an intervention project, our goal was to initiate a series of actions focused on community participation and, ultimately, some form of permanence or, as it is typically called in global health, "sustainability." Fostering participation, however, has not proven to be an easy task. We found that Girardot's sense of itself – of belonging and the realities of inclusion and exclusion that accompany it – played an important, defining role in shaping our efforts. Belonging is a major topic of conversation these days in Girardot, on the street, in the market and in the comfort of the home where people chat, gossip and debate about institutions, municipal leaders, neighbors and community leaders. These private conversations shape public health efforts.

From a town to a city: The biography of a city

The city of Girardot, located 120 kilometers southwest from Bogotá, Colombia's capital, has an average tropical annual temperature of 33°C. This entails an interesting paradox in that the city's climatic and ecological conditions are a perfect breeding ground for vector reproduction and virus circulation but also tourists from distant cities, such as Bogotá, who come searching for rest and fun. With a population of just over 100,000 people, Girardot is an example of a city influenced by conurbation processes, where urban growth links up previously discreet small towns and (slowly) transforms the rural countryside into urban sprawl. In the case of Girardot, this meant the growth of residential, recreational and commercial infrastructure and services. The city is the largest urban center in the department of Cundinamarca but shares its administrative limits (the important Magdalena River) with the department of Tolima. Girardot, however, is not a forgotten city; it has an important history as a regional center. This changed from the 1970s onwards, as a centralization of finance, services and administrative power became more consolidated around Bogotá, and reduced the urban growth of the cities within its zone of influence, such as Girardot (Molina et al., 2003; UNCRD & UNDESA, 2005) (Figure 8.1).

The history of Girardot, as an urban physical space, is both ecological and socio-political. As with much of Latin America, it begins with European conquest and colonial subjugation. The first known human inhabitants of modern-day Girardot were the *Panches* tribe, known for their agriculture, fishing and trading networks. Spanish soldiers, having arrived in what is now Bogotá in 1537, heard of the wealth and riches of the *Panches* and soon began a military campaign to conquer their land. This ended in 1544 with the destruction of the *Panches* indigenous group, the control of their territory and the founding of a new Spanish urban

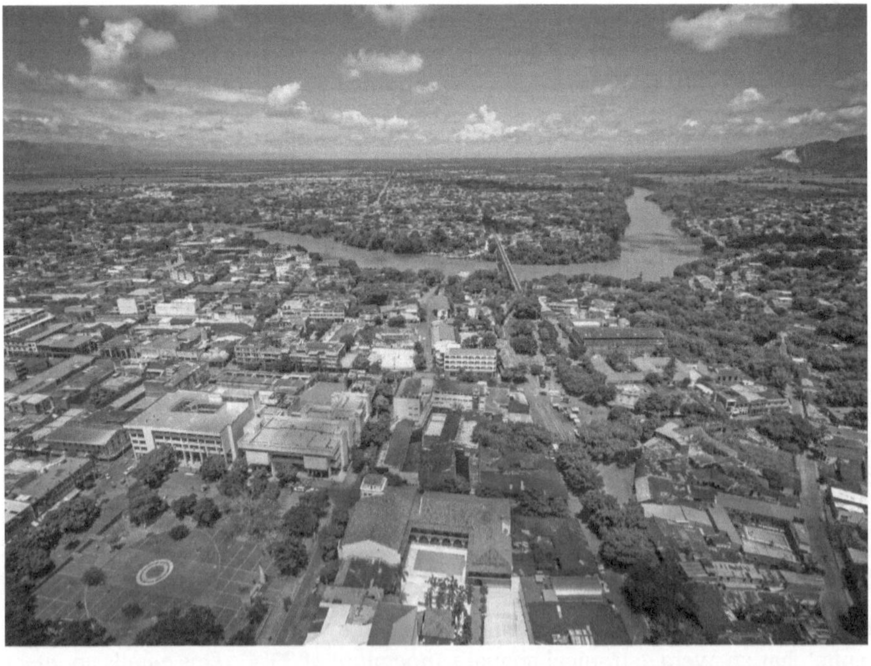

Figure 8.1 The urban ecosystem of Girardot, Colombia. Photo by Gabriel Leaño.

settlement, called Tocaima. Girardot was only founded later, in 1852, as a fluvial port; nevertheless, it quickly gained regional importance when the national railway, coming from Bogotá, reached the port. Soon the city was considered a hub for important communication and transport infrastructure in Colombia, a crossroads due to its location on the Magdalena River. This river is one of Colombia's most important fluvial arteries, connecting the center of the country with the North, passing through eleven departments and flowing into the Caribbean Sea at Barranquilla's commercial port. Combining the fluvial port with the railway meant that Girardot was in the middle of important economic exchanges between Bogotá and the rest of the country.

The city's development was certainly influenced by the railway that connected half of the country with Bogotá in 1881 (Banrep, 2011). The fluvial port and its link with the railway influenced the city's physical growth; more houses, businesses, schools, churches and streets were developed for the city's growing port and attendant commerce. However, the railway of Girardot was a truncated project from its beginning. A lack of technical capacity for construction, corruption in budgeting, a national civil war from 1899 to 1902 (between conservative and liberal national political parties), low railway productivity and high fees for transport all influenced the railway crisis during these years (Benavides & Escobar, 2014). In 1970, the railway closed due to administrative issues, nationwide highway construction, low profitability and the introduction of air transport (Benavides & Escobar, 2014; Correa, 2014).

This city has undergone several demographic changes due to both external and internal migrations. In the 1880s, the warm climate, nearby coffee and tobacco farms, a burgeoning textile industry and railway and fluvial port construction drove migration into the city. Furthermore, international migration of Lebanese communities into Colombia took-up home in Girardot, adding a new cultural group. Two new factors also helped to enhance the economy and importance of Girardot: a major annual livestock fair (beginning in 1908) and beauty contests that began in the 1950s. Both strengthened Girardot as a commercial and tourist center. This history of transitions, migrations and movements, combined with the failure of Girardot's railway and fluvial port, shifted the city's development ambitions. As stated by the Urban Development Pilot Plan of Girardot, published in 1972:

> Girardot does not have a life of its own. The agricultural sector is not located in its jurisdiction, so it has no other alternatives for its commercialization and obtaining services; industrialization is almost impossible, trading is highly competitive due to its proximity to Bogota and the emergence of expansion of urban centers in areas of special agricultural affluence, and the services sector has a deficient and unprepared infrastructure – both material and human – on which to capitalize. Perhaps the only medium-term perspective that the city appears to have is tourism.
>
> (IGAC, Urban Development Pilot Plan of Girardot, 1972)

In many ways, Girardot has followed a general pattern for growing Colombian cities, where agricultural and industrial activities have gradually been abandoned and replaced with service, retail and recreational industries. In this long transit, Girardot has also physically grown from its initial placement around the fluvial port into the mainland, spreading northwards away from the Magdalena River. In 1880, the limit of the urbanized area of Girardot was less than 700 meters away from the river (now the city center). In 1930, the city spread 1.5 kilometers away from the river. By 2017, this distance reached 3.4 kilometers, while the city was also about 6 kilometers from the port to the northeast, where a massive second residence complex of 900 houses (with a golf course and lake) had been built in the 1980s.

Over the last two decades, the city has experienced rapid urbanization due to a growth in tourism that has created new housing types (serviced, self-catering, second residence complexes) and shopping centers. The principal economic activity of Girardot is retail (58%), and services (principally restaurants and bars (36.5%) and hotels and hostels (10%) (Camara de Comercio de Bogotá & Facultad de Ciencias Universidad Nacional, 2007). Due to its favorable climate, Girardot has become known as a "tourist city," mainly for residents of greater Bogotá. During small periods, like long weekends and vacation periods, the population can triple its normal size.

As many Latin American countries, government decentralization policies became the norm in the 1980s (Duque Cante, 2017). Cities in Colombia are classified into six categories that define the level of local decision making over health and education, based on institutional capacity and financial and administrative autonomy (Portal de alcaldes y gobernadores de Colombia, n.d.). Girardot's classification was updated in 2018 to a category one city, giving it a high level of autonomy in, and responsibility for, public health and vector control activities.

Girardot's initial growth was deeply dependent on external forces imposed by commerce and transportation development. Now, as a larger modern city, the official discourse is that tourism is the main opportunity for socio-economic development. But at the same time, the municipal government struggles to face structural problems typical of Colombian cities, such as unemployment, insecurity, transport (informal use of motorcycles as taxis) and informal economic activities (that do not provide taxes). As we will see, this shift from a town to a city has also brought with it a new corpus of psycho-social anxieties for local residents, as they struggle to feel at home in an expanding urban space.

Girardot and *Aedes aegypti*–transmitted diseases

In the 1860s, several febrile disease epidemics were documented along the Magdalena River valley, following the commercial trading and workers' migration routes related to tobacco and Indigo dye production. These "fevers," as they were reported at the time, were likely different diseases: typhoid, pneumonia, dysenteric, smallpox, cholera and yellow fever (García, 2007). The origin of these epidemics was attributed to warm and unhygienic environments and uncivilized populations, an interpretative heritage left over from the Spanish conquerors (García, 2007; García, 2012). Two examples of how economic growth, transportation and fevers were related in Girardot can be found in historical documents. The first involves the fact that, two months after the beginning of railway construction, in October 1881, a yellow fever epidemic hit Girardot, killing some railway staff. The second is an article about the sanitary issues of the port in 1927, which argues that "the complete abandonment of sanitation in the port has increased the mosquito plague" (El Tiempo, 1927). This exemplifies the local coexistence of *Aedes aegypti*–transmitted diseases and city development.

The threat of *Aedes aegypti*, first with yellow fever and then with Dengue, has been linked with the expansion of international trade, economic interests and commercial ports in tropical countries. At the beginning of the 20th century, the control of yellow fever was one of the main concerns of the United States for the expansion and intensification of trade and great efforts were aimed at achieving the continental eradication of *Ae aegypti* in infested countries (Padilla et al., 2012). Several attempts were made for the eradication of the mosquito, for example in the 1950s the continental-wide use of DDT, achieving important but unsustainable results. These costly national programs were abandoned, and within a few years a massive re-infestation of *Aedes aegypti* took place and lead to the reappearance of two epidemics and the introduction of a new Dengue serotype in 1977 (Padilla et al., 2012). In Colombia, the Ministry of Health has since documented regular Dengue epidemics in 1971–1972, 1975, 1977–1978, 1983, 1987, 1990, 1995, 1998, 2001–2002, 2005, 2009–2010 and 2014. In all of these, the region of the Magdalena River valley and, in particular, Girardot, has been affected.

Project challenges: How to make it "*their*" project?

As researchers, we are always thinking about the next step and thus the sustainability of any public health intervention. From our perspective and given the eco-bio-social and Ecohealth approaches used for the *Girardot Aedes-Free* project, the key is convincing local actors and the community in general that this is *their* project. Scaling-up processes require the identification of key actors, understanding the user experience and contextual elements and the creation of empowerment mechanisms like knowledge transfer, social networking, considering community priorities and promoting problem-solving. These are done through focus groups, stakeholder collaborations, local leadership development and the inclusion of participants across all social groups, for diversity and equity.

While community involvement is essential for integrated Dengue control strategies (Caprara et al., 2015), it is also one of the major limitations in current Dengue vector control services (Horstick et al., 2010). Strengthening community involvement and enhancing interactions with local actors are potential strategies for sustainability (Alfonso-Sierra et al., 2016; Quintero et al., 2017). Conversely, social participation can happen in a disorderly and discontinuous manner, from an operational, political or institutional point of view (Caprara et al., 2015). Also, it can be time-consuming and costly, although it is rewarding when actions are sustained over time (although this is never guaranteed!). In Colombia, vector control programs have been vertical and limited, with institutional weaknesses and low response capacity (Padilla et al., 2012). Since 2010, however, the traditional program has been shifting towards a new national program that highlights community participation as a transversal pillar (Padilla et al., 2012).

One of the central issues faced by our community-based intervention was social participation. We involved community and local leaders in all project phases from the intervention design through implementation by using participatory research tools. One such tool, during the intervention design phase, was workshops on creating water containers covers. The objective was to incorporate local knowledge (of water use practices and preferences for water storage innovations) to allow us to construct and install the best water container covers, adapted to the needs and expectations of Girardot residents (García-Betancourt et al., 2014).

In community-based interventions, the consultation process can be time-consuming; problems are inevitable as negotiating participation and navigating different interests and expectations are a major part of the intervention itself (Alfonso-Sierra et al., 2016). In Girardot, some problems related to local participation, such as a lack of attendance at community and local leader meetings, low commitment by municipality personnel and a breach of contract by local suppliers causing delays on the delivery and installation of container covers (García-Betancourt et al., 2014).

To evaluate the community's acceptance and participation in the project, we explored three main questions: (1) What are the residents' perception of Girardot? (2) Is Dengue a central concern for the community and its leaders? and (3) How can we achieve intervention buy-in and project sustainability? Our ethnographic findings[3] showed that the answers to these questions were related to two principal themes: *belonging* and *identity*. Being born and living in a certain place can determine our feelings and sense of belonging (Licari, 2011), and the city in its architecture, history, politics and culture shapes this human experience (Raffaetà & Duff, 2013). As La Cecla (2011) states:

> The map of the house, the rules of residence, the neighborhoods of the village, altars, public places, the division of the territory, correspond for everyone to a set of possibilities, rules and prohibitions with a spatial, social, identitarian, and historic content at the same time.

Space and territories are places of dialogue (Licari, 2011), that create certain types of relationships, and inhibit others from taking place. Identifying how the city shapes local etiologies of belonging and identity is an important method to appreciate what limits or enhances community participation in mosquito control.

Perceptions: Instability and individual interests

Our exploration of residents' perception of Girardot focused heavily on *instability* in governance, confidence and a commitment to collective welfare. These elements were related to individual feelings of place-belongingness or attachment towards the city, although this was not always reflected in commitment to be involved in community well-being or participatory processes. In other words, an absence of a sense of community was widely reported. As a teacher told us during an interview in 2017:

> I would say that Girardot is a confused society. It has immense potential, a wonderful climate, spectacular geography, wonderful hydrography and a privileged location. But I think it's a confused society that stands on only one foot ... because the system doesn't provide opportunities and there are two options: to stay under this socio political condition or go to another city and take a risk.

As the quote suggests, some positive attributes are identified but also a feeling of instability related to the "system," and linked to political processes, corruption, unemployment and lack of governance.

Institutional and governance instability

The perception of instability, as a defining sentiment about the identity of Girardot City, was overwhelmingly explained in reference to institutions and governance, predominately as a lack of confidence in municipal authorities. Insufficient urban development was reported in connection with a loss of confidence in local leaders, due to corruption and the social cost of extensive political chicanery.

Corruption, defined as the "abuse of positions of power or trust, for particular profit, carried out through offerings or requests, delivered or received in money or in kind, in services or benefits, in exchange for actions, decisions or omissions" (Copello & Ejecutivo, 2011), was often linked with a failure of economic growth. Corruption has permeated public and private life: daily bribery, direct appropriation of public goods, vote buying, manipulation on decision-making processes and nepotism are examples of corruption in Girardot. These dynamics determine the relationships between governments and citizens (Langbein & Sanabria, 2013), and can weaken already fragile governance structures.

Colombia scored 37 (out of 100) on the corruption perception index in 2017 (zero being highly corrupt and 100 very transparent). Based on the Global Corruption Barometer, 61% agree that the level of corruption has increased over the last few decades (Transparency International, 2017). Since the 1990s, national administrations have developed strategies for establishing anticorruption policies at the national level, but corruption dynamics are also present locally. Cities and towns appear to be less concerned with designing particular policies and programs to deter corruption (Copello & Ejecutivo, 2011). Girardot is one of these cities, with a history going back to the nineteenth-century experience with railway construction where administrative mismanagement, contractual errors, delays on the construction and unnecessary spend resources were rampant. Actually, corruption is a common front-page news issue; in 2016 the mayor and the ex-mayor of

Girardot were arrested by the attorney general for using municipal resources with the goal of helping their political campaigns (Fiscalía general de la Nación, 2016).

In Girardot, political chicanery and vote-buying are also present. Affiliation with a particular candidate can help people obtain a job, at least for the four-year term that politicians serve. Nepotism is also related to government contracts for roads and infrastructure construction, creating a large power network based on favors that control decision making. Generally, corruption is a normalized event, with deep cultural roots. Residents view candidates as people who seek and attain power largely to achieve personal objectives, such as money or even higher levels of power. In addition, there is a quick turnover rate for many public positions, while campaign promises are seen, in the public imagination, as rhetoric and not something that will be carried out necessarily.

These examples represent both political instability and a lack of community confidence in the municipal authorities. Corruption, politicking, unemployment and delinquency, with all their social costs, are interconnected events that represent, at their core, a lack of belonging that drives underdevelopment and a fragile cohesiveness. Corruption discredits the government and limits its capacity, both reflecting and creating a lack of personal attachment to the city.

Problems of community participation

To understand social participation, it is fundamental to appreciate the demographics of Girardot. This municipality is predominately urban (97%), and its population is young, with a high concentration of people aged 5–19 and 35–44 years (Girardot, 2016). In 2005, 39% of Girardot's population was self-reported to be of Afro-descent (raizal, palenquero, negro and mulato) and only 0.1% as indigenous. Migration due to the Colombian internal armed conflict has influenced mobility into Girardot; in 2015, 1,531 residents had been affected by armed conflict (Girardot, 2016). Households are an average of four members and more than 95% have a connection to electricity, water and sewage (DANE, 2008). Although shortages are not common these days, water storage is seen by the community as a way to avoid unanticipated water supply interruptions, connected to a cultural tradition of water storage based on difficulties in intra-domiciliary water services and provision:

> Water storage is basically a custom [in Girardot], because our parents and grandparents did not have piped water … they began to store water out of need and to avoid travelling to the river every day, and these customs remain … it has proven to be a hard habit to break.
>
> (Community member, 2014)

Religion also plays an important role in the municipality, with 94% of the population self-professed believers (Beltrán, 2012). Faith, however, goes beyond the personal level; in Girardot it reaches the public agenda. Recently, a decree was issued that establishes that "the city of Girardot is consecrated to God"

(Alcaldía de Girardot, 2015). In the actual government development plan (2016–2019), "faith" is presented as a central policy and principle: "All our acts of government and our life are placed in God's hands. Our faith is the basis of trust in the search for good government." Although Colombia is a laical country, this should not astonish us, considering that the evangelization process, construction of churches and the establishment of religious values in social programs has been present since before 1900 (Figure 8.2).

Community participation, through local representatives, is promoted by the national constitution (Rocha et al., 2011). While churches support various community programs (Guarnizo, 2008a), some have also been developed by the local government, focused mainly on family support, youth populations and women. These programs have various structures but are typically run by community action boards (JAC), local management boards (JAL) and community participation committees (CPC). In 2017, Girardot had 108 presidents of community action board, local leaders that act as government and community mediators (Guarnizo, 2008b). The actions of these leaders, however, are often constrained by a lack of administrative support, lack of community support and fragmentation between the boards themselves (Guarnizo, 2008b). We found that many residents (although not all) in Girardot had lost confidence in these local committees and boards, largely due to their involvement in election campaigns (Guarnizo, 2008b). With a dominant perception of an absent government, actions and community behavior has become almost entirely based on considerations of personal benefit and advancement. At the community level, residents and local leaders stressed the fact that people only

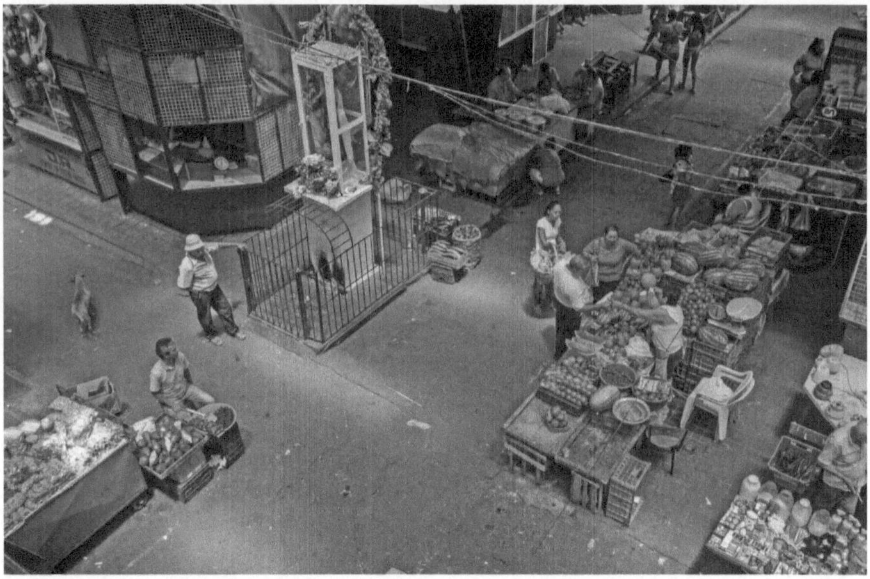

Figure 8.2 Integration of religion, social interaction and commerce in Girardot. Photo by Gabriel Leaño.

attend community meetings or assemblies when they can receive some form of benefit, such as free food or gifts. A community leader told us:

> As we speak of politicians, we also have to talk about the community. For example, you offer an invitation, but if you don't tell them, 'We're going to eat this, we're going to give this,' people don't help. So, people get used to their individual benefit, not a general benefit. Sometimes no one attends an assembly because people have no interest or love for their community … because they are used to paternalism, injected into us many years ago.
>
> (Community leader, 2017)

In Girardot, people are suspicious of altruistic motives and see any motivation for community participation as something that is linked, in some form, with a drive for individual benefits. This is discussed as a lack of interest or love for the community, sentiments that are related to feelings of unstable local governance and the transience of a tourism economy but also paternal expectations – that the government and religious organizations will address community needs. In this case, paternalism should be understood as a behavior based on receiving and asking for benefits rather than collectively organizing to address them.

Motivation for collective action, beyond those with a selfish or material dimension, were noted and found. These were often motivated by the language of "the common good," frequently connected to religious beliefs and ideologies but also the drive to be recognized, to gain prestige, in efforts to link individual benefit with wider social benefit. Individual benefits cannot be completely or casually demonized; it is necessary to understand how individual benefits can connect with a common good and how a project, such as the *Girardot Aedes-Free* project, can articulate and create synergies between individual expectations and these broader sentiments of collective responsibility. Taking this into account, we tried to understand the intersection between *Aedes aegypti*–transmitted diseases and ideas of individual and community action.

The importance of *Aedes aegypti*–borne diseases for the community

Dengue is a common disease in Girardot, given its status as an endemic city.[4] From 1999 to 2010, 6,205 cases were reported in Girardot, with an average of 563 cases per year, in a population of about 100,000 people (Padilla et al., 2012). Residents are, therefore, used to living with the virus and its vector, although perceptions and responses are generally dismissive of its importance, outside major epidemics (M. García, 2012). During non-epidemic periods, for example, Dengue is underestimated and considered a simple "flu":

> I think few people see this disease as a priority. More guidance is needed because this disease kills … [but] many people, perhaps from lack of

education or because of their beliefs, think that nothing will ever happen to them.

(Vector control staff, 2017)

On the other hand, in an outbreak or when case fatalities occur from severe Dengue, attention increases significantly as the media, politicians, health authorities, community leaders and families raise awareness, often leading to an increase in prevention and control actions. As soon as an epidemic or death is reported, Dengue acquires this high-profile status. The spotlight ebbs and flows according to the epidemiological chart. In this sense, residents' motivation, especially for household-level practices, adjusts in parallel to epidemic dynamics. In Girardot, as with Colombia more generally, Dengue outbreaks occur every three or four years,[5] and Dengue only really becomes important to residents during these outbreaks. This cyclical behavior initially changed with a Chikungunya outbreak in 2014 and later with a Zika outbreak in 2016, which became a critical juncture, or policy window, for *Aedes aegypti*–transmitted diseases. The regular cycle had changed. Health services were overwhelmed, especially with Chikungunya, which had never before been reported in the country. These parallel epidemics increased the profile of vector control, through additional information and communication campaigns, enhanced epidemiological surveillance, staff training activities and greater emphasis on addressing water storage risk behaviors (Ministerio de Salud y Protección Social, 2016b):

> We had an exclusive emergency service [in 2014] only for chikungunya cases … and it was overwhelmed. … Initially, we didn't know about the disease, so the government and the Ministry of Health sent in experts, which in a certain way appeased the desperation of the health system. What was the result? Companies' workers were sick for 15 days or even months, which was total chaos. In the health sector, staff were also ill for months – that was complicated – like a three months' crisis. Then, people were trained and the situation calmed down. … With Zika, it was no longer as difficult because people were already informed.
>
> (Health service staff, 2017)

Government actions were not responsible for controlling Chikungunya; rather, the virus only stopped because of herd immunity, when a large percentage of the population was exposed. The health system in Girardot very nearly collapsed due to the increased influx of patients.[6] During the Zika outbreak, things were different. The health services were not strained in the same extreme way due to the virus' asymptomatic and mild symptoms but also from better planning and preparedness.

Due to the magnitude of the Chikungunya epidemic, and its chronic phase of disability and pain (WHO, 2008), the perception of *Aedes aegypti*–transmitted diseases as temporal and "flu-like" changed. This outbreak in Girardot reduced hotel occupancy rates and impacted the local economy. The fact that tourists from

Bogotá decided not to travel to endemic zones like Girardot motivated the municipal authorities to re-think prevention actions. The Zika outbreak, and the threat of microcephaly, also increased prevention activities, eventually becoming a national government concern. This materialized in a national campaign entitled "*Vuelta a Colombia contra el Zika*," in which the media and health sector were trained in vector control behavior change and communication techniques (Ministerio de Salud y Protección Social, 2016c), and surveillance was enhanced in the public health system (Ministerio de Salud y Protección Social, 2016a). In Girardot, 1,936 cases of Zika where reported between September 2015 and January 2016, with an overall attack rate of 18 cases per 1,000 residents. Sixteen pregnant women with Zika virus were reported, although none gave birth to any cases of microcephaly (Rojas et al., 2016). Ongoing studies are being conducted to assess the incidence of Zika and its effects in birth conditions and neurological disorders in Colombia.[7]

Temporality is a central issue in understanding Dengue actions in Girardot. Based on the crisis of governance, and the instability of civic identities, attention to Dengue has been based on crises: sometimes Dengue matters and sometimes it does not. Perceptions of time play an important role in health promotion behaviors, as does ideas of risk and long-term consequences of infection (Hall & Fong, 2007; Kreuter et al., 2003). Both Chikungunya and Zika have, due to their chronic and long-term consequences, changed these perceptions. Furthermore, because both outbreaks caused noticeable economic crises in Girardot, affecting tourism-related income (services and hotels), these new arboviral diseases served as "moments of opportunity" for shaping collaborations, knowledge, participation and vector-control measures. As Horton (2016) discussed this:

> Epidemics change governments … Epidemics change the relationship between doctors and the state … Epidemics change the public conception of disease … Epidemics reshape knowledge … Epidemics change the public … Epidemics change societies.

Both Girardot and our project were affected by the heightened awareness to mosquitoes. National entities such as the Ministry of Health, the media and even political figures such as Colombia's First Lady, Maria Clemencia Rodriguez, launched "*Vuelta a Colombia contra el Zika*" campaign to control Dengue, Chikungunya and Zika. Girardot, and our project, were visited as part of this prevention campaign (Presencia de la República, n.d.). In the context of these events, the project changed its original name from "Dengue-Free" to "*Aedes*-Free."

Likewise, inter-sectoral activities were strengthened. Since 2014, our project had planned to build a municipal inter-sectoral action group to tackle vector-borne diseases. In partnership with several local actors, we proposed an intervention plan based on educational and research activities that included the scaling-up of the covers within the local vector-borne disease plan. An inter-sectoral committee was created, which involved different public and private institutions including from education, transit, social development secretaries, health service institutions, churches, local universities, public schools and public service companies. At the beginning, the research team led meetings and proposed actions. This included, making the committee official through a municipal decree, different education activities with local media and tourists, and conducting research on how Dengue, Chikungunya and Zika impact Girardot's population (Figure 8.3).

At the end of 2016, the municipal council approved the committee based on a municipal agreement led by the Health Secretary. This was an important milestone in the project, as it signaled that our efforts at coordination were, to some degree, working. During the first year of the committee, educational activities were conducted, including information bulletins for tourist and training activities with local students, as well as the creation of a local research group of interested public health staff and community-based recycling and cleaning activities. To ensure that members felt valued, we sought clear objectives and to disseminate results in ways that promoted the actions of the committee and enhanced social recognition. This is important because there are many challenges that limit member commitment: lack of financial resources, time and availability, changes in government authorities and constant rotation of committee members. Enhancing members' responsibility by aligning their own institutional goals with those of particular committee activities has been our main strategy.

Intervention buy-in and project sustainability

Understanding structural level factors such as the political context, governance, resident motivation and risk perceptions are necessary for developing effective mosquito control interventions. But achieving this requires that the knowledge generated by the research team, as well as the social learning acquired by key

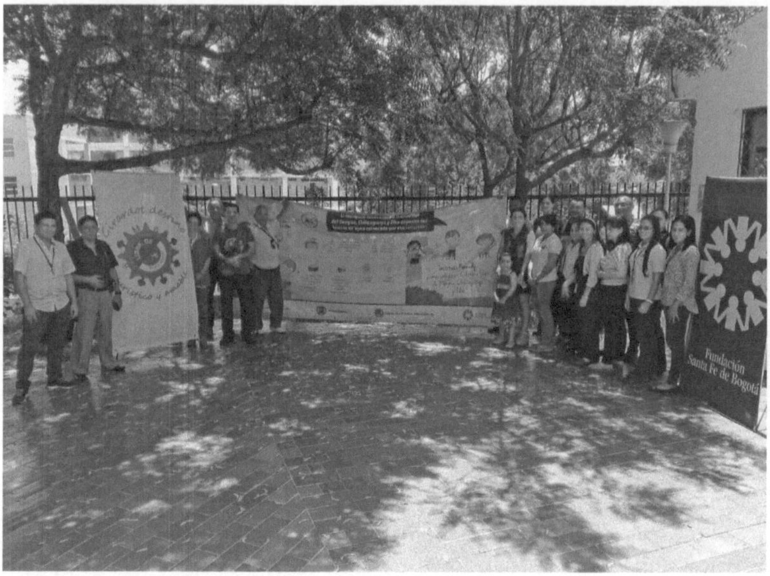

Figure 8.3 Members of the intersectoral committee, Girardot.

stakeholders (during participatory workshops, the implementation process and in reflections on challenges encountered in the field) are somehow integrated into vector control activities, plans and policies. In general, our insecticide-treated cover intervention was widely accepted, but when we evaluated specific usage patterns, we found that some covers were removed, and others were damaged, with holes in the fabric and many completely destroyed. The central question became: why did people remove their covers or fail to fix the covers when needed (Figure 8.4)?

Literature on repairing insecticide-treated bed nets, mainly for malaria, has addressed this question (Panter-Brick et al., 2006). Enabling factors such as awareness, community priorities, repaid skills, access to material, readiness to change and motivation have all been reported. Factors that limit the maintenance of mosquito nets include the opposite of these factors, such as a lack of access to resources, time constrains, issues of cost and household social dynamics (Panter-Brick et al., 2006). Some of these elements were important to the use (and misuse) of covers and their (non) repair in Girardot. Placing heavy objects above the cover was common and led to the net breaking or the frame being damaged in ways that would still allow mosquitos inside. This practice was related to the common saying, "*If something is free, I don't really care about it.*" This kind of expression was the typical explanation given by residents about misusing or discarding the covers. However, there is a paradox, because if the covers are given for free, people do not care for them, but they also would not pay for them:

> Why do people not take care of the covers? Maybe because they didn't pay for them. Maybe when they pay, they take care. … But if you charge, it would be worse because people will not install it.
>
> (Resident, 2017)

> Everything is now subsidized and begging has been promoted. So, why should I work, if I will receive things for free or at half price? As the old expression goes, you will win your bread with your forehead sweat, not with

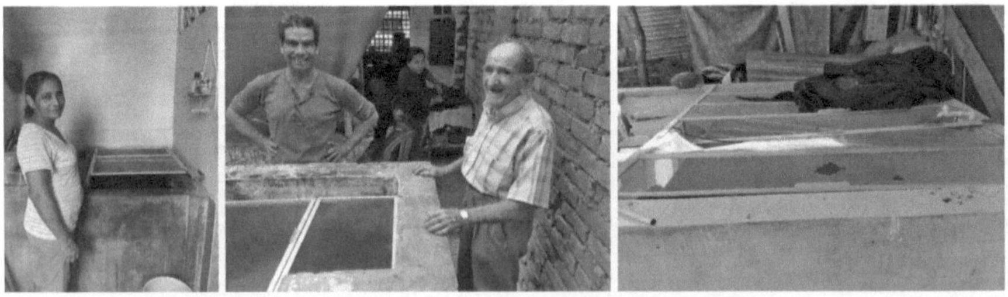

Figure 8.4 Water container covers, Girardot. The photo to the left is the installation process of a cover in Girardot. Some water containers are big deposits placed in the backyard. The photo to the middle is a cover that was installed in 2015, which was still functioning in 2018 because she has been careful with it. The photo to the right is an image of a misused cover that had not been well maintained. Photos by the authors.

> the effort of others. Because of subsidies and assistance, logically people do not progress. This has driven laziness. Where does this begin? First with the Catholic church and second the political parties; we give so much to the poorest that we have impoverished them, taking away the power to progress.
>
> (Resident, 2017)

The root of this behavior was explained as a form of "paternalism," as understood and discussed by residents. Paternalism is seen, here, as a historically-based dynamic known to affect the poorest people or communities that lack resources and is carried out by power elites like political parties or even religious groups through their charity work. In this case paternalism has been linked to the impoverishment of community action and a dilution of a sense of responsibility. It is an ideology of passivity that is reinforced by economic destitution, a lack of educational opportunities and weak sentiments of belonging, among other things. Paternalism, as an action of "giving-for-free" is related to clientelism. Eric Wolf (1996) describes clientelism as an exchange and reciprocal relationship between a client and a boss, based on unequal social terms and structures (Rodríguez, 2002). This concept has also been defined using other descriptors: informal, voluntary, unequal and unconditional. It is based on a patron-client relationship influenced by a postcolonial context (Rodríguez, 2002).

This pattern has repeated itself in new area of social life in contemporary Colombian society. Scarce public resources like job positions, access to social programs and other benefits have become exchangeable goods (Rodríguez, 2002), which in some cases means linking votes with corruption. In others, it means that hierarchical power relationships have permeated public behaviors; people in Girardot revealed that they have become accustomed to "receiving everything for free," as groceries, even houses have become distributed in social benefit programs.[8] This social context has reinforced this behavior, linked to paternalism, clientelism, corruption and a lack of community empowerment.

In the second quote above, a well-known priest from the Catholic Church, with decades of experience working with the community, commented on how social programs in Girardot have perverted community action. The city administrations have historically developed social programs based on subsidies, for example free housing for prioritized populations (Ministerio de Vivienda, 2015), education subsidies (Secretaría de Educación Girardot, 2002), housing improvements (Alcaldia de Girardot, 2017) and subsidies for elderly population (Hsbnoticias, 2017). The priest argued that such subsidies and assistance have influenced residents' laziness and impoverished them, as it creates an expectation of "free" and "easy" goods and services. This is a strong position and it is unclear just how generalizable it really is, but maybe it can explain why some residents do not care about water tank covers.

Not fixing the covers, when they were broken, was often related to lack of knowledge on how to fix them. The community believed that the cover was the "property of the project," so that they were not supposed to fix or change the covers in any way. As one household member expressed:

> The cover usually fell down. … Have I thought about repairing it? No, we haven't made those modifications because we respect how project has placed them. Maybe later you will say that we damaged the cover because we manipulated it.

Some people, however, also removed their covers or failed to fix even small holes. Others did repair and alter their covers, sewing-up holes and changing the fabric. Using the covers is, ultimately, based on the end user's perception of its utility, which are related largely to ideas of disease risk. The literature shows that awareness and community priorities are important here (Panter-Brick et al., 2006). In Girardot, we found that specific types of people tended to have higher disease risk perceptions. These were naturally more "careful" people groups: elderly women and small families of only two or three members. Despite some obvious problems, in general the community supported the project and took care of the covers:

> What was the level of acceptance? It depends on what people think; if they think that the cover is useful they will take care of it. … I think that based on the first follow-up, 80% of the people liked the covers, and if they liked the covers, they will take care of them and the intervention can be sustained.
>
> (Field staff, 2017)

The goal of the project, however, was to create a sense of ownership and, hence, sustainability. There were a couple of important issues to consider here. While the physical barriers and insecticides on the covers prevented mosquito oviposition, the cover design and its installation were also perceived as a general household improvement:

> The cover is functional; it protects the tank and controls the mosquitos. But people also say that the advantage of the cover was that the house looks pretty; now, it was more than a water tank.
>
> (Field staff, 2017)

The fact that the cover provided some decorative value increased residents' care and value for the covers. This has also been reported in other Ecohealth initiatives; for example, in Central America, the walls and floors of rural houses were improved using local materials to prevent Chagas disease, and in Mexico, insecticide-treated nets were used to build window screens. In both cases, apart from controlling vector infestation, these interventions also helped improve the quality of housing, which positively affected community acceptability of the intervention (Monroy et al., 2011; Vazquez-Prokopec et al., 2016).

Ownership and sustainability is also influenced by context-based strategies. Residents argued for the importance of "spreading the word" via person-to-person information dissemination. This type of dissemination is a natural form of information diffusion, although in many cases public health interventions often focus much more on "material" (like printed information sheets) and formal meetings.

Recognizing that most health information is disseminated in casual conversations with friends, family and neighbors, taking this seriously required a shift in how "risk messages" are understood and disseminated. In our project, we found that information about the intervention and its benefits was rapidly disseminated through neighbor-to-neighbor conversation. People started to ask us for covers before they were installed, something that was likely influenced by our inclusion of students in all project activities.

The covers have been installed in Girardot, and local authorities have assumed the leadership of the project. Now our role (as engaged researchers) is to continue to be participants of the intersectoral committee, and to watch what happens. Local suppliers of the covers and seamstresses have the capacity to replicate the intervention. We will have to see what happens…

Discussion and conclusions

This chapter has explored the social and physical landscape of a Colombian city, and how mosquitoes and water cover, to prevent their breeding, exemplifies the importance of assessing local notions of belonging in participatory health programs.

Our research approach was meant to maintain a wide perspective on the complex interactions between social and ecological systems. Nevertheless, the richness and complexity of Girardot's urban space surpassed our expectations, leading us to explore and appreciate the influence of historical, social and emotional forces in this *Aedes*-endemic city. Focusing only on epidemiological characteristics hides these complexities, especially in post-colonial settings. Since the founding of the Republic of Colombia in 1886, society has undergone important transformations with the creation and growth of modern cities, transport networks and government institutions. In Girardot, all of these changes have created new pathogenic opportunities due to a domiciled vector (*Aedes aegypti*), susceptible populations (for example, tourists from Bogotá), urban growth and the circulation of new arboviruses from Africa and Asia (Powell & Tabachnick, 2013; Sorre, 1933). The lack of belonging, driven by weak community bonds and the instability of the political system, has added challenges for controlling mosquitoes.

This took time for us to understand in Girardot. Our role, as outsiders, was to offer tools, promote community empowerment and leave enough space for natural adaptations. This included, as we discussed above, the creation of the intersectoral committee and its work in engaging residents, leaders and students in project activities. National guidelines based on integrated vector management (IVM) are a suitable starting point for these types of projects but designing and applying this approach also means engaging in the interface between spatial and psychosocial realities. In this case, insecticide treated covers were found to be a suitable prevention strategy targeting the most productive *Aedes* breeding sites in Girardot. But translating this into long-term change is much more challenging than we originally assumed, impacted by the relationships between, and cognitive frameworks of, residents, authorities and local leaders. In 2018, our research activities have now formally ended. Our final activity was to present the results of our 10 years of work to local authorities and other key actors, as a final step in transferring leadership to local stakeholders.

In conclusion: a city, as the physical setting of the drama between vectors, viruses and humans, should never be understood as an immutable place (Gregoric Bon, 2010); rather, it is a configuration of social, material, and affective practices. Feelings of belonging, or their opposite, an anxiety of displacement, transience and uneasy social conflicts, are often invisible mediators of this urban territory, with its water containers and mosquito reproduction. Such emotional attachments are not a static surface but instead are dynamic meeting-places between ecologies and histories in the making, with particular relevance for public health.

Notes

1 This project was developed based on several grants over the years from TDR-WHO, IDRC and Colciencias. We are grateful to our local project staff (especially Oneida Arboleda), local leaders and residents that took time for our many interviews, and provided noteworthy insights that assisted us greatly with the analysis that appears in this chapter.
2 Our approach lined up with national policies, specific with the National Integrated Management Strategy (Estrategia de Gestion Integrada) that aims to enhance intersectoral actions and promote sociocultural and technical adaptation of policies and guidelines for the prevention and control of communicable diseases (MSPS, 2012). Our challenge was to use formative research to adapt interventions to the specific context of Girardot.
3 To untangle them, we conducted team discussions, fieldwork interviews with different local actors, focus groups, and participant observations between 2014 and 2017.
4 Girardot is one of the 18 municipalities that account for 50% of Dengue cases in Colombia between 1999 and 2010 (Padilla et al., 2012).
5 This is related to the circulation of all Dengue serotypes, the accumulation of exposed individuals, the infestation of the vector and the nature of local urban ecosystems (Padilla et al., 2012).
6 Officially, there were 8,955 cases of Chikungunya reported in Girardot in 2014 and 2015, although many cases were also not reported due to self-medication and high demand of health services at the time (Pacheco et al., 2017).
7 This includes collaborations between the US CDC and the Colombian National Health Institute to investigate the longer-term effects of Zika virus infection during pregnancy (CDC, 2016).
8 The "Mi casa ya" Gobern National Program has provided free houses to 100,000 households in Colombia. In Girardot, 467 families have benefited from this program (Vivienda, 2013).

References

Alcaldía de Girardot. 2015, 'Decreto 206 de 2015: por medio del cual se consagra la ciudad de Girardot a Dios y se dictan otras disposiciones', http://www.girardot-cundinamarca.gov.co/Transparencia/Normatividad/Decretos/2015/Decreto N%C2%BA 206 de 2015.pdf

Alcaldia de Girardot. 2017, *Dirección de Vivienda: Informe Ejecutivo Avances Plan de Desarrollo "GIRARDOT PARA SEGUIR AVANZANADO" 2016–2019*. http://girardot-cundinamarca.gov.co/Transparencia/Informes/Informe de gestion de Vivienda - 2017.pdf

Alfonso-Sierra, E., Basso, C., Beltrán-Ayala, E., Mitchell-Foster, K., Quintero, J., Cortés, S., et al. 2016, 'Innovative dengue vector control interventions in Latin America: what do they cost?' *Pathogens and Global Health*, vol. 110, pp. 14–24. DOI:10.1080/20477724.2016.1142057.

Antonsich, M. 2010, 'Searching for belonging- an analytical framework', *Geography Compass*, vol. 4, no. 6, pp. 644–659. DOI:10.1111/j.1749–8198.2009.00317.x.

Banrep. 2011, 'Ferrocarriles en Colombia 18361930'. http://www.banrepcultural.org/biblioteca-virtual/credencial-historia/numero-257

Bauböck, R. 2005, 'Theorizing identity politics, belonging modes and citizenship', in Sicakkan, H. G., & Lithman, Y. (eds.), *Preface*, Edwin Mellen Press, New York, pp. iii–vii.

Beltrán, W. M. 2012, 'Descripción cuantitativa de la pluralización religiosa en Colombia', *Universitas Humanistica*, vol. 73, no. 201206, pp. 201–137. http://www.scielo.org.co/pdf/unih/n73/n73a08.pdf%5Cnhttps://scholar.google.es/scholar?start=10&q=religiones+en+bogota&hl=es&as_sdt=0,5

Benavides, D., & Escobar, H. A. 2014, 'El ferrocarril de girardot el gigante que no pudo con la corrupcion', *Revista Dimensión Empresarial*, vol. 12, no. 1, pp. 98–110.

Camara de Comercio de Bogotá, & Facultad de Ciencias Universidad Nacional. 2007, *Plan de competitividad de girardot 20072019* (Camara de). Bogotá DC.

Caprara, A., Lima, J. W. D. O., Peixoto, A. C. R., Motta, C. M. V., Nobre, J. M. S., Sommerfeld, J., et al. 2015, 'Entomological impact and social participation in dengue control: a cluster randomized trial in Fortaleza, Brazil', *Transactions of the Royal Society of Tropical Medicine and Hygiene*, vol. 109, no. 2, pp. 99–105. DOI:10.1093/trstmh/tru187.

CDC. 2016, CDC and the Instituto Nacional de Salud of Colombia collaborate to understand long-term effects of Zika virus infection during pregnancy.

Copello, A. M., & Ejecutivo, R. 2011, La lucha contra la corrupción en Colombia : la carencia de una política integral.

Correa, J. S. 2014, 'El rio Magdalena y sus Ferrorcarriles', *Credencial Historia*, vol. 290. http://www.banrepcultural.org/biblioteca-virtual/credencial-historia/numero-290/el-rio-magdalena-y-sus-ferrocarriles

DANE. 2008, *Estadística las principales variables demográficas y socioeconómicas del Censo 2005 Informe final.*

Duque Cante, N. 2017, 'Importancia de la categorización territorial para la descentralización y las relaciones intergubernamentales Importance of territorial categorization for decentralization and intergovernmental relations in Colombia', *Revista Derecho Del Estado*, 67–95. DOI:10.18601/01229893.n38.03.

El Tiempo. 1927, El ferrocarril de Girardot. 22 September.

Fiscalía general de la Nación. 2016, 'Primer gran golpe contra la corrupción: Fiscalía capturó al alcalde y al exalcalde de Girardot (Cundinamarca)'. http://www.fiscalia.gov.co/colombia/noticias/primer-gran-golpe-contra-la-corrupcion-fiscalia-capturo-al-alcalde-y-al-exalcalde-de-girardot-cundinamarca/

García, C. M. 2007, 'Las "fiebres del Magdalena": medicina y sociedad en la construcción de una noción médica colombiana, 18591886,' *História, Ciências, Saúde – Manguinhos*, vol. 14, no. 132, pp. 63–89.

García, M. 2012, 'Geografía médica , bacteriología y el caso las fiebres en Colombia en el siglo XIX', *Historia Critica*, vol. 46, no. 2012, pp. 66–87.

García-Betancourt, T., González-Uribe, C., Quintero, J., & Carrasquilla, G. 2014, 'Ecobiosocial community intervention for improved aedes aegypti control using water container covers to prevent dengue: lessons learned from Girardot Colombia. *EcoHealth*, vol. 11, no. 3, pp. 434–438. DOI:10.1007/s10393–014–0953–8.

García-Betancourt, T., Higuera-Mendieta, D.R., González-Uribe, C., Cortés, S., Quintero, J. 2015. 'Understanding water storage practices of urban residents of an endemic dengue area in Colombia: perceptions, rationale and socio-demographic characteristics', *PLoS ONE*, vol. 10, no. 6, pp. e0129054. DOI:10.1371/journal.pone.0129054.

Girardot, A. de. 2016, Plan de Desarrollo. Municipio de Girardot 2016-2019.

Gregoric Bon, N. 2010, 'Migrant routes and local roots: negotiating property in Dhermi/ Drimades of Southern Albania', in B. Boenisch-Brednich & C. Trundle (eds.), *Local lives: migration and the politics of place*, Routledge: Surrey, UK.

Guarnizo, N. 2008a, *Diagnóstico participativo de las dinamicas comunales entre las juntas de acción comunal de Girardot en torno del desarrollo social.* Uniminuto. http://repository.uniminuto.edu:8080/xmlui/bitstream/handle/10656/392/TC_GuarnizoSerranoNohora_08.pdf?sequence=1

Guarnizo, N. 2008b, *Diagnóstico participativo de las dinamicas comunales entre las juntas de acción comunal de Girardot en torno del desarrollo social.* Uniminuto.

Hall, P. A., & Fong, G. T. 2007, 'Temporal self-regulation theory : a model for individual health behavior', *Health Psychology Review*, vol. 1, no. 1, pp. 6–52. DOI:10.1080/17437190701492437.

Horstick, O., Runge-Ranzinger, S., Nathan, M. B., & Kroeger, A. 2010, 'Dengue vector-control services: how do they work? A systematic literature review and country case studies', *Transactions of the Royal Society of Tropical Medicine and Hygiene*, vol. 104, no. 6, pp. 379–86. DOI:10.1016/j.trstmh.2009.07.027

Hsbnoticias. 2017, 'En Girardot, abuelitos de "Colombia Mayor" ya pueden reclamar su subsidio,' http://hsbnoticias.com/noticias/local/en-girardot-abuelitos-de-colombia-mayor-ya-pueden-reclamar-s-323876

Jones, P. R., & Krzyzanowski, M. 2007. 'Identity, belonging and migration: beyond describing 'others,' in G. Delanty, R. Wodak, & P. R. Jones (eds.), *Identity, belonging and migration.* Liverpool University Press: Liverpool.

Kreuter, M. W., Lukwago, S. N., Bucholtz, D. C., & Clark, E. M. 2003, 'Achieving cultural appropriateness in health promotion programs : targeted and tailored approaches', *Health Education & Behavior*, vol. 30, pp. 133–146. DOI:10.1177/1090198102251021.

Krzyzanowski, M., & Wodak, R. 2007, 'Multiple identities, migration and belonging: "Voices of migrants"', in Caldas-Coulthard, C., & Iedema, R. (eds.), *Identity troubles*, pp. 95–119 Routledge.

La Cecla, F. 2011, 'Losing Oneself. Man without environment. Editori Laterza.

Langbein, L., & Sanabria, P. 2013, 'The shape of corruption: Colombia as a case study', *Journal of Development Studies*, vol. 49, no. 11, pp. 1500–1513. DOI:10.1080/00220388.2013.800858.

Licari, G. 2011, 'Anthropology of urban space: identities and places in the postmodern city', *World Futures: Journal of General Evolution*, vol. 67, no. 1, pp. 47–57. DOI:10.1080/02604027.2010.533583.

Ministerio de Salud y Protección Social. 2016a, Circular 000053: instrucciones para la implementación y seguimiento a la ejecución de los lineamientos clínicos de atención para condiciones de salud por virus de zika y fortalecimiento de las acciones de vigilancia en salud pública para dengue. https://www.minsalud.gov.co/sites/rid/Lists/BibliotecaDigital/RIDE/DE/DIJ/circular-0053-de-2016.pdf

Ministerio de Salud y Protección Social. 2016b, 'Vuelta a Colombia contra el Zika, la estrategia gubernamental contra la enfermedad.' https://www.minsalud.gov.co/sites/rid/Lists/BibliotecaDigital/RIDE/DE/COM/enlace-minsalud-78-vueltacol.pdf

Ministerio de Salud y Protección Social. 2016c, 'Vuelta a Colombia contra el Zika, la estrategia gubernamental contra la enfermedad.'

Ministerio de Vivienda. 2015, 'Minvivienda llega a Girardot mañana para entregar casa propia a 384 familias.' http://www.minvivienda.gov.co/sala-de-prensa/noticias/2015/diciembre/minvivienda-llega-a-girardot-manana-para-entregar-casa-propia-a-384-familias

Molina, H., Rueda, J. O., Sarmiento, A., & Pardo, M. 2003, 'Dinámica demográfica y estructura funcional de la región Bogotá-Cundinamarca 19732020', http://www.sdp.gov.co/portal/page/portal/PortalSDP/SeguimientoPoliticas/politicaIntegracionRegional/Documentos/PA002–1DinamicaDemografica.pdf

Monroy, C., Castro, X., Bustamante, D. M., Pineda, S. S., Rodas, A., Quiñonez, B., et al. 2011, 'An ecosystem approach for the prevention of Chagas disease in rural Guatemala', in *Ecohealth research in practice: innovative applications of an ecosystem approach to health*, Springer, pp. 153–162. DOI:10.1007/978–1-4614–0517–7_14.

MSPS. 2012, 'Plan Decenal de Salud Pública 2012–2021 Dimensión vida saludable y enfermedades transmisibles'. https://www.minsalud.gov.co/plandecenal/Documents/dimensiones/dimension-vidasaludable-yenfermedades-transmisibles.pdf

Pacheco, O., Martinez, M., Alarcón, A., Bonilla, M., Caycedo, A., Valbuena, T., et al. 2017, 'Publicación anticipada en linea', *Biomedica*, vol. 37, no. 4.

Padilla, J., Rojas, D., & Sáenz- Gómez, R. 2012, *Dengue en Colombia: epidemiología de la reemergencia a la hiperendemia.* (C.Hernández, Ed.). Guías de Impresión Ltda: Bogotá DC.

Panter-Brick, C., Clarke, S. E., Lomas, H., Pinder, M., & Lindsay, S. W. 2006, 'Culturally compelling strategies for behaviour change: a social ecology model and case study in malaria prevention', *Social Science and Medicine*, vol. 62, no. 11, pp. 2810–2825. DOI:10.1016/j.socscimed.2005.10.009.

Portal de alcaldes y gobernadores de Colombia. n.d., '¿Cuáles son las categorías y los criterios de categorización de los municipios en Colombia? Y ¿cuántos municipios están clasificados dentro de cada categoría?' http://www.portalterritorial.gov.co/preguntas.shtml?apc=oax;x;x;x39-&x=80241

Powell, J. R., & Tabachnick, W. J. 2013, 'No history of domestication and spread of Aedes aegypti - a review', *Memórias Do Instituto Oswaldo Cruz*, vol. 108: 11–17.

Presencia de la República. n.d., 'Gobierno reitera llamado a los colombianos a trabajar unidos para fortalecer la lucha contra el zika'. http://es.presidencia.gov.co/noticia/Gobierno-reitera-llamado-a-los-colombianos-a-trabajar-unidos-para-fortalecer-la-lucha-contra-el-zika

Quintero, J., Brochero, H., Manrique-saide, P., Barrera-pérez, M., Basso, C., Romero, S., et al. 2014, 'Ecological, biological and social dimensions of dengue vector breeding in five urban settings of Latin America : a multi-country study', *BMC Infectious Diseases*, vol. 14, pp. 1–13.

Quintero, J., García-Betancourt, T., Caprara, A., Basso, C., Garcia, E., Manrique-Saide, P., et al. 2017, 'Taking innovative vector control interventions in urban Latin America to scale : lessons learnt from multi-country implementation research Taking innovative vector control interventions in urban Latin America to scale', *Pathogens and Global Health*, vol. 7724, no. August, pp. 1–11. DOI:10.1080/20477724.2017.1361563

Quintero, J., García-Betancourt, T., Cortés, S., García, D., Alcalá, L., González-Uribe, C., et al. 2015, 'Effectiveness and feasibility of long-lasting insecticide-treated curtains and water container covers for dengue vector control in Colombia: a cluster randomised trial', *Transactions of the Royal Society of Tropical Medicine and Hygiene*, vol. 109, no. 2, pp. 116–25. DOI:10.1093/trstmh/tru208.

Raffaetà, R., & Duff, C. 2013, 'Putting belonging into place: place experience and sense of belonging among ecuadorian migrants in an Italian Alpine Region', *City and Society*, vol. 25, no. 3, pp. 328–347. DOI:10.1111/ciso.12025

Rocha, C. A., Moreno, E. Y., Molina, I. J., & Ortiz, G. 2011, 'Redes comunicativas para la construcción del capital social en Agua de Dios y Girardot (Cundinamarca, Colombia)', in J. M. Pereira & A. Cadavid (eds.), *Comunicación, desarrollo y cambio social. Interrelaciones entre comunicación, movimiento ciudadanos y medios* (Pontificia). Redes comunicativas para la construcción del capital social en Agua de Dios y Girardot (Cundinamarca, Colombia), Bogotá DC, pp. 217–239.

Rodríguez, G. F. 2002, 'Clientelismo político y políticas sociales', *Gaceta Laboral*, vol. 8, no. 2, pp. 153–165.

Rojas, D., Dean, N., Yang, Y., Kenah, E., Quintero, J., Tomasi, S., et al. 2016, 'The epidemiology and transmissibility of Zika virus in Girardot and San Andres island, Colombia, September 2015 to January 2016', *Euro Surveill*, vol. 21, no. 28. DOI:10.2807/1560–7917.ES.2016.21.28.30283.

Secretaría de Educación Girardot. 2002, 'Requisitos para beneficiarios del subsidio,' http://girardot-cundinamarca.gov.co/Transparencia/BancoDocumentos/Requisitos para beneficiarios del subsidio.pdf

Sorre, M. 1933, 'Complexes pathogènes et géographie médicale', *Annales de Géographie*, 42(235) 1–18.

TDR. 2011, 'Dengue vector control research completed in Asia. 5 year initiative focused on eco-bio-social strategies'. http://www.who.int/tdr/news/2011/dengue-control/en/

Transparency International. 2017, *People and corruption: Latin America and the Carribean*. Global Corruption Barometer.

UNCRD, & UNDESA. 2005, *De las ciudades a las regiones desarrollo regional integrado en Bogotá-Cundinamarca*. Mesa de Planificación Regional Bogotá-Cundinamarca, Bogota.

Universidad Externado de Colombia. 2007, *Ciudad, espacio y población: el proceso de urbanización en Colombia*. Bogotá. https://www.uexternado.edu.co/wp-content/uploads/2017/04/Ciudad_espacio_y_poblacion._El_proceso_de-Urbanizacion.pdf

Vazquez-Prokopec, G. M., Lenhart, A., & Manrique-Saide, P. 2016, 'Housing improvement: a novel paradigm for urban vector-borne disease control?' *Transactions of the Royal Society of Tropical Medicine and Hygiene*, vol. 110, no. 10, pp. 567–569.

Vivienda, M. de. 2013, '467 familias de Girardot ganan en sorteo público su casa gratis'. http://www.minvivienda.gov.co/sala-de-prensa/noticias/2013/julio/467-familias-de-girardot-ganan-en-sorteo-público-su-casa-gratis

WHO. 2008, 'Guidelines on Clinical Management of Chikungunya Fever', http://www.wpro.who.int/mvp/topics/ntd/Clinical_Mgnt_Chikungunya_WHO_SEARO.pdf

WHO. 2010, *Global forum on urbanization and health 1517 November, 2010 Kobe, Japan*. Retrieved from http://www.who.int/kobe_centre/publications/global_forum_report_2010/en/

9 Reinventing mosquito control

Experimental trials and nonscalable relations in the Florida Keys

Priscilla Bennett

> Americans and people all over the world are paying a horrible price for the knowledge-oblivious anxiety about modern genetic technology in plants, animals, and now mosquitoes.
>
> (Milloy, 2016)

This quote came from an opinion piece published in the *Tallahassee Democrat* (a popular Floridian newspaper), entitled "Technology Can Save Us from Zika" (Milloy, 2016). After a Dengue fever outbreak struck the island of Key West, at the tip of the Florida Keys, between 2009 and 2010, plans were proposed for an experimental trial of OX513A, a genetically modified mosquito. Few had heard of the OX513A mosquito or of the UK-based company, Oxitec, that had developed it when plans for the trial were made public in 2011 (Araújo et al. 2015). Targeting *Aedes aegypti,* and based on precepts of the Sterile Insect Technique (SIT), the product was originally advertised as a solution to Dengue fever, the most common arboviral disease, causing an estimated 390 million annual infections worldwide (Powers and Waterman 2017).[1] Once described as an "environmental plague for the new millennium" (Lennox and Arata 1999), Dengue is the most widespread and rapidly spreading vector-borne disease (Gubler, 2002: 332). It is also not an easy disease to control; *Aedes* mosquitoes breed in multiple sources of clean domestic water sources ("even in a bottle cap," as health promotion materials often state), a biological characteristic that has earned them the prerogative title of the "cockroaches" of the mosquito world. Rapidly increasing Dengue rates, together with a lack of confidence in or enthusiasm for current control tools, has been an important driver for increased funding, political commitment and investment in novel vector-control technologies. According to the World Health Organization (WHO 2014:11), we need "to find improved solutions for fighting vectors and the diseases they transmit." Because *Aedes aegypti* is the mosquito responsible for a number of important arboviral "emerging infectious diseases" (EIDs), the technology has garnered considerable attention as cases of Dengue fever, along with Chikungunya, and now Zika have appeared in seemingly unexpected, and yet somewhat predictable, places (Adalja et al. 2016).

In the realm of global health, scholars have long identified the various problems associated with "top down" public health interventions. In the attempt to design programs that are generalizable, strategies tend to overlook the importance of particularity and specificity in local settings (Adams et al. 2014; Biehl and Petryna 2013; Nading 2012). Declaring diseases as "global," writes Alex Nading (2014: 203), "presumes that it matters, materially and semiotically, in the same way from place to place." In the scaling up of global health programs, with narratives of progress and the increased commitment to technological innovation, certain landscapes of disease nevertheless remain dismissed, neglected or simply forgotten (Kelly and Beisel 2011; Lakoff 2010). Such disregard for "the social and political contexts in which people live out their lives," writes Lock and Nguyen (2010: 14), commonly result in inefficiency and unintentional consequences in the long term.

For mosquito-borne illnesses and vector-control programs, ethnographic insights can help refine program efforts through attending to "the political implications and limitations of public health engagement more broadly" (Kelly et al., 2017: 4). Based in Nicaragua, Nading's (2014; 2015; 2017) work on Dengue control shows how a focus on the emergent aspects of what are deemed "global" diseases often obscure the complex, and yet invariably essential, "local" biologies and ecologies that sustain them, mediate public health responses, and can make a difference to program outcomes. Adams et al.'s proposal for "slow research" as a method for improving global health engagement is a useful call to action. In this critical view, differences across local settings are treated "as if they were a kind of background static – a variable, but not necessarily one critical to the design of the research or intervention." The logics and political economy of "scaling-up" together with knowledge norms that prioritize large-scale comparisons facilitate this view (Adams et al., 2014: 180–1). In contrast, more locally grounded, or "slow," approaches promise to improve effective health interventions by paying better attention to biosocial conditions and are increasingly finding sympathetic advocates.

Broadly, these scholars advocate for an analytical framework designed to notice what Tsing (2012; 2015) has described as "nonscalable forms" – those details of a particular site that cannot be extracted from the diversity of their contexts and remain the same. As new and aspiring expansive projects come into contact with such diversity, the transformative connections and relationships that ensue can then produce new agendas. Tsing (2005) has referred to this process as *friction* –"encounters across difference" through which standardization occurs as projects seek to make these diverse forms commensurate. The diversity of local sites is then obscured or lost through the translation process, as project elements are made uniform and expandable. But those nonscalable forms can have meaningful consequences for long-term outcomes, as "scalability is always incomplete" (Tsing 2012: 515).

Oxitec's technology has received a wide variety of criticism. These have included concerns about unknown public health risks, the uncertain environmental impacts it could unleash and the company's conduct in previous trials. But it also includes a suspicion that the OX513A mosquito may be just another "magic bullet" approach that will inevitably fail, like those in the past, to truly solve the dilemma of mosquito-borne disease (Subbaraman 2011; Resnik 2014).[2] In their article "The Five Things To Know about Genetically Modified (GM) Insects for Vector Control," Alphey and Alphey (2014) note that genetic methods are not standalone solutions. The authors reinforce the view that genetic methods should be viewed as powerful additions to integrated vector management programs as they come with both specific strengths and limitations. Oxitec has maintained that their technology is not a means of mosquito eradication, although they insist it will be the most effective *Aedes aegypti* control technique.[3]

In order to develop good, or effective, scalability in large-scale projects (like releasing genetically engineered mosquitoes) global health projects still require some degree of engagement with, or at least acknowledgement of, nonscalable relations. It is only through their interaction with nonscalable phenomena, or the elements that resist standardization in particular settings, that projects solve ways to expand and become portable. But scalability often conceals the variations that allow for this expansion in the first place, as they seek to replicate activities and products in the same way across diverse sites, although they will inevitably be integrated into particular localities and take on new forms and meanings. Rather than putting the emphasis on how incorporating local particularities into policy and practice can improve global health programs, this chapter looks at how local particularities have influenced and shaped the innovation of a new global health technology and its scale-up.[4]

While the project in Key West unfolded, with the goal of releasing the first genetically engineered mosquito on American soil, it faced a number of regulatory hurdles, practical challenges and a good deal of citizen opposition. In the face of such cultural, social and political resistance, Oxitec has had to contend with blending local and global concepts of scalability, as it "moves from small to large without redoing the design" (Tsing, 2012: 507). Although some may consider that, even in this circumstance, such local specificities were not critical to the proof-of-concept of the OX513A mosquito release, local differences still had to be sufficiently incorporated both conceptually and practically in order for the project to expand "to scale." In tracing these nonscalable relations, there are big and small stories to tell.

Envisioning paradise

There is a kind of otherworldliness that casts itself across the island of Key West once the sun goes down on the southernmost tip of the continental United States. Ambient lights illuminate tangles of strangler figs on the front lawns of historic Conch Houses. Tour groups circle the famous Kapok tree that stands outside the courthouse, listening to eerie tales of local legends as Key West "Gypsy" chickens roost in the branches above (Figure 9.1). Down the road, the waters of the Florida Straits wash up against the site of Southernmost Point marked by its iconic

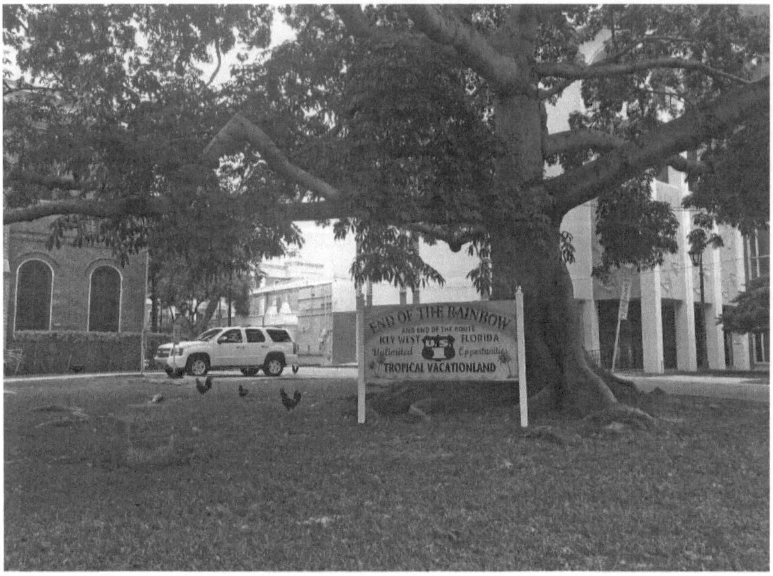

Figure 9.1 The popular Kapok tree on Whitehead Street in front of the Monroe County Courthouse in Key West.

concrete buoy. A bustling tourist stop during daylight hours, stillness settles over the island after the sun goes down, feeling a long way from anywhere as the crowds disperse towards restaurants and bars once frequented by Ernest Hemingway. One is easily "struck," as Barnett (2009: 139) described it, "by [the island's] distinctive sense of place and by its sense of a lingering past" (Figure 9.1).

The Port of Key West is host to over 800,000 cruise ship passengers a year (DOH-Monroe 2017: 13). On any given day, an average of nearly 17,000 visitors are estimated to be in Key West, mingling with its more than 25,000 regular inhabitants.[5] But the now celebrated "Tropical Vacationland" was once a place that inhabitants escaped from. Pestilent diseases such as Dengue and yellow fever and relentless mosquito swarms afflicted the island, as they also once did in many areas of Florida. In his article "Influence and Impact of Mosquito-Borne Diseases on the History of Florida, USA," Hribar (2013: 53) emphasized that "it is only within the last 60 years or so that Florida has become the nation's year round playground." Mosquito control, together with the introduction of modern air conditioning, has played a large role in this transformation. One of the island's popular historical tales offers a glimpse into the region's transformation. A real estate developer, Richter Clyde Perky, who sought to eliminate the hordes of mosquitoes that stood in the way of his fishing retreat's success, constructed two bat towers on Sugarloaf Key in the 1920s. His is one of several attempts to reinvent the Keys as a tropical paradise, which faced the difficult challenge of ridding the region of the mosquitoes that plagued it as both carriers of disease and incessant pests. Reportedly upon opening the bat tower, "the bats took flight and never returned." Documents of the incident allege that Keys inhabitants, known as "Conches," not surprised by this turn of events, "claimed 'that mosquitoes ate the bats'" (Patterson, 2004: 54; McIver 1989).

Toppled by the impacts of Hurricane Irma in September, 2017, the last surviving tower had stood for over 80 years on a site where drones were deployed in 2015 for what was called "reconnaissance" for mosquito breeding areas (Filosa, 2015): a lasting testament to how far the Keys have come in mosquito control operations. Yet mosquitoes continue to be a part of life in the Keys, where living with, or more accurately, avoiding them, requires a fair amount of daily management. But historical accounts depict what seemed at the time to be an insurmountable struggle of thick swarms and disease outbreaks that emerged alongside military and commercial expansion on the island. The sportswriter George Washington Sears, in the late 19th century, once described the "key mosquito" as "poisonous, virulent, persistent, and oh, so numerous," that rendered the Florida Keys "uninhabitable" (Nessmuk, 1886: 282). Repeated epidemics of yellow fever afflicted Key West almost every year throughout the second half of the 19th century (Hardy and Pynchon, 1964: 8). Albert W. Diddle, writing in the 1940s, highlighted the "trials and tribulations" of the Keys unique history due to its climate, geographic location, political bureaucracy, epidemics and wars. Illustrating the burden of disease on the Keys community, he described the island's experience of insecurity, as follows:

> The transient nature of the population and the ingress of travelers increased the possibility of outbreaks of disease for several decades. During these periods the citizens often became panicky. Sometimes the sick were abandoned and left to die … where there was a 'hint of the appearance of yellow fever in the city, trunks were hurriedly packed and the first steamer leaving Key West took the family away,' not to return until the 'Northers' blew away 'the poison of disease' in the late fall.
>
> (1946: 19–20)

In Barnett's account of the city's laborious reinvention as today's popular tourist destination, he begins with an evaluation of the many slogans that have sought to capture and help recreate the island's geographic and cultural separation from mainland America. These have tended to "promise a place apart from the rest of the nation" (2009: 139). Key West in the popular American imagination now carries, he argues, nothing like what 19th-century islanders had in mind. As the city grew to become an important commercial port, acting as a hub linking the United States to the Caribbean islands and Central America, the local economy relied almost entirely on its multinational connections. Walter C. Maloney (1876: 17–18), in his dedication address of the new city hall in the late 19th century, declared the island "the Commercial Emporium of the State of Florida" both for its advantageous geographical position and accessible harbor. Incoming foreign vessels required coal and provisions, which supported local businesses, and a flourishing wrecking industry that developed alongside commercial port activities was a main source of income for residents (Stebbins, 2007: 36–7). Despite the city's heightened vulnerability to the oppression of a number of diseases, particularly yellow fever (see Figure 9.2), that arose with the burgeoning industry, Key West was the largest city in Florida in 1890, and, as many of its history tours now advertise, was also once the wealthiest. In their analysis of the culture and economy of Key West, Steinberg and Chapman argued that "the Key's identity and economy were more a result of their proximity to adjacent sea-lanes than their relations with mainland Florida" (2009: 3). As the shipping industry waned and links to the greater part of the state eventually solidified, the city's history of prosperous "ship salvaging, smuggling, sponge diving, cigar rolling, transshipment, and U.S. Naval operations" (while not entirely a thing of the past) are primarily relived through the many historic museums and tours that cater to the island's most important industry today (Steinberg and Chapman, 2009: 2–5) (Figure 9.2).

Although outbreaks of yellow fever were eventually brought under control in Key West at the turn of the century, Dengue fever continued to afflict the island.

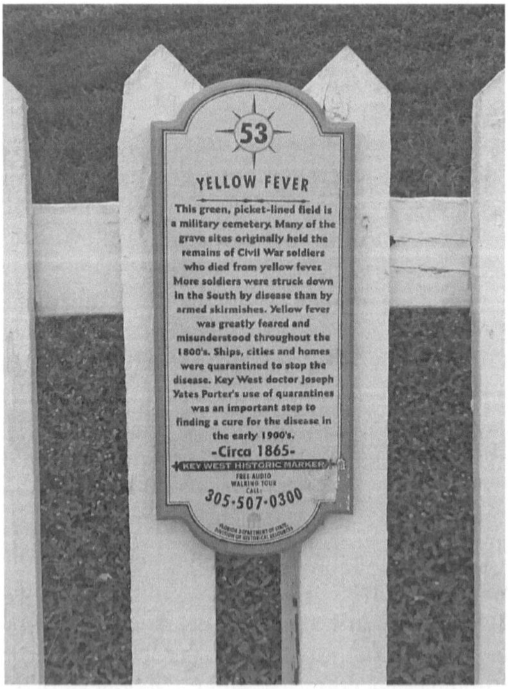

Figure 9.2 "Yellow Fever" historical marker number 53 of the Key West Historic Marker Tour located at 625 White Street.

Criticizing the city for what he considered inadequate measures towards resolving the mosquito problem, a physician and yellow fever expert complained over a century ago:

> Dengue has broke up Key West socially and financially several times, and probably will give us pains and scares again. ... It is proper to say that Key West is doing nothing and perhaps will never do anything to check the mosquito pests.
>
> (Murray, 1903: 1339)

But decades of intense efforts in organizing community leaders and rallying support for a statewide mosquito control program (together with broader scientific advancements in tropical medicine) eventually paid off (Patterson, 2009). Although the economic encumbrance and extensive human suffering caused by epidemics of Dengue fever, yellow fever, and malaria helped to propel the development of a Florida-wide mosquito control program (Hardy and Pynchon, 1964: 32–33), it was tourism that led to the establishment of what many regard today as a top mosquito control program. In its transition from a commerce and production economy throughout the 1930s, tourism development became a top priority for Key West. An article entitled "*Declare war on mosquitoes*" from *The Key West Citizen* in November 1938 announced:

> Good news to Key Westers interested in making this city an ideal resort and vacation center is contained in the announcement by Dr. Charles Williams, assistant surgeon general of the U.S. Public Health Service, that a group of six federal inspectors would work here the entire winter in mosquito eradication activities. ... In summary, it looks as though Key West [is] finally getting some action to rid the city of the cause of most tourist complaints ... a new, brighter and better Key West is arising.

The government's efforts towards eradicating disease were so effective that mosquito-borne illness temporarily slipped into a mostly forgotten past,[6] making the challenge even greater for health officials to foster community awareness when the "final stop on the Overseas Highway" (as Key West is sometimes called) experienced a Dengue fever outbreak after decades of calm. Mosquito control in the Keys had become focused on minimizing the nuisance of insects for visitors and inhabitants, until on September 3, 2009, when Dengue was confirmed in a recent traveler to Key West. It was the first reported autochthonous, or locally acquired, case in Florida since 1934, and in the continental United States since 1945 (CDC, 2010: 580). Active surveillance in 2009 identified 24 cases in addition to the three originally confirmed; further cases began surfacing on April 13, 2010 (Radke et al. 2012). Total reported and confirmed cases came to approximately 93, the last being reported in November 2010.[7] A guest columnist in the local paper called attention to the forgotten possibility of disease when they commented that "although mosquito-borne diseases have been absent from many residents' minds, Keys mosquitoes always have the potential to carry disease like yellow fever, malaria, West Nile virus and dengue – and many more diseases are making their way around the globe" (Fitzsimmons, 2010).

On top of the challenge of controlling the outbreak, a rise in the number of reported cases of Dengue in 2010 also attracted unwanted attention from the media. Speculations grew on how this (re-)emerging disease outbreak may spread to the rest of the country, with some medical experts fearing Dengue could spread across the Eastern Seaboard (Grady and Skipp 2010), and become endemic in the United States (Franco et al. 2010: 273). As a "gateway" for new exotic diseases, it would not be the last incidence of mosquito-borne illness on Key West but rather the first in a series of harsh reminders of the possibility of arbovirus transmission and the many complications involved in its control.

Key West's Dengue problem

Like any typical weeknight in the Keys, bars overflowed with flip flop–clad tourists and live music spilled out into the streets. Out with local friends, I had hoped to spend the evening simply enjoying the aspects of Key West that lure several million visitors there each year. I began to understand the often-overheard complaints from locals about the invasion of tourists. After a few weeks and some hard lessons living on the island, I had taken up the habit of checking the city's cruise ship calendar, avoiding certain areas of Old Town on the days ships were in port, which could sometimes include up to three per day. My local guides often led us away from boozy Duval Street to one of the many tucked away spots in a dense area of bars, restaurants, and entertainment venues. Old Town has a reputation for its littered streets, dirty puddles, filled-to-capacity sidewalks and slow traffic. But what it lacks in comfort and convenience it makes up for in charm. Making our way to one of the many eclectic bars the island is known for, our conversation led (as many in Key West do) to what had lured me to the island in the first place.

There is a reason that Key West often makes it on to top ten lists for "best places to travel solo," "top destinations for singles" or "favorite islands with a laid-back atmosphere." Conversations with strangers come rather easily in a place with a constant flow of people and one of the highest numbers of alcoholic beverage licenses per capita (DOH-Monroe 2017). I found that people were often enthusiastic about sharing their personal experiences and perspectives on mosquitoes. A couple from Alabama seated next to me one evening expressed their disbelief of the swarms they fought off during a previous golfing trip in the Upper Keys. A local, joining the conversation, questioned me in a casual tone on the hazardous nature "of that stuff they're spraying." While most people were well aware of mosquitoes' presence, few of my friends who worked outside of the public sector had heard about Dengue, even those employed in the service industry.

Moments like this highlighted the different experiences of disease not only across large geographical distances, but also within communities, as experiences of illness often hold "different significance in different spaces and for different actors" (Beisel et al., 2016: 8). Responses to the transmission of Dengue fever in the 2009–2010 outbreak exposed the many challenges involved in the organization and coordination of community-based vector control programs. Due to differing systems of management, understandings, and priorities involved in disease response, approaches and opinions across agencies clashed on who held responsibility. The official newsletter of the Florida Mosquito Control Association (FMCA), documented the outbreak as it unfolded in Key West. In a column written by entomologist Walter Tabachnick (2009: 13), the Florida Keys Mosquito Control District's (FKMCD) response was first described as both effective and impressive, commended for conducting "aggressive mosquito control … brought to bear in an attempt to reduce human cases and protect public health." As more cases of Dengue were reported in 2010, mounting criticism targeted state and local institutions for failing to adequately publicize the event (Grady and Skipp 2010). Reports claimed the outbreak "could have been stopped in 2010 with the active participation of the public in control efforts" (Tabachnick, 2010:6).

In a study assessing multi-level decision-maker responses to the Key West outbreak, Hayden et al. (2015) found that local and federal stakeholders considered the "lack of perceived severity of risk" to be the main obstacle for better public involvement in vector control and disease prevention. One respondent claimed it was due to "a large failure in effectively communicating a message they are ready to listen to and act upon" (Hayden et al., 2015: 398). One of the central challenges health officials faced was figuring out the best methods for delivering effective risk communication and health promotion during the outbreak. Community leaders and stakeholders were well aware of the important implications of the outbreak, with the major focus falling on reduced tourist dollars. But disagreement surfaced over how best to articulate and convey "dengue control and prevention messaging." While some health authorities claimed that "widely disseminated information" was necessary in curbing disease transmission, other city officials and community leaders argued the events were being sensationalized by the FKMCD to influence their budget. Ensuring the health of tourists and residents, while at the same time maintaining the island's image as a carefree paradise proved to be a delicate balancing act, particularly as the two interdependent qualities came into direct conflict.

Stakeholders focused their attention on protecting what was also labeled a major risk factor for the reemergence of mosquito-borne illness: global travel. Although the specific time and route of the Dengue introduction to Key West was not identified, a recurring narrative I encountered focused the blame on visitors and immigrants from Latin American and Caribbean countries (see also Kelly et al. 2017). Reports uncovered the existing concern over travelers returning from Dengue-endemic regions, as well as immigrants from these same countries, as potential sources for reintroduction (Radke et al. 2012). A senior employee with the mosquito control district commented at a town hall meeting in December 2014:

> We are a densely populated island … a mostly urbanized area … an ideal location for the *Aedes aegypti* mosquito. … With a high number of tourists regularly visiting the island of just under twenty-five thousand people, a lot of people come in and out and that has a big effect on any mosquito-borne issue.

While Key West was being criticized as a site "where the importance of the tourist industry to the local economy creates an automatic resistance to publicity of any factor, such as a disease outbreak, that could negatively impact tourism" (Rey, 2014: 996), the FKMCD came under scrutiny for using the Dengue outbreak to their advantage – "There's no glory in prevention" a doctor of infectious disease reasoned to me. Having an already contentiously sizable budget (O'Hara, 2011b), an editorial in the local paper in 2010 accused the district of "hyping dengue to justify a big tax increase. This appears to smack of the current political genre: 'You never want a serious crisis to go to waste.'" Bad press wasn't the only concern, but the editorial also revealed disagreements on who carried the responsibility for public health:

> The Mosquito Control District has 71 Full-time and 26 part-time employees – an air, land and sea mosquito attack force – whose jobs it is to swat the Florida Keys' Population of the dengue fever mosquito. … We thought the current annual $10 million budget was to prevent such an occurrence.

There seemed to be no right answer for the mosquito control district. They were, as Tabachnick (2010: 7) described it, in a "Catch-22": denounced for inciting public alarm in their urge for public participation against a perilous situation, and accused of budgetary opportunism, while also being criticized for ineffective measures against the outbreak, which others charged was the sole responsibility of the district.

In response, the FKMCD and the Florida Department of Health-Monroe County (DOH-Monroe)[8] launched the *Action to Break the Cycle of Dengue* (ABCD), a campaign that was centered on community involvement some insisted to be necessary to curb the spread of the "new" disease (Adalja et al. 2012). The call "to mobilize the Keys to reduce the breeding of *Aedes aegypti*," included the involvement of multiple government organizations, community partners and residents (Whiteside, 2011). A combination of tactics were enacted: encouraging individuals to dump standing water, organizing neighborhood trash cleanups, creating school educational programs, handing out door-hangers (see Figure 9.3), and using radio spots and editorials to encourage personal protection and control measures (Adalja et al. 2012; Rey 2014; Hayden et al. 2015). During my ethnographic fieldwork, a public health leader in the ABCD campaign, having strongly emphasized community awareness as crucial to its success, expressed reservations about the proposed implementation of genetically engineered (GE) mosquitoes. The possibility of it "taking the responsibility away from the public" was counterintuitive, he argued, to an effective and sustainable (community-based) mosquito control program.

The ABCD campaign was based on what Kelly and Lezaun (2014: 380) have described as an attempt to "rejoin disease control with the tasks of urban maintenance." An estimated 1,935 seasonal housing units were documented as occupied by part-time residents in 2010, limiting access to domestic inspectors who have

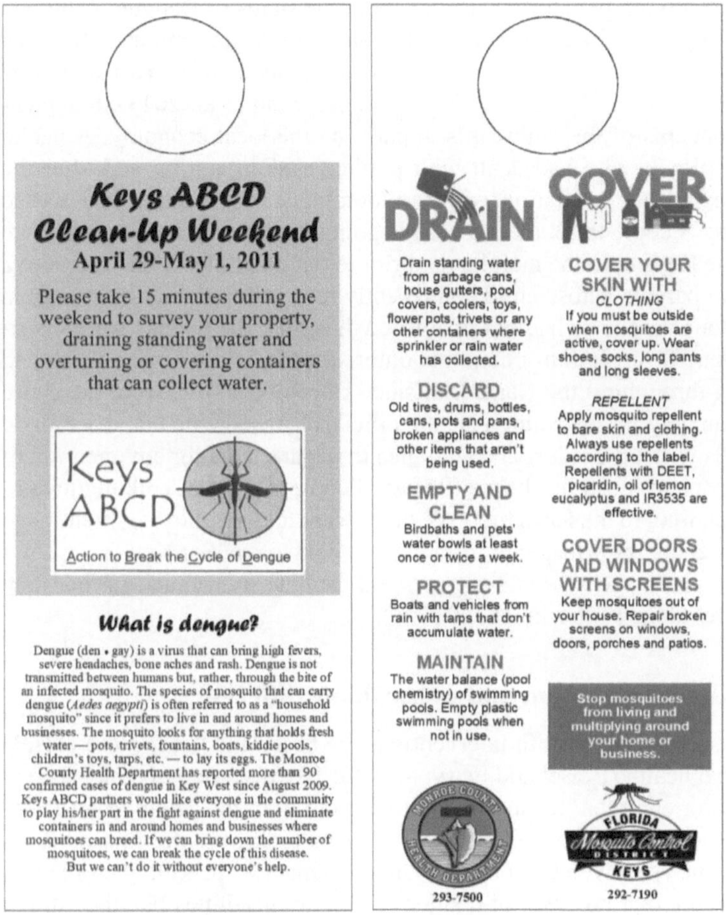

Figure 9.3 ABCD Campaign flyer (front and back) issued to residents and local businesses by MCHD (now DOH-Monroe) and the FKMCD in 2011.

close to 9,400 households to cover.[9] Densely situated housing throughout the city, known and unknown cisterns, unkempt swimming pools, and residents who are forgetful, absent, or reluctant to take action (as I experienced personally with my own landlords), pose a significant challenge to urban maintenance. Domestic inspectors can only manage to visit individual households about once a month, leaving them, as one inspector emphasized, to rely on residents to maintain their own homes (Figure 9.3).

Monroe County was not the only area affected by Dengue fever following the initial case in 2009. Infections were reported across several other Floridian counties into 2012 (Añez and Rios 2013). As Florida became depicted as "a gateway" to mosquito-borne disease (Bouri et al. 2012), Key West felt like the beginning of the route. Almost four years since the last confirmed case, the health department was still receiving phone calls asking about the status of Dengue. Although no cases were reported since 2011, the outbreak had a lasting impact. Research later found that the particular Dengue virus strains isolated in Key West suggested endemic transmission in Monroe County (Muñoz-Jordan et al. 2013), heightening ongoing concerns of the outbreak's impacts on the local economy. A health department employee who had dealt with public relations during and after the outbreak expressed his frustration with the looming insecurity that had settled over Key West: "People think that disease is going to show up here and then go marching up the Keys onto the mainland." Prior to our meeting, he had received a phone call from parents whose child had recently returned from summer camp in the Keys. Although a doctor had not diagnosed the child, the parents were insistent it was Dengue fever. It didn't help that outbreaks of Chikungunya, which had been spreading throughout the Caribbean since December 2013, were the cause of heightened anxiety for the county. Health officials listened with bated breath on conference calls with other Florida county health departments for any mention of the Florida Keys and mosquito-borne illness: "People think that chikungunya or any disease is coming to the Keys first. We don't want to hear [the two] mentioned in the same sentence," he whispered from the seat next to me. For Key West, solving the difficult challenge of *Aedes aegypti* and Dengue went much further than mosquito control alone (Tabachnick, 2012: 4).

A global health intervention and nonscalable difference

As experiments and public health interventions are becoming "ever more closely linked" in global health (Beisel and Petryna, 2013: 18), disease outbreaks present an opportunity for emergent technologies. An article from the *Miami New Times* claimed that when a new mosquito control director took over the Florida Keys district in 2011, he was given two orders: "Cut the budget while killing more mosquitoes, and ensure that no cases of dengue fever grab headlines like they did in 2009 and 2010" – headlines which portrayed the Keys as "a way for dengue to get a new foothold, or a re-foothold, in the United States" (Sweeney, 2012). While the outbreak initiated a refocusing of vector control to the forefront of public health initiatives and community-level action (Kelly et al. 2017), it also prompted consideration for new approaches to accomplish the district's goals. This began with a new formulation of a product already widely used throughout the Keys, the larvicide *Bacillus thuringiensis israelenis* (BTI). The district worked with manufacturers to come up with the new technique as "*Aedes aegypti* populations remained at levels high enough to transmit the dengue illness," which some were attributing to, "the insufficiency of collective community action" (Fitzsimmons 2010).

Another more novel method was later announced as a "birth control" project for Dengue mosquitoes (O'Hara, 2011a). A high-profile city with a world-renowned mosquito control program that still couldn't prevent Dengue fever, this was pitched as a golden opportunity (Palmer 2015). Although it is one of several transgenic technologies that target disease vectors, Oxitec's positioning and timing have helped to locate it at the front of the line. In his article "GM Mosquito Trial Alarms Opponents, Strains Ties in Gates-Funded Project," Enserink (2010: 1030) reported, "Few deny that in the race to develop disease-fighting mosquitoes, Oxitec has an impressive lead." First promoted as a solution to curbing the spread of Dengue fever, he stated that: "Oxitec sees a key market in *Ae. aegypti*, the vector for dengue … for which no drugs or vaccines exist."[10] Experimental trials of the OX513A mosquito, carried out in the Cayman Islands and Malaysia, sought to test the effectiveness of the genetically engineered mosquito in reducing the population of *Aedes aegypti* (Harris et al. 2011; Lacroix et al. 2012). Field releases in Brazil, a site of extensive research for Oxitec, showed a marked decrease in the "target wild population" of mosquitoes, the degree of which researchers claimed would be effective in Dengue prevention. Results in Brazil were consistent with the previous Cayman trials, "suggesting that differences between the two locations, including the environment or wild mosquito strain, made little difference" (Carvalho et al., 2015: 2).

The emphasis on the mosquito's ability to suppress populations in spite of ecological or biological differences supported the technology as a feasible method "in preventing epidemic dengue," although the company has yet to demonstrate its effects on disease outcomes (Chakradhar, 2015: 418). While the technology's ability to reduce local *Aedes aegypti* populations (through male OX513A mosquitoes interbreeding with wild ones, and producing unviable offspring) is essential to its success, other differences would prove just as critical to its future as a vector control intervention. Attempts to gain regulatory approval for field trials in Key West quickly exposed that there is more to the OX513A and its trials than just the technical aspects of performance. In her history of yellow fever control, Stepan (1978: 398) highlighted that while the evidential side of science is critical to its own advancement, "external factors often play an important role," particularly when it comes to the political and economic factors that attach degrees of urgency to a disease, and the priority given to the research and application of a solution. Expected to continue its "world-class operation" (DOH-Monroe, 2017: 31), the FKMCD proposed experimental trials of the OX513A as a way to overcome the multiple political and technical challenges of controlling both the vector and engaging its (human) urban public:

> Unlike insecticides traditionally used for vector control, Oxitec mosquitoes can easily get inside private properties, where much of the vector problem persists. 'The male mosquito will always find the female. It doesn't have to ask permission to enter the house.'
>
> (Waltz, 2016: 221)

Project plans for Key West came shortly after the company's first open-field trial in Grand Cayman in the fall of 2009 (Subbaraman 2011), which was met with stark criticism for its perceived lack of public consultation. One report claimed, "There were no town hall meetings or public debates because the government of the Cayman Islands didn't deem them necessary" (Enserink 2010: 1030).

Supporters and critics alike stressed public engagement as a pivotal factor in the level of anticipated success for Oxitec across diverse global sites of engagement. Brazil has been cited as one such success due to "the result of a stronger effort to engage that community" (Storr 2014). But there has been no shortage of engagement efforts in Key West, with Oxitec and the FKMCD recalibrating their moves more than once.

There is a lot to be gained for Oxitec in conducting field trials in Key West. When trials were first undergoing consideration, the occurrence of disease seemed ample justification, while the district's considerable funding, the local ecosystem and geographical features and the infrastructure and resources already available, were beneficial to collecting valuable data (Kolbe and Ngai 2016). The advantages were clear – trials in Key West seemed both feasible and advantageous to the future of the product, as one lead research team member from Oxitec explained, with regulatory approval and testing in the United States, the product could be improved and made more affordable, and other countries without regulatory frameworks would look to the US Food and Drug Administration (FDA) (the lead regulatory agency at the time) for guidance in adopting the new technology. But the regulatory process for experimental releases was unclear at best when trials were first proposed for Key West (Pérez 2016). The FDA eventually asserted jurisdiction over genetically engineered mosquitoes interpreting the technology as a "new animal drug" under the Federal Food, Drug and Cosmetic Act, a designation that was later challenged (FDA 2017; see also Lin 2017).[11] After trials in Key Haven were rejected by residents and local government officials decided to cancel experimental trials in the suburb community, Oxitec resubmitted an application for a new site in the Florida Keys. In October 2017, the FDA issued final guidance clarifying that mosquito-related products, that function as pesticides, would be regulated by the Environmental Protection Agency (EPA). A few publications in the local paper expressed satisfaction over the change in regulatory oversight, but little more was publicly discussed.

Public engagement proved a central element in helping to guide the regulatory process, with the FDA opening up and extending public comment periods "before determining its next steps" (FDA 2016). Yet public forums hosted by the FKMCD and Oxitec to "inform the public" about the planned trial in Key Haven became more of an opportunity for attendants to demonstrate dissent. Opponents argued against the genetically engineered qualities of the technology, the "undemocratic nature" of the experiment, and the unknown environmental and legal ramifications that the technology's approval might unleash (i.e. establishing a precedent for releasing more genetically modified organisms in the future) (see Kolbe and Ngai 2016; Ernst et al. 2015; Tabachnick 2012). Others expressed distrust in for-profit public health: "Hurricanes, bring them on; long-timers here seldom evacuate. Mosquitoes, well, that's the price of paradise. Zika, this too shall pass, like dengue. But science and government, I'm not so sure about" (Alvarez 2016).

The Keys have a history of suspicion about American state power. Steinberg and Chapman (2009) described the emergence and legacy of the short-lived "Conch Republic" in 1982 as the Florida Keys tried to secede from the United

States in response to a government-imposed roadblock to control illegal immigration. In their analysis, the authors reconsider the notion of sovereignty as "less about the power to isolate and exclude than it is about the right to maintain some degree of control, or at least dignity, in a world of connections, inclusions, and fragmented, unstable identities" (Steinberg and Chapman, 2009: 1). Early public health interventions imposed by the Florida State Board of Health were originally met with "enmity," as documented by Hardy and Pynchon (1964: 15), in the development of regulations and procedures for quarantines due to "government supervisions and restrictions which the people view as imposed more for the benefit of other communities than for Key West." Reactions to the proposed trials by a portion of the local community revealed a similar stance. A commentator at a town hall meeting in 2014 protested, "Because we are a small area, and a minimally populated area, and Key Haven suites you perfectly, we object to that. We really do, because we are humans and we don't like being treated like guinea pigs."

Making "knowledge, landscapes, and projects scalable," as Tsing (2012: 523) argues, is a difficult endeavor. Defined by moments of both success and failure, scalable projects by design attempt to cover up and block what Tsing (2012) identifies as "the transformative diversity of social relations." For experimental trials set for Key West, solving the nonscalable elements involved a continued effort in solving the public health aspect of alarm. Conducting public engagement required confronting not only the ecological, political and economic complexities in which publics are situated, but also the culturally informed values and multiple, competing narratives of epidemics that came to influence intervention and response. It became clear from the activities in Key West that expansive projects such as the OX513A rely not only on their technical performance in particular sites, but also their ability to contend with local differences to justify their technology as an appropriate intervention in the first place.

Meyerson and Reaser (2003: 307–8) argue that it is often a "formidable challenge to convince policy makers, industry, and the public to adopt a comprehensive approach to biological security … when imminent threats and tangible benefits from protection are not readily apparent." Challenges in implementing many public health interventions often "revolve around conflicts between local needs and these universal solutions" (Beisel et al., 2016: 8). Opponents in the Keys saw the "unknown risks" of the technology to outweigh those of the disease:

> In a way, the mosquito control district's progress has undermined the effort. The district moved quickly, and with success, to control a dengue outbreak in 2009 and 2010, mostly through a large aerial spraying effort and by sending workers door to door to inspect properties and spray them. If that worked, why do they need mutant mosquitoes?
>
> (Alvarez 2016)

In response, Oxitec aligned their approach "with a humanitarian impulse to privilege solutions to a common crisis over gains for individuals" (Reeves et al., 2012:

11), linking "local well-being" to "global well-being." Key West became representative of global circumstances, a version of the future that other regions currently unaffected by, but with the conditions for Dengue, could soon face (Nading, 2015).

As part of that technique, the OX513A as a public health intervention became framed in practices of securitization. In this "tale of conflict," Alex Nading (2015: 26) writes, "both support for Oxitec and criticism of it hinge upon 'scalar narratives' that anticipate crisis": the OX513A as a solution to an emerging global health threat, or the source of a potential global environmental threat. Before trials could get underway for the collection of data necessary for eventually commercializing the product in the United States, the company has had to try to situate Key West as a global site, an example of the future for emergent infectious disease and a possible solution to it. It is an example of what Adams et al. (2014: 184) argue to be "the global in situ … always itself a local phenomenon." A common orientation in contemporary global health, so Nading points out, is to impede anticipated pandemics. This discourse of emergence turns diseases into security issues, and classifying them as global, "presumes a level playing field – a 'standardizable body' – that simply does not exist" (2014: 204). Large-scale framings centered on preparedness have the adverse effect of extracting diseases from their historical, political, social, and economic contexts and lures us into thinking of them as predictable and ahistorical.

Emphasizing its biological vulnerability, such practices helped turn Key West into a site demanding health intervention and technological innovation, positioning it at the border of its own security along with the future of the rest of the nation's (Anderson 2010). But as efforts are made to standardize a tool (in this case, OX513A) for disease control, emergence becomes a foundation for justifying scalability. The focus is not necessarily on the disease itself; rather, OX513A can scale because it is bound to the threat of a malicious and dynamic disease vector (*Aedes aegypti*), which means that it can scale, conceivably, everywhere the mosquito is found. Making trials work in accordance with local difference does not contribute to Oxitec's project everywhere, but will influence it nonetheless, as it moves forward in Key West and elsewhere. This is the kind of articulation "between scalable and nonscalable elements" Tsing (2012: 515) argues is fundamental in the making of a portable commodity.

Discussion and conclusions

"Don't forget about Zika," read the title of an editorial in *The Key West Citizen* on June 16, 2017: "It's quiet now, but no one knows for how long." Barely more than a year prior, in May 2016, Oxitec delivered a statement before the US House Committee on Science, Space and Technology during the hearing titled "Science of Zika: The DNA of an Epidemic." The company spoke on the ongoing Zika crisis in Puerto Rico, urging members:

> In view of that urgent health need … to give the FDA all your support and encouragement so they can expedite the approval of our application … the

> FDA needs more tools at its disposal in order to help protect Americans. We want to make this technology available in the coming months rather than the coming years.

Soon after this meeting, the CDC reported locally acquired cases of Zika in the United States on June 15, 2016, in Miami-Dade County (Valentine et al., 2016: 1129). By that August, Oxitec had been awarded regulatory approval for trial releases in the Keys. Being such a controversial issue, an initiative to gauge support was held during the 2016 presidential election. Two nonbinding referenda were held on the November ballot for Key Haven residents and residents of wider Monroe County. Voters from Key Haven, a suburb of Key West and the designated trial site, voted overwhelmingly in opposition to releases. Residents expressed a variety of objections to the release, particularly public health risks of human exposure to GM mosquitoes, inadequate regulatory review, possible environmental ramifications, and the negative impact the trials could have on property values. One resident was quoted in a report published by the public radio station (FONSI) after the FDA released a preliminary safety report: "We're concerned that this is being shoved down our throat. … If 90 percent of Key Haven had dengue or Zika, I would be the first on here listening to a solution to a problem. … We don't have a problem" (Klingener 2016).

In response to majority approval by the wider Monroe County residents, the mosquito control board of commissioners gave their consent to move forward with releases of the OX513A pending approval, but under the condition of relocating the trial site. As of early 2018, Oxitec was actively campaigning for support from city councils and county commissioners as they anticipated EPA approval in the near future. The release site would be determined following approval through collaborative decision-making between the mosquito control district and Oxitec.

In a study on the implementation and use of mobile malaria rapid diagnostic tests (RDTs), Beisel and authors demonstrate that rendering RDTs effective as mobile and suitable technological solutions involves more than just the practical design features of the product: "A key aspiration for these technologies," the authors describe, "is to make them as universal as possible – so usable across many different places and by different people" (2016: 8). Through the analytical lens of co-construction, the authors identify that standardization does not come prepackaged, rather, the "ease and speed" these technologies hope to deliver are only ever achievable in practice, as users and technologies interact. The end result is a heterogeneous standardization that is only achieved through "tricky moral negotiation" in particular settings, bringing new uncertainties along with them.

Oxitec has similar ambitions motivating their attempts to conduct trials in multiple sites across the globe. The universal aspect of the technology is dependent on the framing of mosquito-borne illnesses as emergent, which situates its portability and applicability within the mosquito that the company targets. As the disease vector spreads across the globe (and climate change threats to increase its population), the implementation of the OX513A would ideally follow. Beisel et al.'s analysis shows that health interventions often frame perceptions of illness, making them "technical and intervenable in ways that can be counted, evaluated and targeted" (2016: 8). The simplicity of technologies is often taken for granted as a result, made to seem appropriate for application across an array of settings, but complexities inevitably emerge as their execution and subsequent interactions with local particularities expose that processes of disease transmission and infection are not so easily "knowable, stable, and bounded" (Nading, 2013: 69). Disease often unfolds in ways that defy expectations, operating instead as Lowe (2010: 644) best illustrates, "through infections and re-assortments that are coincidental, responsive, opportunistic, and often non-rational."

The particular circumstances of Key West that become integrated into such projects of scale, either apparent or obscured, will undoubtedly influence the outcome(s). The questions we are left with are: which ones and how? Eventually, Tsing argues, those nonscalable effects "that once could be swept under the rug" will make a difference (2012: 523). As the OX513A has already shaped how we envision the future for disease response, we should consider what it might take for these technologies to effectively engage with local circumstances, while also giving attention to the multiple factors that render places vulnerable to disease in the first place.

Aspiring global projects face both complications and advantages in their development within local settings. Key West has shaped both the OX513A as a public health intervention as well as the regulatory pathway and reception for genetically engineered pest technologies more broadly. The project has incited both old and new questions regarding the role of the public in scientific endeavors, challenging the meaning and practice of responsible innovation, and framing the broader conversation in terms of the future role of genetic technologies for the prevention of mosquito-borne illness. Importantly, the negotiation process that continues to unfold has provided some degree of democratic decision making in this high-profile experimental trial that could certainly come to set a precedent for future projects.

Notes

1 The Release of Insects carrying a Dominant Lethal (RIDL®) gene system technology was developed before the OX513A was conceived as a product. The *Aedes aegypti* was chosen as one of the first mosquitoes for which to develop this technology as researchers sought to target a widespread and economically significant vector species (Thomas et al. 2000).

2 The OX513A has become a magic bullet approach in the public imagination, a narrative that developed as the technology itself attracted attention as a solution to global mosquito control challenges, one that could be implemented at scale anywhere around the world.

3 While the OX513A is considered one of the most successful demonstrations of RIDL technology, other strains can be designed for a number of vector species with specific sterility-inducing transgenes considered suitable to different settings and circumstances (Gabrieli et al. 2014).

4 I would like to thank the community of Key West for inviting me to participate in several enlightening gatherings and events that informed this chapter. Thank you also to

members of Oxitec, the staff at the Florida Department of Health in Monroe County, the Florida Keys Mosquito Control District and other government officials and local advocates for spending time with me and discussing their perspectives on mosquito control, public health, activities for the anticipated experimental trials, and life in the Florida Keys. A special thank you to Josh Reno for his insights into the broader implications of this research and suggested revisions, and to Kevin Bardosh for inviting me to be a part of the SULID network.

5 The FCRC Consensus Center's City of Key West Comprehensive Plan data and analysis 2012 report estimated an average of 14,241 overnight visitors with an additional average of 2,734 day-trip visitors in Key West. Close to three million visitors pass through Monroe County each year, and account for nearly 60% of the total local economy (DOH-Monroe 2017).

6 Three human cases of West Nile virus were reported in Monroe County in 2001 but were quickly contained (Hribar et al. 2003).

7 See the Florida Department of Health website: http://www.floridahealth.gov/diseases-and-conditions/dengue/index.html

8 It was previously the Monroe County Department of Health (MCDH).

9 According to DOH-Monroe (2017), there is also an undocumented number of seasonal residents occupying the island in recreational vehicles each year.

10 Currently one Dengue vaccine, Dengvaxia (CYD-TDV) by Sanofi Pasteur, is licensed in several countries, beginning with Mexico in December 2015 (WHO 2016), with five additional candidates under evaluation.

11 The FDA issued draft guidance #236 in January 2017 in an effort to clarify circumstances under which mosquito-related products will be regulated:

https://www.fda.gov/downloads/AnimalVeterinary/GuidanceComplianceEnforcement/GuidanceforIndustry/UCM533600.pdf

References

Adalja, A. A., Sell, T. K., Bouri, N., & Franco, C. 2012, 'Lessons learned during dengue outbreaks in the United States, 2001–2011', *Emerging Infectious Diseases*, vol. 18, no. 4, pp. 608–614.

Adalja, A., Sell, T. K., McGinty, M., & Boddie, C. 2016, 'Genetically modified (GM) mosquito use to reduce mosquito-transmitted disease in the US: a community opinion survey', *PLoS Currents*, vol. 25, no. 8. DOI:10.1371/currents.outbreaks.1c39ec05a743d41ee39391ed0f2ed8d3.

Adams, V., Burke, N. J., & Whitmarsh, I. 2014, 'Slow research: thoughts for a movement in global health', *Medical Anthropology*, vol. 33, no. 3, pp. 179–197.

Albert, W. D. 1946, 'Medical events in the history of Key West', *Tequesta*, vol. 6, pp. 14–37.

Alphey, L., & Alphey, N. 2014, 'Five things to know about genetically modified (GM) insects for vector control', *PLoS Pathogens*, vol. 10, no. 3. DOI:10.1371/journal.ppat.1003909.

Alvarez, L. 2016, 'In Florida Keys, some worry about 'science and government' more than zika', *New York Times*, 25 August, p. A9.

Anderson, B. 2010, 'Security and the future: anticipating the event of terror', *Geoforum*, vol. 41, no. 2, pp. 227–235.

Añez, G., & Rios, M. 2013, 'Dengue in the United States of America: a worsening scenario?' *BioMed Research International*. DOI:10.1155/2013/678645.

Araújo, H. R., Carvalho, D. O., Ioshino, R. S., Costa-da-Silva, A. L., & Capurro, M. L. 2015, '*Aedes aegypti* control strategies in Brazil: incorporation of new technologies to overcome the persistence of dengue epidemics', *Insects*, vol. 6, no. 2, pp. 576–594.

Barnett, W. C., & Barnet, W. C. 2009, 'Inventing the Conch Republic: the creation of Key West as an escape from modern America', *The Florida Historical Quarterly*, vol. 88, no. 2, pp. 139–172.

Beisel, U., Umlauf, R., Hutchinson, E., & Chandler, C. I. 2016, 'The complexities of simple technologies: re-imagining the role of rapid diagnostic tests in malaria control efforts', *Malaria Journal*, vol. 15, no. 1, pp. 64.

Biehl , J., & Petryna, A. 2013, 'Critical global health', in J. Biehl, & A. Petryna (eds.), *When people come first: critical studies in global health*. Princeton University Press, Princeton, NJ, pp. 1–20.

Bouri, N., Sell, T. K., Franco, C., Adalja, A. A., Henderson, D. A., & Hynes, N. A. 2012, 'Return of epidemic dengue in the United States: implications for the public health practitioner', *Public Health Reports*, vol. 127, no. 3, pp. 259–266.

Carvalho, D. O., McKemey, A. R., Garziera, L., Lacroix, R., Donnelly, C. A., Alphey, L., et al. 2015, 'Suppression of a field population of *Aedes aegypti* in Brazil by sustained release of transgenic male mosquitoes', *PLoS Neglected Tropical Diseases*, vol. 9, no. 7. DOI:10.1371/journal.pntd.0003864

Centers for Disease Control and Prevention (CDC). 2010, 'Locally acquired dengue—Key West, Florida, 2009–2010', *MMWR. Morbidity and Mortality Weekly Report*, vol. 59, no. 19, pp. 577–581.

Chakradhar, S. 2015, 'Buzzkill: regulatory uncertainty plagues rollout of genetically modified mosquitoes', *Nature Medicine*, vol. 21, no. 5, pp. 416–418. DOI:10.1038/nm0515–416.

Enserink, M. 2010, 'GM mosquito trial alarms opponents, strains ties in gates-funded project', *Science*, vol. 330, no. 6007, pp. 1030–1031.

Ernst, K. C., Haenchen, S., Dickinson, K., Doyle, M. S., Walker, K., Monaghan, A. J., et al. 2015, 'Awareness and support of release of genetically modified "sterile" mosquitoes, Key West, Florida, USA', *Emerging Infectious Diseases*, vol. 21, no. 2, pp. 320–324.

Filosa, G. 2015, 'Rural bug reconnaissance', *The Key West Citizen*, 24 January, p. 1A.

Fitzsimmons, C. 2010, 'Public participation is vital to controlling disease-carrying mosquitoes', *The Key West Citizen*, 18 February, p. 4A.

Florida Department of Health in Monroe County (DOH-Monroe). 2017, *Monroe county community health almanac*. http://monroe.floridahealth.gov/programs-and-services/community-health-planning-and-statistics/almanac/2017almanac1.pdf

Food and Drug Administration (FDA). 2016, *FDA releases final environment assessment for genetically engineered mosquito*. https://www.fda.gov/animalveterinary/newsevents/cvmupdates/ucm490246.htm

Food and Drug Administration (FDA). 2017, *Guidance for industry regulation of mosquito-related products*. https://www.fda.gov/downloads/AnimalVeterinary/GuidanceComplianceEnforcement/GuidanceforIndustry/UCM533600.pdf

Franco, C., Hynes, N. A., Bouri, N., & Henderson, D. A. 2010, 'The dengue threat to the united states', *Biosecurity and Bioterrorism: Biodefense Strategy, Practice, and Science*, vol. 8, no. 3, pp. 273–276.

Gabrieli, P., Smidler, A., & Catteruccia, F. 2014, 'Engineering the control of mosquito-borne infectious diseases', *Genome Biology*, vol. 15, no. 11, 535.

Grady, D., & Skipp, C. 2010, 'Dengue fever? What about it, Key West says', *The New York Times*, 24 July, p. A1.

Gubler, D. J. 2002, 'The global emergence/resurgence of arboviral diseases as public health problems', *Archives of Medical Research*, vol. 33, no. 4, pp. 330–342.

Hardy, A. V., & Pynchon, M. 1964, *Millstones and milestones: Florida's public health from 1889*. https://archive.org/stream/millstonesmilest00hard/millstonesmilest00hard_djvu.txt

Harris, A. F., Nimmo, D., McKemey, A. R., Kelly, N., Scaife, S., Donnelly, C. A., et al. 2011, 'Field performance of engineered male mosquitoes', *Nature Biotechnology*, vol. 29, no. 11, pp. 1034–1037.

Hayden, M. H., Cavanaugh, J. L., Tittel, C., Butterworth, M., Haenchen, S., Dickinson, K., et al. 2015, 'Post outbreak review: dengue preparedness and response in Key West, Florida', *The American Journal of Tropical Medicine and Hygiene*, vol. 93, no. 2, pp. 397–400.

Hribar, L. G. 2013, 'Influence and impact of mosquito-borne diseases on the history of Florida, USA', *Life: The Excitement of Biology*, vol. 1, 53–68.

Hribar, L. J., Vlach, J. J., Demay, D. J., Stark, L. M., Stoner, R. L., Godsey, M. S., et al. 2003, 'Mosquitoes infected with West Nile virus in the Florida Keys, Monroe County, Florida, USA', *Journal of Medical Entomology*, vol. 40, no. 3, pp. 361–363.

Jordan, J. L. M., Santiago, G. A., Margolis, H., & Stark, L. 2013, 'Genetic relatedness of dengue viruses in Key West, Florida, USA, 2009–2010', *Emerging Infectious Diseases*, vol. 19, no. 4, pp. 652–654.

Kelly, A. H., & Beisel, U. 2011, 'Neglected malarias: the frontlines and back alleys of global health', *Biosocieties*, vol. 6, no. 1, pp. 71–87.

Kelly, A. H., Koudakossi, H. N. B., & Moore, S. J. 2017, 'Repellents and new "spaces of concern" in global health', *Medical Anthropology*, vol. 36, no. 5, pp. 464–478.

Kelly, A. H., & Lezaun, J. 2014, 'Urban mosquitoes, situational publics, and the pursuit of interspecies separation in Dar es Salaam', *American Ethnologist*, vol. 41, no.2, pp. 368–383.

Klingener, N. 2016, 'Key haven residents oppose gmo mosquito test', *WLRN*, 11 April. http://www.wlrn.org/

Kolbe, L., & Ngai, V. 2016, 'Once bitten: fighting dengue fever in Key West and San Juan', *Virginia Quarterly Review*, vol. 92, no. 3, pp. 114–127.

Lacroix, R., McKemey, A. R., Raduan, N., Wee, L. K., Ming, W. H., Ney, T. G., et al. 2012, 'Open field release of genetically engineered sterile male *Aedes aegypti* in Malaysia'. *PloS one*, vol. 7, no. 8. DOI:10.1371/journal.pone.0042771.

Lakoff, A. 2010, 'Epidemic intelligence and the technopolitics of global health', in *Berkeley workshop on environmental politics*, pp. 1–35. http://globetrotter.berkeley.edu/bwep/colloquium/papers/lakoff_BWEP.pdf

Lennox, R.W., & Arata, A.A. 1999, January, *Dengue fever: an environmental plague for the new millennium?* https://www.ircwash.org/sites/default/files/Lennox-1999-Dengue.pdf

Lin, A. C. 2017, 'Mismatched regulation: genetically modified mosquitoes and the coordinated framework for biotechnology', *UC Davis Law Review*, vol. 51, no. 1, pp. 205–232.

Lock, M., & Nguyen, V. K. 2010, *An anthropology of biomedicine*. Wiley-Blackwell, Malden, MA.

Lowe, C. 2010, 'Viral clouds: becoming H5N1 in Indonesia', *Cultural Anthropology*, vol. 25, no. 4, 625649.

Maloney, W. C. 1876, *A sketch of the history of Key West*. Advertiser Printing House, Newark, NJ.

McIver, S. 1989, *True tales of the everglades*. Florida Flair Books, Miami, FL.

Meyerson, L. A., & Reaser, J. K. 2003, 'Bioinvasions, bioterrorism, and biosecurity', *Frontiers in Ecology and the Environment*, vol. 1,, no. 6, pp. 307–314.

Milloy, S. 2016, 'Technology can save us from Zika', *Tallahassee Democrat*, 1 April. https://www.tallahassee.com/

Murray, R. D. 1903, 'Malaria in Key West, Florida', *The Alkaloidal Clinic*, vol. 10, no. 1, pp. 1337–1339.

Nading, A. M. 2012, 'Dengue mosquitoes are single mothers: biopolitics meets ecological aesthetics in Nicaraguan community health work', *Cultural Anthropology*, vol. 27, no. 4, pp. 572–596.

Nading, A. M. 2013, 'Humans, animals, and health: from ecology to entanglement', *Environment and Society*, vol. 4, no. 1, pp. 60–78.

Nading, A. M. 2014, *Mosquito trails: ecology, health, and the politics of entanglement*. University of California Press, Oakland, CA.

Nading, A. M. 2015, 'The lively ethics of global health GMOs: the case of the Oxitec mosquito', *Biosocieties*, vol. 10, no. 1, pp. 24–47.

Nading, A. M. 2017, 'Local biologies, leaky things, and the chemical infrastructure of global health', *Medical Anthropology*, vol. 36, no. 2, pp. 141–156.

Nessmuk. 1886, May 6, 'A night among the keys', *Forest and Stream: A Weekly Journal of The Rod and Gun*. http://www.biodiversitylibrary.org/item/137754#page/291/mode/1up.

O'Hara, T. 2011a, 'Battling the bugs', *The Key West Citizen*, 24 February, p. 1A.

O'Hara, T. 2011b, 'Cutting budget top priority in 2011', *The Key West Citizen*, 2 January, pp. 1A, 8A.

Palmer, L. 2015, 'Genetically modified mosquito sparks a Controversy in Florida', *Yale Environment 360*, 4 June. https://e360.yale.edu/

Patterson, G. 2004, *The mosquito wars: a history of control in Florida*. University Press of Florida, Gainesville, FL.

Patterson, G. 2009, *The mosquito crusades: a history of the American anti-mosquito movement from the Reed Commission to the first Earth Day*. Rutgers University Press, New Brunswick, NJ.

Pérez, D. R., 2016, May, *Public interest comment on the food and drug administration's public availability of draft environmental assessment and preliminary finding of no significant impact concerning investigational use of Oxitec OX513A mosquitoes*. https://regulatorystudies.columbian.gwu.edu/public-comment-fda%E2%80%99s-public-availability-draft-environmental-assessment-and-preliminary-finding-no.

Powers, A. M., & Waterman, S. H. 2017, 'A decade of arboviral activity – Lessons learned from the trenches', *PLoS Neglected Tropical Diseases*, vol. 11, no. 4, pp .e0005421.

Radke, E. G., Gregory, C. J., Kintziger, K. W., Sauber-Schatz, E. K., Hunsperger, E. A., Gallagher, G. R., et al. 2012, 'Dengue outbreak in Key West, Florida, USA, 2009', *Emerging Infectious Diseases*, vol. 18, no. 1, pp. 135–137.

Reeves, R. G., Denton, J. A., Santucci, F., Bryk, J., & Reed, F. A. 2012, 'Scientific standards and the regulation of genetically modified insects', *PLoS Neglected Tropical Diseases*, vol. 6, no. 1. DOI: 10.1371/journal.pntd.0001502.

Resnik, D. B. 2014, 'Ethical issues in field trials of genetically modified disease-resistant mosquitoes', *Developing World Bioethics*, vol. 14, no. 1, pp. 37–46.

Rey, J. R. 2014, 'Dengue in Florida (USA)', *Insects*, vol. 5, no. 4, pp. 991–1000.

Stebbins, C. E. 2007, *City of intrigue, nest of revolution: a documentary history of Key West in the nineteenth century*. University Press of Florida, Gainesville, FL.

Steinberg, P. E., & Chapman, T. E. 2009, 'Key West's Conch Republic: building sovereignties of connection', *Political Geography*, vol. 28, no. 5, pp. 283–295.

Stepan, N. 1978, 'The interplay between socio-economic factors and medical science: yellow fever research, Cuba and the United States', *Social Studies of Science*, vol. 8, no. 4, pp. 397–423.

Storr, K. A. 2014, 'When science bites back', *Scienceline*. March. http://scienceline.org/2014/03/when-science-bites-back/

Subbaraman, N. 2011, 'Science snipes at Oxitec transgenic-mosquito trial', *Nature Biotechnology*, vol. 29, pp. 9–11.

Sweeney, C. 2012, 'Can genetically modified mosquitoes keep dengue fever away from Key West?' *Miami New Times*, 31 May. http://www.miaminewtimes.com/news/can-genetically-modified-mosquitoes-keep-dengue-fever-away-from-key-west-6386995

Tabachnick, W. J. 2009, 'Dengue in Key West, 2009: Florida Keys mosquito control and the Florida Department of Health swing into action', *Buzzwords*, vol. 9, no. 5, pp. 12–13. http://mosquito.ifas.ufl.edu/BuzzWords.htm

Tabachnick, W.J. 2010, 'Dengue in Key West: the perfect storm', *BuzzWords*, vol. 10, no. 5, pp. 6–7. http://mosquito.ifas.ufl.edu/BuzzWords.htm

Tabachnick, W.J. 2012, 'Moving forward in the battle against *aedes aegypti* and dengue in Key West, Florida', *BuzzWords* vol. 12, no. 2, pp. 3–5. http://mosquito.ifas.ufl.edu/BuzzWords.htm

Thomas, D. D., Donnelly, C. A., Wood, R. J., & Alphey, L. S. 2000, 'Insect population control using a dominant, repressible, lethal genetic system', *Science*, vol. 287, no. 5462, pp. 2474–2476.

Tsing, A. L. 2005, *Friction: an ethnography of global connection*, Princeton University Press, Princeton, NJ.

Tsing, A. L. 2012, 'On nonscalability: the living world is not amenable to precision-nested scales', *Common Knowledge*, vol. 18, no. 3, pp. 505–524.

Tsing, A. L. 2015, *The mushroom at the end of the world: on the possibility of life in capitalist ruins*. Princeton University Press, Princeton, NJ.

Valentine, G., Marquez, L., & Pammi, M. 2016, 'Zika virus epidemic: an update', *Expert Review of Anti-Infective Therapy*, vol. 14, no. 12, 1127–1138.

Waltz, E. 2016, 'GM mosquitoes fire first salvo against Zika virus', *Nature Biotechnology*, vol. 34, no. 3, pp. 221–222.

Whiteside, M. 2011, 'With the public's help, we can break the cycle of dengue fever in Key West', *The Key West Citizen*, 15 March, p. 4A.

World Health Organization (WHO). 2014. *A Global brief on vector-borne diseases*. http://apps.who.int/iris/bitstream/handle/10665/111008/WHO_DCO_WHD_2014.1_eng.pdf?sequence=1

World Health Organization (WHO). 2016, 'Dengue vaccine: WHO position paper – July 2016', *Weekly Epidemiological Record*, vol. 91, no. 30, pp. 349–364.

Index

Page numbers in **bold** indicate tables. Page numbers in *italics* indicate figures.